PRACTICAL STATISTICS FOR NURSING USING SPSS®

Dedicated to my choir directors,
Mr. Campbell and Mr. Waddell,
who taught me precision through persistence.

PRACTICAL STATISTICS FOR NURSING USING SPSS®

HERSCHEL KNAPP

University of Southern California

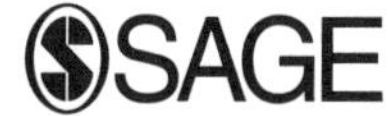

Los Angeles | London | New Delhi
Singapore | Washington DC | Melbourne

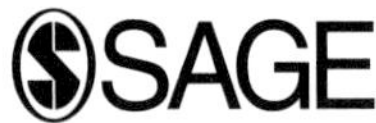

FOR INFORMATION:

SAGE Publications, Inc.
2455 Teller Road
Thousand Oaks, California 91320
E-mail: order@sagepub.com

SAGE Publications Ltd.
1 Oliver's Yard
55 City Road
London, EC1Y 1SP
United Kingdom

SAGE Publications India Pvt. Ltd.
B 1/I 1 Mohan Cooperative Industrial Area
Mathura Road, New Delhi 110 044
India

SAGE Publications Asia-Pacific Pte. Ltd.
3 Church Street
#10-04 Samsung Hub
Singapore 049483

Acquisitions Editor: Helen Salmon
eLearning Editor: Katie Ancheta
Editorial Assistant: Anna Villarruel
Production Editor: Libby Larson
Copy Editor: Gillian Dickens
Typesetter: C&M Digitals (P) Ltd.
Proofreader: Jen Grubba
Indexer: Will Ragsdale
Cover Designer: Janet Kiesel
Marketing Manager: Susannah Goldes

Printed in the United States of America

Library of Congress Cataloging-in-Publication Data

Names: Knapp, Herschel, author.

Title: Practical statistics for nursing using SPSS / Herschel Knapp.

Description: Los Angeles : SAGE, [2017] | Includes index.

Identifiers: LCCN 2015042923 |
ISBN 9781506325675 (pbk. : alk. paper)

Subjects: | MESH: SPSS (Computer file) | Statistics as Topic—Nurses' Instruction.

Classification: LCC RT68 | NLM WA 950 | DDC 610.73072/7—dc23 LC record available at http://lccn.loc.gov/2015042923

This book is printed on acid-free paper.

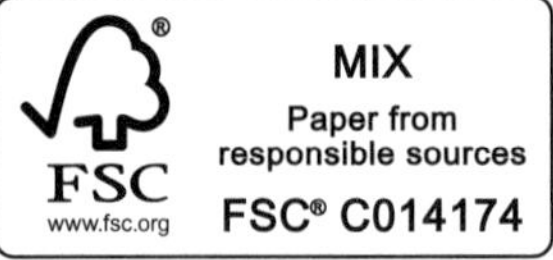

16 17 18 19 20 10 9 8 7 6 5 4 3 2 1

Brief Contents

Detailed Contents

Preface

Somewhere, something incredible is waiting to be known.

– Carl Sagan

DOWNLOADABLE DIGITAL LEARNING RESOURCES

Download (and unzip) the digital learning resources for this book from the website **study.sagepub.com/statsfornursing**. This website contains tutorial videos, prepared data sets, and the solutions to all of the odd-numbered exercises. These resources will be discussed in further detail toward the end of the Preface.

OVERVIEW OF BOOK

This book covers the statistical functions most frequently used in nursing science publications; this should not be considered a complete compendium of useful statistics, however, since in other technological fields that you are likely already familiar with (e.g., word processing, spreadsheet, presentation software, etc.), you have probably discovered that the "90/10 rule" applies: You can get 90% of your work done using only 10% of the functions. For example, if you were to thoroughly explore each submenu of your word processor, you would likely discover more than 100 functions and options; however, in terms of actual productivity, 90% of the time, you are probably using only about 10% of them to get your work done (e.g., load, save, copy, delete, paste, font, tab, center, print, spell check). Back to statistics: If you can master the statistical processes contained in this text, it is expected that this will arm you with what you need to effectively analyze the majority of your own data and confidently interpret the statistical publications of others.

This book is not about abstract statistical theory or the derivation or memorization of statistical formulas; rather, it is about *applied* statistics. This book is designed to provide you with practical answers to the following questions: (1) *What statistical test should I use for this kind of data?* (2) *How do I set up the data?* (3) *What parameters should I specify when ordering the test?* and (4) *How do I interpret the results?*

In terms of performing the actual statistical calculations, we will be using IBM® SPSS® Statistics*, an efficient statistical processing software package. This facilitates speed and

*SPSS is a registered trademark of International Business Machines Corporation.

accuracy when it comes to producing quality statistical results in the form of tables and graphs, but SPSS is not an automatic program. In the same way that your word processor does not write your papers for you, SPSS does not know what you want done with your data until you tell it. Fortunately, those instructions are issued through clear menus. Your job will be to learn what statistical procedure suits which circumstance, to configure the data properly, to order the appropriate tests, and to mindfully interpret the output reports.

The 14 chapters are grouped into six parts:

BRIEF TABLE OF CONTENTS

Part I: Statistical Principles

This set of chapters provides the basis for working in statistics:

Chapter 1: Research Principles focuses on foundational statistical concepts, delineating what statistics are, what they do, and what they do not do.

Chapter 2: Sampling identifies the rationale and methods for gathering a relatively small bundle of data to better comprehend the larger population or a specialized subpopulation.

Chapter 3: Working in SPSS orients you to the SPSS (also known as PASW—Predictive Analytics Software) environment, so that you can competently load existing data sets or configure it to contain a new data set.

Part II: Summarizing Variables

This chapter explains how to explore variables on an individual basis.

Chapter 4: Descriptive Statistics provides guidance on comprehending the values contained in continuous and categorical variables.

Part III: Measuring Differences Between Groups

These chapters provide tests for detecting differences between groups that involve continuous variables.

Chapter 5: *t* Test and Mann-Whitney *U* Test: The ***t* test** is used in two-group designs (e.g., control vs. experimental) to detect if one group significantly outperformed the other. In the event that the data are not fully suitable to run a ***t* test,** the **Mann-Whitney *U* test** provides an alternative.

Chapter 6: ANOVA and Kruskal-Wallis Test: ANOVA is similar to the ***t* test**, but it is capable of processing *more than two groups*. In the event that the data are not fully suitable to run an **ANOVA,** the **Kruskal-Wallis test** provides an alternative.

Chapter 7: ANCOVA is similar to **ANOVA,** but it is capable of including a *covariate*, which adjusts the results to account for the influences of a potentially identified confounding variable.

Chapter 8: MANOVA is similar to **ANOVA,** but it is capable of processing *more than one* outcome (dependent) variable.

Part IV: Measuring Differences Over Time

These chapters provide statistics for detecting change(s) in a continuous variable over time using a single group.

Chapter 9: Paired *t* Test and Wilcoxon Test: The **paired *t* test** is generally used to gather data on a variable before and after an intervention to determine if the performance on the posttest is significantly better than the pretest. In the event that the data are not fully suitable to run a **paired *t* test,** the **Wilcoxon test** provides an alternative.

Chapter 10: ANOVA Repeated Measures is similar to the **paired *t* test,** but it is capable of assessing a variable over *more than two time points.*

Part V: Measuring Relationship Between Variables

These chapters compute statistics that describe the nature of the relationship(s) between the variables.

Chapter 11: Correlation and Regression uses the **Spearman** statistic to assess the relationship between two continuous variables. Similarly, the **Spearman** statistic is generally used to assess the relationship between two ordered lists.

Chapter 12: Chi-Square assesses the relationship between categorical variables.

Chapter 13: Logistic Regression predicts the odds of a dichotomous outcome occurring (or not) based on data from continuous and/or categorical predictors.

Part VI: Data Handling

This chapter demonstrates supplemental techniques in SPSS to enhance your capabilities, versatility, and data processing efficiency.

Chapter 14: Supplemental SPSS Operations explains how to generate random numbers, sort and select cases, recode variables, import non-SPSS data, and practice appropriate data storage protocols.

After you have completed Chapters 4 through 13, the following table will help you navigate this book to efficiently select the statistical test(s) best suited to your (data) situation. For now, it is advised that you skip this table, as it contains statistical terminology that will be covered thoroughly in the chapters that follow.

Overview of Statistical Functions

Chapter	Statistic	When to Use	Results
4	Descriptive statistics	Any continuous or categorical variable	Generates a summary of a variable using figures and graphs
5	*t* Test and Mann-Whitney *U* test	Two groups with continuous variables	Indicates if there is a statistically significant difference between the two groups (G_1:G_2)
6	ANOVA and Kruskal-Wallis test	Similar to the *t* test, except it is used when there are more than two groups	Similar to the *t* test, except it compares all pairs of groups (G_1:G_2, G_1:G_3, G_2:G_3)
7	ANCOVA	Similar to ANOVA but adjusts results per known confounding variable	Similar to ANOVA, except results are adjusted per the identified confounding variable
8	MANOVA	Similar to ANOVA, but processes two or more dependent (outcome) variables	Similar to ANOVA, except instead of results revealing between-group differences for one (outcome) variable, the results reflect differences between groups for two or more outcome variables
9	Paired *t* test and Wilcoxon test	Compares pretest to posttest (continuous variables within one group)	Indicates if there is a statistically significant difference between the pretest and posttest (T_1:T_2)
10	ANOVA repeated measures	Similar to the paired *t* test, except it is used when there are more than two time points	Similar to the paired *t* test, except it compares scores from all pairs of time points (T_1:T_2, T_2:T_3, T_1:T_3)
11	Correlation and regression	Two continuous variables for each subject/record, or two ranked lists	Indicates the strength and direction of the relationship between two variables
12	Chi-square	Two categorical variables	Indicates if there is a statistically significant difference between two categories
13	Logistic regression	Determine the likelihood(s) of a dichotomous outcome	Indicates the odds that a variable predicts one of two possible outcomes

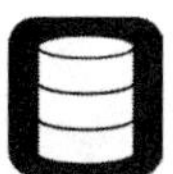

LAYERED LEARNING

This book has six parts. Parts III and IV use *Layered Learning* to explain similar concepts in a cumulative fashion. For example, **Part III: Measuring Differences Between Groups** contains four conceptually connected chapters: **Chapter 5: *t* Test** shows how to determine if one group outperformed the other (e.g., Treatment : Control). **Chapter 6: ANOVA** builds on the concept of the *t* Test, but instead of comparing just two groups to each other (e.g., Treatment : Control), ANOVA can compare three or more groups to each other (e.g., Treatment_1 : Treatment_2 : Control). Essentially, ANOVA is just one step up from what you will already understand from having mastered the *t* test, so the learning curve is not as steep. **Chapter 7: ANCOVA** is essentially the same as an ANOVA test, but it adjusts the results based on the values of an identified confounding variable. **Chapter 8: MANOVA** is the last chapter in Part III, which is just one more variation in this set. The point is, you will not be starting from *square one* in each of these chapters—as you enter Chapters 6, 7, and 8, you will see that you are already more than halfway there to understanding the new statistic, based on your comprehension of the prior chatper(s). This form of Layered Learning is akin to simply adding one more layer to an *already existing* cake (hence the layer cake icon).

Similarly, **Part IV: Measuring Differences Over Time** contains two chapters: **Chapter 9: Paired *t* Test and Wilcoxon Test** is used to compare the scores from two time points (e.g., Pretest : Posttest); **Chapter 10: ANOVA Repeated Measures** builds on this concept, but instead of assessing scores from (only) two time points, ANOVA repeated measures can compare scores spanning more than two time points (e.g., score at day 1, score at day 30, score at day 60, etc.).

DIGITAL LEARNING RESOURCES

The exercises in **Chapter 3: Working in SPSS** include the data definitions (codebooks) and corresponding concise data sets printed in the text for manual entry; this will enable you to learn how to set up SPSS from the ground up. This is an essential skill for conducting original research.

Chapters 4 through 13 teach each statistical process using an appropriate example and corresponding data set. The practice exercises at the end of these chapters provide you with the opportunity to master each statistical process by analyzing actual data sets. For convenience and accuracy, these prepared SPSS data sets are available for download.

The website for this book is **study.sagepub.com/statsfornursing**, which contains the following resources:

VIDEOS

The (.mp4) videos provide an overview of each statistical process, directions for processing the pretest checklist criteria, ordering the statistical test, and interpreting the results.

DATA SET

The downloadable file also contains prepared data sets for each example and exercise to facilitate prompt and accurate processing. Additionally, it contains the documented solutions to odd-numbered exercises to check the quality of your learning.

The examples and exercises in this text were processed using Version 18 of the software and should be compatible with most other versions.

RESOURCES FOR INSTRUCTORS

Password-protected instructor resources are available on the website for this book at **study.sagepub.com/statsfornursing** and include the following:

- All student resources (listed above)
- Editable PowerPoint presentations for each chapter

MARGIN ICONS

The following four icons are used on an as-needed basis:

REFERENCE POINT—This point is referenced elsewhere in the text (think of this as a bookmark)

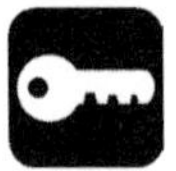

KEY POINT—Important fact

TECHNICAL TIP—Helpful data processing technique

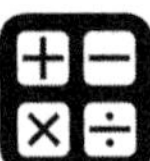

FORMULA—Useful formula that SPSS does not perform but can be easily processed on any calculator

The following icons provide navigation in each chapter (in this order):

VIDEO*—Tutorial video demonstrating the **PRETEST CHECKLIST** and **TEST RUN**

LAYERED LEARNING—Identifies chapters that are conceptually connected

OVERVIEW—Summary of what statistics does and when it should be used

DATA SET*—Specifies which prepared example/exercise data set to load

PRETEST CHECKLIST—Instructions to check that the data meet the criteria necessary to run a statistical test

TEST RUN—Procedures and parameters for running a statistical test

RESULTS—Interpreting the output from the **TEST RUN**

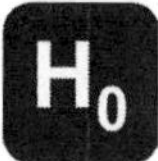

HYPOTHESIS RESOLUTION—Accepting/rejecting hypotheses based on the **RESULTS**

DOCUMENTING RESULTS—Write-up based on the **HYPOTHESIS RESOLUTION**

*Go to **study.sagepub.com/statsfornursing** and download the tutorial videos, prepared data sets, and solutions to all of the odd-numbered exercises.

Acknowledgments

SAGE and the author acknowledge and thank the following reviewers whose feedback contributed to the development of this text:

Todd Franke, University of California, Los Angeles

Heather Carter-Templeton, The University of Alabama

Jennell P. Charles, Clayton State University

Daniel Rodriguez, La Salle University

We extend special thanks to Ann D. Bagchi for her skillful technical proofreading, to better insure the precision to this text.

We also gratefully acknowledge the contribution of Dean Cameron, whose cartoons enliven this book.

About the Author

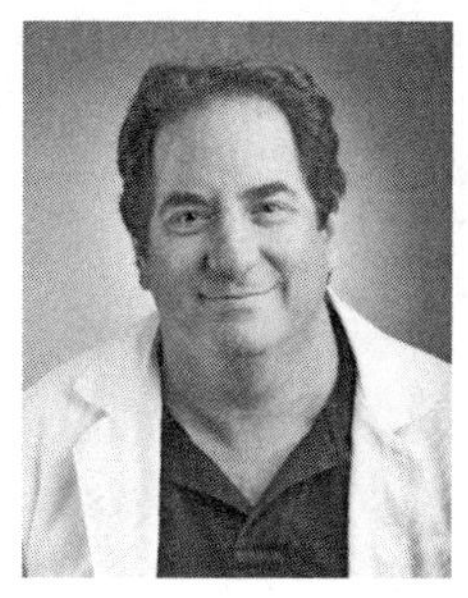

Herschel Knapp, PhD, MSSW, has more than 20 years of experience as a health science researcher; he has provided project management for innovative implementations designed to improve the quality of patient care via multisite, health science implementations. He teaches master's-level courses at the University of Southern California; he has also taught at the University of California, Los Angeles and California State University, Los Angeles. Dr. Knapp has served as the lead statistician on a longitudinal cancer research project and managed the program evaluation metrics for a multisite, nonprofit children's center. His clinical work includes emergency/trauma therapy in hospital settings. The author of numerous articles in peer-reviewed health science journals, he is also the author of *Introductory Statistics Using SPSS* (2013), *Therapeutic Communication: Developing Professional Skills* (2nd ed., 2014), and *Introduction to Social Work Practice: A Practical Workbook* (2010). Dr. Knapp has developed and implemented innovative telehealth systems, utilizing videoconferencing technology to facilitate optimal health care service delivery to remote patients and to coordinate specialty consultations among health care providers, including interventions to diagnose and treat people with HIV and hepatitis, with special outreach to the homeless. He is currently providing research and analytic services to promote excellence within a health care system.

PART I

Statistical Principles

This set of chapters provides the basis for working in statistics:

Chapter 1: Research Principles focuses on foundational statistical concepts, delineating what statistics are, what they do, and what they do not do.

Chapter 2: Sampling identifies the rationale and methods for gathering a relatively small bundle of data to better comprehend the larger population or a specialized subpopulation.

Chapter 3: Working in SPSS orients you to the SPSS (sometimes referred to as PASW—Predictive Analytic Software) environment, so that you can competently load existing data sets or configure it to contain a new data set.

CHAPTER 1

Research Principles

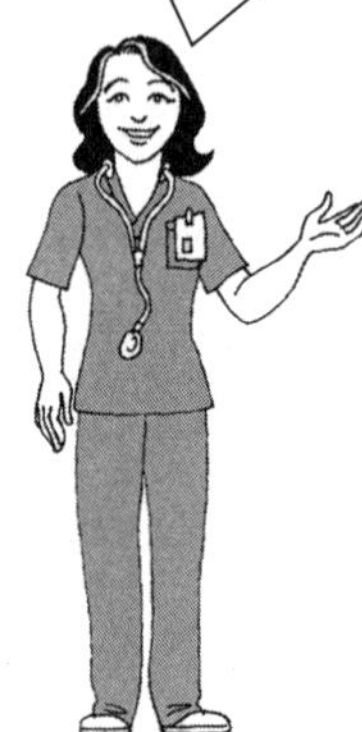
These fundaments
will get things started.

- Research Questions
- Control and Experimental Groups
- Rationale for Random Assignment
- Hypothesis Formulation
- Reading Statistical Outcomes
- Accept/Reject Hypothesis
- Levels of Measure
- Types of Variables

The scientific mind does not so much provide the right answers as ask the right questions.

—Claude Levi-Strauss

LEARNING OBJECTIVES

Upon completing this chapter, you will be able to:

- Identify various forms of research questions
- Differentiate between *control* and *experimental* groups
- Comprehend the rationale for random assignment
- Understand the basis for hypothesis formulation
- Understand the fundamentals of reading statistical outcomes
- Appropriately accept/reject hypotheses based on statistical outcomes
- Understand the four levels of measure
- Determine the variable type: *categorical* or *continuous*

OVERVIEW—RESEARCH PRINCIPLES

This chapter introduces statistical concepts that will be used throughout this book. Applying statistics involves more than just processing tables of numbers; it involves being curious and assembling mindful questions in an attempt to better understand what is going on in a setting. As you will see, statistics extends far beyond simple averages and headcounts. Just as a toolbox contains a variety of tools to accomplish a variety of diverse tasks (e.g., screwdriver to place or remove screws, saw to cut materials, etc.), there are a variety of statistical tests, each suited to address a different type of research question.

RESEARCH QUESTIONS

A statistician colleague of mine once said, "I want the numbers to tell me a story." Those nine words elegantly describe the mission of statistics. Naturally, the story depends on the nature of the statistical question. Some statistical questions render descriptive (summary) statistics, such as: How many nursing students are there? How many nurses are female and how many are male? What is the average age of students at a school? How many accidents have occurred at an intersection? What percentage of the people in a geographical region have a particular disease? What is the average income per household in a community? What percentage of seniors opt for a flu shot? Attempting to comprehend such figures simply by inspecting them visually may work for a few dozen numbers, but visual inspection of these figures would not be feasible if there were hundreds or even thousands of numbers to consider. To get a reasonable idea of the nature of these numbers, we can mathematically and graphically summarize them and thereby better understand any amount of figures using **Descriptive Statistics,** as detailed in Chapter 4.

Another form of research question involves comparisons; often this takes the form of an experimental outcome. Some questions may involve comparisons of scores between two groups, such as: Is a drug equally effective for both females and males? Do smokers sleep more than nonsmokers? Do students whose parents are in health care professions have better test scores than students whose parents are not? In a two-group clinical trial, one group was given a new drug to lower blood pressure, and the other group was given a placebo (e.g., a sugar pill); did the drug outperform the placebo? These sorts of questions, involving scores from two groups, are answered using the ***t* test,** which is covered in Chapter 5.

Research questions and their corresponding designs may involve more than two groups. For example, three clinics use different handwashing protocols; is there a statistically significant difference in infection rates from one clinic to another? Another example could be a clinical trial aimed at discovering the optimal dosage of a new antihypertensive medication; Group 1 gets a placebo, Group 2 gets the drug at a 10-mg dose, and Group 3 gets the drug at a 15-mg dose; is there a statistically significant difference in the blood pressure among these three groups? Questions involving analyzing these sorts of scores from more than two groups are processed using **ANOVA** (analysis of variance), which is covered in Chapter 6.

Occasionally, the outcome of a study may be influenced by an identifiable extraneous factor. Suppose in the above blood pressure medication clinical trial example, we identify that some of the participants in this study smoke; since we know that smoking can raise blood pressure, we can tell the analysis of covariance (ANCOVA) processor how many cigarettes each participant smokes per day. This will enable the results to be adjusted accordingly. **ANCOVA** is covered in Chapter 7.

There may be times when a single intervention may affect more than one thing. For example, consider a three-group study designed to reduce depression; Group 1 gets a placebo, Group 2 gets 10 mg of the drug, and Group 3 gets 20 mg of the drug. Naturally, we would want to measure depression among these groups, but we may also want to measure self-esteem. Furthermore, we may want to determine if there is a synergistic relationship between depression and self-esteem across these groups. This can be determined using multivariate analysis of variance **(MANOVA),** as detailed in Chapter 8.

Some research questions involve assessing the effectiveness of a treatment measured over a period of time using a single group. For example, suppose we want to determine if meditation is effective in reducing stress. Before administering the meditation training, we record the resting pulse rate of each participant—this would be the *pretest,* next we would provide the meditation workshop, and finally, after the participants actually do the meditation, we would measure their *posttest* pulse rate. The question is: Is there a statistically significant difference between the test scores *before and after* the treatment? Questions involving before-and-after scores within a (single) group are processed with the **paired *t* test**, which is covered in Chapter 9.

As useful as the pretest/posttest design is, there are occasions when we want to track an outcome over more than just two time points (pretest and posttest); for example, a pretest/posttest design for a smoking cessation intervention may gather pretest data (number of cigarettes smoked daily), then implement the smoking cessation intervention, and gather posttest data 30 days later. Suppose the findings indicate that participants were able to reduce their smoking by 60%. Instead of stopping there, we could continue to follow these participants and gather smoking data on a monthly basis to see what happens to smoking rates over time. Whereas the paired *t* test enables us to determine the change spanning (only) two time points (pretest : posttest), we may want to (statistically) measure the participant's progress several times over a longer time period (e.g., Day 1, Day 30, Day 60, Day 90, etc.). This would reveal if smoking rates go back up, level off, or continue to reduce over time. The statistic for assessing progress over time is the **ANOVA repeated measures,** which is covered in Chapter 10.

Researchers are often interested in how one variable relates to another. We might ask, What is the relationship between exercise and weight (if exercise goes up, does weight go down)? What is the relationship between mood and hours of sleep per night (when mood is low, do people sleep more or less)? Questions involving the correlation between two (continuous) scores are processed using **correlation and regression,** which are covered in Chapter 11.

Research questions may involve comparisons between categories. For example, we may want to know if men tend to take the day off work more often than women when sick or vice versa. In other words, we may want to know if gender has any bearing on going to work while sick. Questions involving comparisons among categories are processed using **chi-square** (*chi* is pronounced *k-eye*), which is covered in Chapter 12.

Some health science research focuses on comprehending the odds of an outcome occurring (or not). For example, it would be useful to know who is most likely to contract a particular disease. Such findings may reveal that the odds of contracting a particular disease are four times higher among those who work outdoors, compared to those who work indoors. These results are derived using **logistic regression,** which is covered in Chapter 13.

As you can see, even at this point, a variety of statistical questions can be asked and answered. An important part of knowing which statistical test to reach for involves understanding the nature of the question and the type of data at hand (categorical/continuous).

The answers to these statistical questions can be used to facilitate evidence-based practice, wherein facts and figures are used to identify and adopt interventions that have a scientifically successful track record. Strategically using such findings helps to take the guesswork out of the decision-making process when it comes to assembling proposals for new health care services, modifying existing services, formulating optimal policies and practice guidelines, and evaluating the effectiveness of programs.

CONTROL AND EXPERIMENTAL GROUPS

Even if you are new to statistics, you have probably heard of *control* and *experimental* groups. To understand the rationale for using this two-group system, consider an investigation that uses an experimental group *only.*

Suppose you conducted a one-group study and collected information only on people who received a flu shot, and you discover that 99% of those individuals remained healthy throughout the entire flu season. In isolation, this 99% finding seems fairly impressive. Now consider an enhanced design, where in addition to surveying people who *had the flu shot,* you also gather data on those who *did not have a flu shot,* and you discover that 99% of those who did not get a flu shot remained healthy throughout the flu season as well. Now suddenly that flu shot is starting to look considerably less impressive. Having the second (control) group gives you a baseline to compare with the experimental group. Intuitively, to determine the effectiveness of an intervention, you are looking for *substantial differences in the performance between the two groups*—is there a significant difference between the results of those in the experimental group compared with the control group? The statistical tests covered in this text focus on different types of procedures for evaluating the difference(s) between groups (experimental : control) to help determine the effect of the intervention—whether the experimental group significantly outperformed the control group.

RATIONALE FOR RANDOM ASSIGNMENT

Understanding the utility of randomly assigning subjects to experimental/control groups is best explained by example: A nurse in charge of a research program has designed an experiment to test a new antihypertensive drug. Participants are recruited and 100 people qualify for this study, which involves treating half of the participants with Drug A (the new drug) and the other half with Drug B, the leading antihypertensive treatment. At the conclusion of the study, the nurse will measure the blood pressure from each participant and compare the systolic scores to determine if Drug A outperformed Drug B. The question is: *How should the 100 participants be divided into two groups?* This is not such a simple question. If the participants are divided into females and males, this may influence the outcome; gender may be a relevant factor in how the drug(s) work—if by chance we send the gender who is more susceptible to the drug to receive Drug A, this may serve to inflate those scores. Alternatively, suppose we decided to slice the group in half by seating, presuming all of the participants are called to the facility at the same time—this introduces a different potential confound; what if the half who sits near the front of the room are naturally more amenable to the treatment adherence than those who sit in the back half of the room? Again, this grouping method may confound the findings of the study. Finally, suppose the researcher splits the group by age; this can present yet another potential confound—maybe Drug A is more effective in younger people; this could corrupt our findings. In addition, it is unwise to allow participants to self-select which group they want to be in; it may be that the more health-conscious participants may systemically opt for the Drug A group, thereby potentially influencing the outcome. Through this simple example, it should be clear that the act of selectively assigning subjects to (control/experimental) groups can unintentionally affect the outcome of a study; it is for this reason that we often opt for *random assignment* to assemble such groups.

In this example, the nurse uses a coin flip to assign participants to each of the two groups: Heads assigns the participant to the Drug A (experimental) group, and tails assigns a participant to the Drug B (control/treatment as usual) group. This random assignment method ultimately means that regardless of factors such as gender, seating position, age, motivation, and so on, each participant will have an equal (50/50) chance of being assigned to either group. The process of random assignment will generally result in roughly the same proportion of women and men, the same proportion of front- and back-of-the-room sitting participants, and the same proportion of older and younger participants being assigned to each group. If done properly, random assignment helps to cancel out factors endemic in subjects that may have otherwise tipped the findings one way or another.

HYPOTHESIS FORMULATION

Everyone has heard of the word *hypothesis;* hypotheses simply spell out each of the anticipated possible outcomes of an experiment. In simplest terms, we need one hypothesis that states that nothing notable happened, because sometimes experiments fail. This would be the null hypothesis (H_0), basically meaning that the experiment had a null effect—nothing notable happened; the experimental group performed about the same as the control group. Another possibility is that something notable *did* happen (the experiment worked), so we would need an alternate hypothesis that accounts for this (H_1). Continuing with the antihypertension drug example, we first construct the null hypothesis (H_0); as expected, the null hypothesis states that the experiment produced *null* results—basically, the experimental group (the group that got Drug A) and the control group (the group that got Drug B) performed about the same; essentially, that would mean that Drug A was no more effective than the traditional medication, Drug B. The test hypothesis (H_1) is phrased indicating that the experimental (Drug A) group outperformed the control (Drug B) group. Hypotheses are typically written in this fashion:

H_0: Drug A and Drug B produced equivalent (systolic) blood pressure results.

H_1: Drug A produced lower (systolic) blood pressure results than Drug B.

When the results are in, we would then know which hypothesis to reject and which to accept; from there, we can document and discuss our findings.

To summarize: In simplest terms, the statistics that we will be processing are designed to answer the following question: *Do the members of the experimental group (that get the innovative treatment) significantly outperform the members of the control group (who get no treatment, a placebo, or treatment as usual)?* As such, the hypotheses need to reflect each plausible outcome. In this simple example, H_0 states that there is *no* significant difference in the blood pressure of the experimental group compared to the control group, suggesting that *the treatment was ineffective.* On the other hand, we need another hypothesis that anticipates that the treatment will significantly outperform the control condition; as such, H_1 states that there *is* a statistically significant difference in the blood pressure between the experimental and control conditions, suggesting that *the treatment was effective.* The outcome of the statistical test will point us to which hypothesis to keep and which to reject.

READING STATISTICAL OUTCOMES

Statistical tests vary substantially in terms of the types of research questions each are designed to address, the format of the source data, their respective equations, and the content of their results, which can include figures, tables, and graphs. Although there are some similarities in reading statistical outcomes (e.g., means, alpha [α] level, *p* value), these concepts are best explained in the context of working examples; as such, discussion of how to read statistical outcomes will be thoroughly explained as each emerges in Chapters 4 through 13.

ACCEPT/REJECT HYPOTHESES

As is the case with reading statistical outcomes, the decision to accept or reject a hypothesis depends on the nature of the test and, of course, the results: the alpha (α) level, *p* value, and, in some cases, the means. Just as with reading statistical outcomes, instructions for accepting/rejecting hypotheses for each test are best discussed in the context of actual working examples; these concepts will be covered in Chapters 5 through 13.

VARIABLE TYPES/LEVELS OF MEASURE

Comprehending the types of variables involved in a data set or research design is essential when it comes to properly selecting, running, and documenting the results of statistical tests. There are two types of variables: continuous and categorical. Each has two levels of measure; continuous variables may be either interval or ratio, and categorical variables may be either nominal or ordinal.

Continuous

Continuous variables contain the kinds of numbers that you are accustomed to dealing with in counting and mathematics. A continuous variable may be either interval or ratio.

Interval

Interval variables consist of numbers that have equal spacing between them, such as numbers on a number line, ranging from $-\infty$ to $+\infty$; the distance between 1 and 2 is the same as the distance between 2 and 3, which is the same as the distance between 3 and 4, and so on. Some additional examples of interval variables are bank account balance (which could be negative) and temperature (°C or °F). Interval variables are considered continuous variables.

Ratio

Ratio variables are similar to interval variables, except that interval variables can have negative values, whereas ratio variables cannot be less than zero. Ratio variables include measurements such as height, weight, pulse rate, calories, number of pills in a bottle, number of siblings, or number of members in a group. Ratio variables are considered continuous variables.

Learning tip: Notice that the word *ratio* ends in *o*, which looks like a *zero*.

Categorical

Categorical variables (also known as *discrete* variables) involve assigning a number to an item in a category. A categorical variable may be either nominal or ordinal.

Nominal

Nominal variables are used to represent categories that defy ordering. For example, suppose you wish to code eye color, and there are six choices: amber, blue, brown, gray, green, and hazel. There is really no way to put these in any order; for coding and computing purposes, we could assign 1 = amber, 2 = blue, 3 = brown, 4 = gray, 5 = green, and 6 = hazel. Since order does not matter among nominal variables, these eye colors could have just as well been coded 1 = blue, 2 = green, 3 = hazel, 4 = gray, 5 = amber, and 6 = brown. Nominal variables may be used to represent categorical variables such as gender (1 = female, 2 = male), agreement (1 = yes, 2 = no), religion (1 = atheist, 2 = Buddhist, 3 = Catholic, 4 = Hindu, 5 = Jewish, 6 = Taoist, etc.), or marital status (1 = single, 2 = married, 3 = separated, 4 = divorced, 5 = widow/widower).

Since the numbers are arbitrarily assigned to labels within a category, it would be inappropriate to perform traditional arithmetic calculations on such numbers. For example, it would be foolish to compute the average *marital status* (e.g., would 1.5 indicate a *single married* person?). The same principle applies to other nominal variables such as religion or gender. There are, however, appropriate statistical operations for processing nominal variables that will be discussed in **Chapter 4: Descriptive Statistics.** In terms of statistical tests, nominal variables are considered categorical variables.

> **Learning tip:** There is no order among the categories in a nominal variable; notice that the word *nominal* starts with *no,* as in *no order.*

Ordinal

Ordinal variables are similar to nominal variables in that numbers are assigned to represent items within a category. Whereas nominal variables have no real rank order to them (e.g., amber, blue, brown, gray, green, hazel), the values in an ordinal variable *can* be placed in a ranked order. For example, there is an order to educational degrees (1 = high school diploma, 2 = associate's degree, 3 = bachelor's degree, 4 = master's degree, 5 = doctorate degree). Other examples of ordinal variables include military rank (1 = private, 2 = corporal, 3 = sergeant, etc.) and meals (1 = breakfast, 2 = brunch, 3 = lunch, 4 = dinner, 5 = late-night snack). In terms of statistical tests, ordinal variables are considered categorical variables.

> **Learning tip:** Notice that the root of the word *ordinal* is *order,* suggesting that the categories have a meaningful *order* to them.

GOOD COMMON SENSE

As we explore the results of multiple statistics throughout this text, keep in mind that no matter how precisely we proceed, the process of statistics is not perfect. Our findings do not *prove* or *disprove* anything; rather, statistics helps us to reduce uncertainty—to help us better comprehend the nature of those that we study.

Additionally, what we learn from statistical findings speaks to the *group* that we studied on an *overall basis,* not any one *individual.* For instance, suppose we find that the average pulse rate within a group is 100; this does not mean that we can point to any one person in that group and presume that his or her pulse rate is 100.

Key Concepts

- Research question
- Control group
- Experimental group
- Random assignment
- Hypotheses
- Statistical outcomes
- Accepting/rejecting hypotheses
- Types of data (continuous, categorical)
- Level of data (continuous: interval, ratio; categorical: nominal, ordinal)

Practice Exercises

Exercise 1.1

Each of the following exercises describes the basis for an experiment that would render data that could be processed statistically.

1. In an effort to fight childhood obesity, the nurse at an elementary school implements an aerobic square dance club that meets for 30 minutes each lunch hour for a month.
   a. State the research question.
   b. Identify the control and experimental group(s).
   c. Explain how you would randomly assign participants to groups.
   d. State the hypotheses (H_0 and H_1).
   e. Discuss the criteria for accepting/rejecting the hypotheses.

2. Recent findings suggest that nursing home residents may experience fewer depressive symptoms when they participate in pet therapy with certified dogs for 30 minutes per day.
   a. State the research question.
   b. Identify the control and experimental group(s).

c. Explain how you would randomly assign participants to groups.
d. State the hypotheses (H_0 and H_1).
e. Discuss the criteria for accepting/rejecting the hypotheses.

Hint: You may implement the Acme Depression Scale, which renders a score from 0 (no depression) to 10 (high depression).

3. A physical therapy clinic wants to determine if sending patients a text message reminder the day before appointments reduces no-shows.

   a. State the research question.
   b. Identify the control and experimental group(s).
   c. Explain how you would randomly assign participants to groups.
   d. State the hypotheses (H_0 and H_1).
   e. Discuss the criteria for accepting/rejecting the hypotheses.

4. Anytown Community wants to determine if handwashing education in the schools helps to reduce illness.

   a. State the research question.
   b. Identify the control and experimental group(s).
   c. Explain how you would randomly assign participants to groups.
   d. State the hypotheses (H_0 and H_1).
   e. Discuss the criteria for accepting/rejecting the hypotheses.

5. Employees at Acme Healthcare Systems, consisting of four separate hospitals, are chronically late. The nurse manager is considering implementing a *get out of Friday free* lottery; each day an employee is on time, he or she gets one token entered into the weekly lottery.

   a. State the research question.
   b. Identify the control and experimental group(s).
   c. Explain how you would randomly assign participants to groups.
   d. State the hypotheses (H_0 and H_1).
   e. Discuss the criteria for accepting/rejecting the hypotheses.

6. The Acme Herbal Tea Company advertises that their product is "the tea that relaxes."

   a. State the research question.
   b. Identify the control and experimental group(s).
   c. Explain how you would randomly assign participants to groups.
   d. State the hypotheses (H_0 and H_1).
   e. Discuss the criteria for accepting/rejecting the hypotheses.

Hint: You may implement the Acme Stress Index, which renders a score from 0 (no stress) to 10 (high stress).

7. A nurse in a geriatric ward has a theory that singing improves memory.
    a. State the research question.
    b. Identify the control and experimental group(s).
    c. Explain how you would randomly assign participants to groups.
    d. State the hypotheses (H_0 and H_1).
    e. Discuss the criteria for accepting/rejecting the hypotheses.

Hint: You may implement the Acme Memory Acuity Test, which renders a score from 0 (low recall) to 10 (high recall).

8. A pharmacy manager wants to find out if printing labels in 16-point font will result in better dosage adherence than the usual 10-point font.
    a. State the research question.
    b. Identify the control and experimental group(s).
    c. Explain how you would randomly assign participants to groups.
    d. State the hypotheses (H_0 and H_1).
    e. Discuss the criteria for accepting/rejecting the hypotheses.

9. Nurse Able wants to determine if including wireless Internet access (WIFI) in waiting rooms reduces patient anxiety.
    a. State the research question.
    b. Identify the control and experimental group(s).
    c. Explain how you would randomly assign participants to groups.
    d. State the hypotheses (H_0 and H_1).
    e. Discuss the criteria for accepting/rejecting the hypotheses.

10. Nurse Baker wants to determine if a brief video promoting flu shots is more effective than providing a pamphlet containing the same information.
    a. State the research question.
    b. Identify the control and experimental group(s).
    c. Explain how you would randomly assign participants to groups.
    d. State the hypotheses (H_0 and H_1).
    e. Discuss the criteria for accepting/rejecting the hypotheses.

CHAPTER 2

Sampling

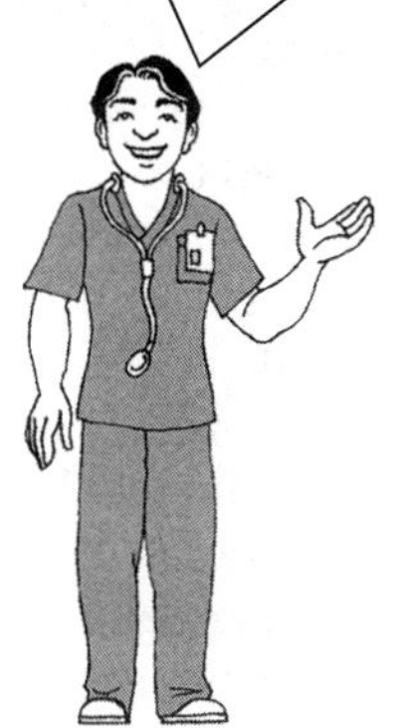
Who needs the whole population when a **sample** will do nicely?

- Rationale for Sampling
- Sampling Terminology
- Representative Sample
- Probability Sampling
- Nonprobability Sampling
- Sampling Bias

Ya gots to work with what you gots to work with.

—Stevie Wonder

LEARNING OBJECTIVES

Upon completing this chapter, you will be able to:

- Comprehend the rationale for sampling: time, cost, feasibility, extrapolation
- Understand essential sampling terminology: population, sample frame, sample
- Derive a representative sample to facilitate external validity
- Select an appropriate method to conduct probability sampling: simple random sampling, stratified sampling, proportionate sampling, disproportionate sampling, systemic sampling, area sampling
- Select an appropriate method to conduct nonprobability sampling: convenience sampling, purposive sampling, quota sampling, snowball sampling
- Understand techniques for detecting and reducing sample bias
- Optimal sample size

OVERVIEW—SAMPLING

Statistics is about processing numbers in a way to produce concise, readily consumable information. One statistic that you are probably already familiar with is the average. Suppose you wanted to know the average age of students in a classroom; the task would be fairly simple—you could ask each person to write down his or her age on a slip of paper and then proceed with the calculations. In the relatively small setting of a classroom, it is possible to promptly gather the data on everyone, but what if you wanted to know the age of all enrolled students or all students in a community? Now the mission becomes more time-consuming, complex, and probably expensive. Instead of trying to gather data on *everyone,* as in the U.S. census survey, another option is to gather a *sample*. Gathering a sample of a population is quicker, easier, and more cost-effective than gathering data on everyone, and if done properly, the findings from your sample can provide you with quality information about the overall population.

You may not realize it, but critical decisions are made based on samples all the time. Laboratories process thousands of blood samples every day. On the basis of the small amount of blood contained in the test tube, a qualified health care professional can make determinations about the overall health status of the patient from whom the blood was drawn. Think about that for a moment: A few CCs (cubic centimeters) of blood are sufficient to carry out the tests to make quality determinations; the laboratory did not need to drain the entire blood supply from the patient, which would be time-consuming, complicated, expensive, and totally impractical—it would kill the patient. Just as a small sample of blood is sufficient to represent the status of the entire blood supply, proper sampling enables us to gather a small and manageable bundle of data from a population of interest, statistically process that data, and reasonably comprehend the larger population from which it was drawn.

RATIONALE FOR SAMPLING

Moving beyond the realm of a statistics course, statistics takes place in the real world to answer real-world questions. As with most things in the real world, gathering data involves the utilization of scarce resources; key concerns involve the time, cost, and feasibility associated with gathering quality data. With these very real constraints in mind, it is a relief to know that it is not necessary to gather *all* of the data available; in fact, it is rare that a statistical data set consists of figures from the entire population (such as the U.S. census). Typically, we proceed with a viable sample and extrapolate what we need to know to better comprehend the larger population from which that sample was drawn. Let us take a closer look at each of these factors.

Time

Some consider time to be the most valuable asset; time cannot be manufactured or stored—it can only be used. Time spent doing one thing means that other things must wait. Spending an exorbitant amount of time gathering data from an entire population precludes the accomplishment of other vital activities. For example, suppose you are interested in people's opinions on (getting or not getting) the flu shot for a paper that you are drafting for a course. Every minute you spend gathering data postpones your ability to proceed with the completion of the paper, and that paper has a firm due date. Additionally, there are other demands competing for your time (e.g., other courses, work, family, friends, rest, recreation, etc.). Sampling reduces the amount of time involved in gathering data, enabling you to statistically process the data more promptly and proceed with the completion of the project within the allotted time.

Another aspect of time is that some (statistical) answers are time sensitive. Political pollsters must use sampling to gather information in a prompt fashion, hence leaving sufficient time to interpret the findings and fine-tune campaign strategies prior to the election; they simply do not have time to poll all registered voters—a well-drawn sample is sufficient.

Cost

Not all data are readily available (for free). Some statistical data may be derived from experiments or interviews, which involves multiple costs, including a recruitment advertising budget, paying staff to screen and process participants, providing reasonable financial compensation to study participants, facility expenses, and so on. Surveys are not free either; expenses may include photocopying, postage, website implementation charges, telephone equipment, and financial compensation to study participants and staff. Considering the costs associated with data collection, one can see the rationale for resorting to sampling as opposed to attempting to gather data from an entire population.

Feasibility

Data gathering takes place in the real world—hence, real-world constraints must be reckoned with when embarking on such research. Due to time and budgetary constraints, it is seldom feasible or necessary to gather data on a population-wide basis; sampling is a viable option. In the case involving the blood sample, clearly it is neither necessary nor feasible to submit the patient's entire blood supply to the lab for testing—quality determinations can be made based on well-drawn samples. In addition, if a research project focuses on a large population (e.g., all of the people who have ever received care within a health care system) or a population spanning a large geographical region, it may not be feasible to gather data on that many people—hence, sampling makes sense.

Extrapolation

It turns out that by sampling properly, it is unnecessary to gather data on an entire population to achieve a reasonable comprehension of it. Extrapolation involves using sampling methods and statistics to analyze the sample of data that was drawn from the population. If done properly, such findings help us to (better) understand not only the smaller (sample) group but also the larger group from which it was drawn.

SAMPLING TERMINOLOGY

As in any scientific endeavor, the realm of sampling has its own language and methods. The following terms and types of sampling methods will help you comprehend the kinds of sampling that you may encounter in scientific literature and provide you with viable options for carrying out your own studies. We will begin with the largest realm (the *population*) and work our way down to the smallest (the *sample*).

Population

The *population* is the entire realm of people (or items) that could be measured or counted. A *population* is not simply all people on the planet; the researcher specifies the population, which consists of the entire domain of interest. For example, the population may be defined as all of the people who have ever received care at a hospital. Additional examples of populations could be all people who reside in a city, all people who belong to a club, all students enrolled at a school, all people who are registered voters in an election district, or all people who work for a company. As you might have surmised, the key word here is *all.*

Sample Frame

If the population that you are interested in is relatively small (e.g., the 5 people in a waiting room, the 16 people who are receiving infusions, etc.), then gathering data from the entire population is potentially doable. More often, the population is larger than you can reasonably accommodate, or you may be unable to attain a complete list of the entire population that you are interested in (e.g., everyone who has ever been a patient at a hospital, everyone living in a city, etc.). The *sample frame,* sometimes referred to as the *sampling frame,* is the part of a *population* that you could potentially access. For example, Acme Clinic maintains a list of patient names and email IDs. If this list included every single patient who has ever been seen at the Acme Clinic, then it would represent the entire (patient) population of the clinic; however, patients have the privilege to opt out of this list, indicating that they do not want to be contacted by the clinic in between visits. Suppose the total population of the clinic consists of 30,000 patients, and 70% opt to have their name appear on this list; this would mean that the sample frame, the list from which you could potentially select study participants, consists of 21,000 patients (30,000 × .70).

Sample

A *sample* is a portion of individuals selected from the *sample frame*. While 21,000 is considerably less than 30,000, that may still be an unwieldy amount for your purposes.

Consider that your investigation involves conducting a 1-hour interview with participants and that each participant will be compensated $10 for his or her time; the participant fee budget for this study would be $210,000, and assuming you conducted back-to-back interviews for 8 hours a day, 7 days a week, you would have your data set in a little over 7 years. Considering the constraints mentioned earlier (time, cost, and feasibility), you can probably already see where this is going: (1) Is a $210,000 budget for subjects really feasible? (2) Do you really have 7 years to gather your findings? (3) Many of the patients on this list may be unreachable 7 years from now—email IDs can change. (4) Memory is not perfect; over time, some memories remain fully intact, whereas some events and

Figure 2.1 Three tiers of sampling: population, sample frame, and sample.

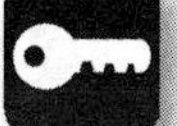

Just to recap: You can think of the *population, sample frame,* and *sample* as a series of subgroups (Figure 2.1):

- The ***population*** is the entire realm of those in a specified set (e.g., every person who has been a patient at a clinic, all people in the waiting room, all people in the infusion center).
- The ***sample frame*** is the sublist of those in the *population* who could potentially be accessed.
- The ***sample*** is the sublist of those selected from the *sample frame* who you will (attempt to) gather data from.

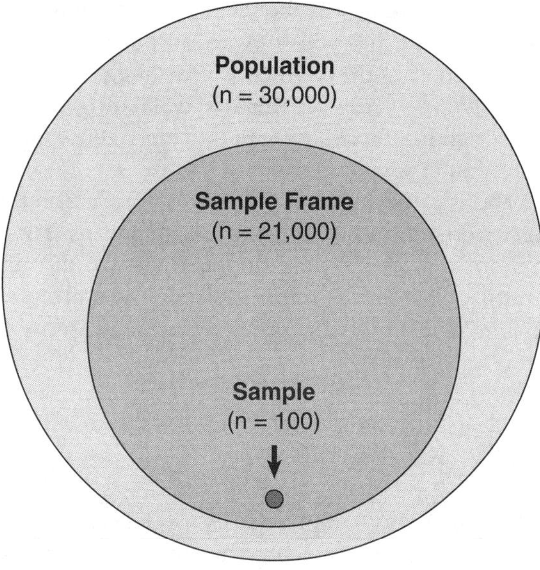

details may be forgotten or (unintentionally) distorted, diminished, or inflated over time. Data gathered later in this 7-year survey cycle may be less accurate.

In this case, accessing the entire *sample frame* is clearly untenable, but the *sample frame* is still useful; instead of attempting to recruit the 21,000 patients, you may choose to gather information from a subset of 100 patients from this *sample frame*. These 100 patients will constitute the *sample*. Selecting a *sample* of 100 patients from the *sample frame* of 21,000 means that your participant fee budget is reduced from $210,000 to $1,000, and instead of taking more than 7 years to gather the data, using the same interviewing schedule, you would have your complete data set in under 2 weeks. In terms of feasibility, sampling is clearly the way to go. As for how to select that sample of 100 patients from among the sample frame of 21,000, there are a variety of techniques covered in the sections on *probability sampling* and *nonprobability sampling*.

REPRESENTATIVE SAMPLE

You may not realize it, but you already understand the notion of a *representative sample*. Suppose you are at a cheese-tasting party, and the host brings out a large wheel of cheese from Acme Dairy. You are served a small morsel of the cheese that is less than 1% of the whole cheese and, based on that, you decide if you like it enough to buy a hunk of it or not. The assumption that you are perhaps unknowingly making is that the whole rest of that big cheese will be exactly like the tiny *sample* that you tasted. You are presuming that the bottom part of the cheese is not harder, that the other side of the cheese is not sharper, that the middle part of the cheese is not runnier, and so on. Essentially, you are assuming that the sample of cheese that you tasted is *representative* of the flavor, color, and consistency of the whole wheel of cheese. This is what a representative sample is all about: The small sample that you drew is proportionally representative of the overall population (or big cheese) from which it was taken. Often, it is the goal of researchers to select a *representative sample,* thereby facilitating external validity—meaning that what you discover about the *sample* can be viably generalized to the overall *population* from which the sample was drawn.

Sampling is about gathering a manageable set of data so that you can learn something about the larger population through statistical analysis. The question remains: How do you get from the *population,* to the *sample frame,* to the actual representative *sample*? Depending on the nature of the information that you are seeking and the availability of viable participants/data, you may opt to employ *probability sampling* or *nonprobability sampling* methods.

PROBABILITY SAMPLING

You can think of probability sampling as *equal-opportunity sampling,* meaning that each potential element (person/data record) has the same chance of being selected for your sample. There are several ways of conducting probability sampling.

Simple Random Sampling

Simple random sampling begins with gathering the largest sample frame possible and then numbering each item/person (1, 2, 3, . . . 60). For this example, let us assume that there are 60 people (30 females and 30 males) on this list and you want to recruit 10 participants (Figure 2.2); you could use SPSS to generate 10 random numbers ranging from 1 to 60. It is not essential that you perform this procedure at this time; Chapter 14 (Supplemental SPSS Operations) has a section that provides step-by-step instructions for generating random numbers to your specifications.

Figure 2.2 Simple random sampling.

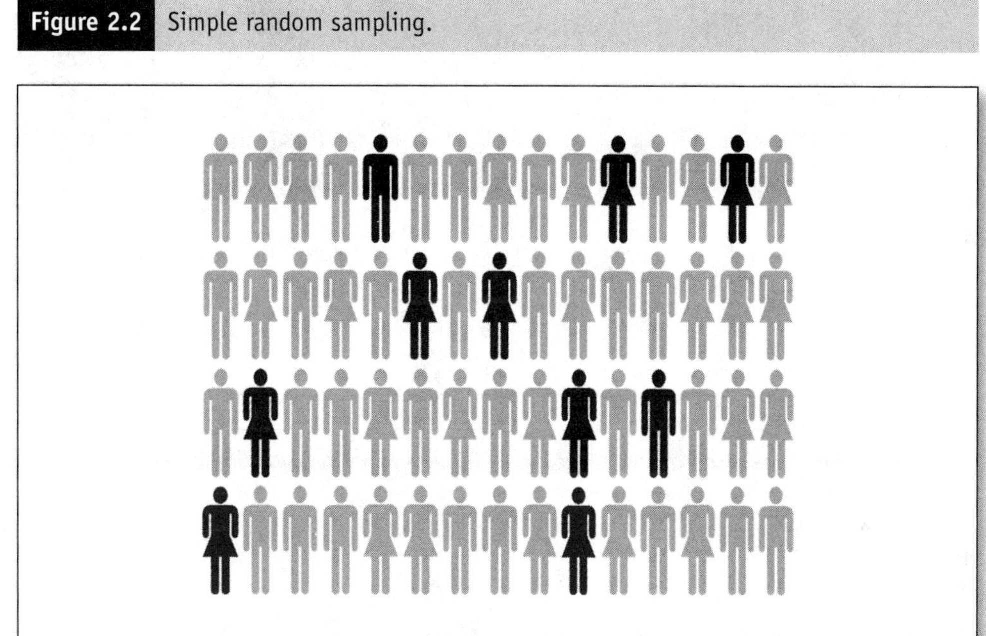

From a *sample frame* of 60, randomly select a *sample* of 10.

Stratified Sampling

In the above example, *simple random sampling* rendered a *sample* consisting of 80% females and 20% males, which may not suit your needs. Suppose you still want a *sample* of 10 from the *sample frame* of 60, but instead of leaving the gender counts to random chance, you want to specifically control for the number of females and males in your *sample; stratified sampling* would ensure that your *sample* is balanced by gender. To draw a *stratified sample* based on gender, divide your sample frame into two lists (strata): female and male. In this case, the initial sample frame of 60 is divided into two separate strata: 30 females and 30 males. Suppose you still want to draw a (total) *sample* of 10; you would use *simple random sampling* to randomly select 5 participants from the female strata and another 5 participants from the male strata (Figure 2.3).

Figure 2.3 Stratified sampling.

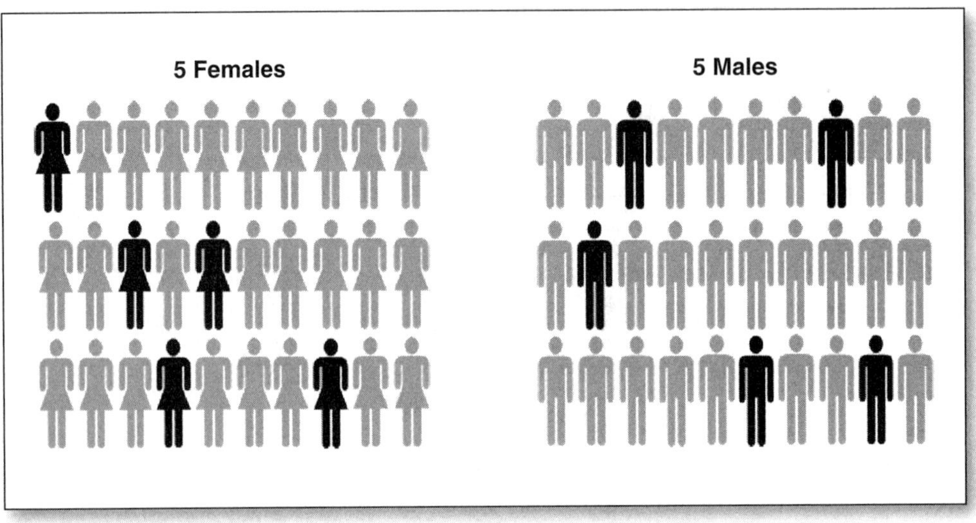

Separate the *sample frame* into two strata: females and males. Randomly select a *sample* of 5 from each strata.

NOTE: *Systemic sampling* (which will be discussed on page **22**) could also be used to make selections within each strata.

Disproportionate/Proportionate Sampling

Within the realm of *stratified sampling,* you can further specify if you want to gather a *proportionate* or *disproportionate* sample. Continuing with the gender stratification example, suppose you were conducting a survey of patients currently at a clinic that consists of 30 females and 10 males, and for purposes of this survey, gender is relevant.

The first step is to split the sample frame into two strata (lists) based on gender: female and male. You then have the option to draw a *proportionate sample* or a *disproportionate sample*. To draw a *proportionate sample,* you would draw the same percentage (in this case, 10%) from each strata: 3 from the 30 in the female strata and 1 from the 10 in the male strata (Figure 2.4).

When the count within one or more strata is relatively low, *proportional sampling* will expectedly produce a sample of the stratum that may be too small to be viable; in the above case, sampling 10% from the 10 in the male strata meant selecting only 1 male participant. In such instances, *disproportionate sampling* may be a better choice.

Figure 2.4 Proportional stratified sampling—same percentage randomly selected from each group.

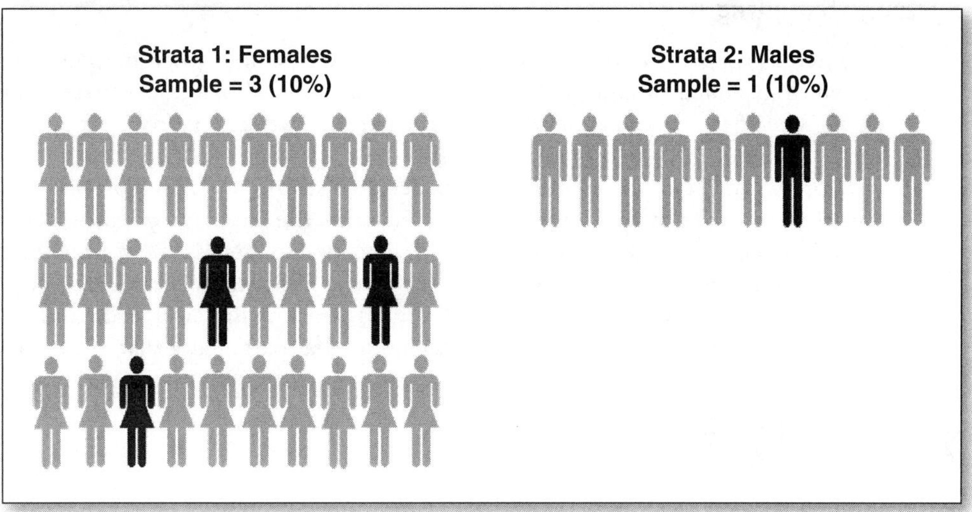

To gather a *disproportionate sample,* randomly select the same amount of participants from each stratum, regardless of the size of each stratum. In this case (Figure 2.5), 3 are being drawn from each stratum: 3 females and 3 males. Although the sample *sizes* from

Figure 2.5 Disproportional stratified sampling—same (total) number randomly selected from each group.

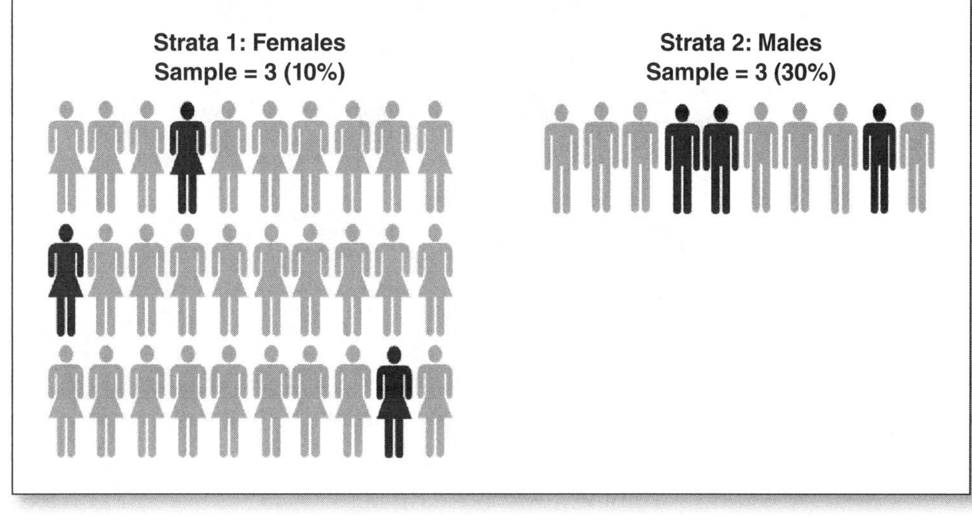

each stratum are now equal (3 from each stratum), the *proportions* are now different; 10% of the females have been selected, whereas 30% of the males have been selected.

Systemic Sampling

Whereas *simple random sampling* may produce a sample wherein the items may be drawn from similar proximity (e.g., several participants who are next to each other may all be selected), *systemic sampling* uses a periodic selection process that draws the *sample* more evenly throughout the *sample frame*.

Suppose you had 60 people and you decide that the target *sample* size will be 15 participants. Begin by dividing the *sample frame* by the target *sample* size (60 ÷ 15 = 4); the solution (4) is the "*k*" or skip term. Next, you need to identify the *start point;* this will be a random number between 1 and *k;* for this example, suppose the randomly derived *start* point number is 3. The process begins with selecting the 3rd person and then skips ahead *k* (4) people at a time to select each additional participant that will comprise the

Figure 2.6 Systemic sampling.

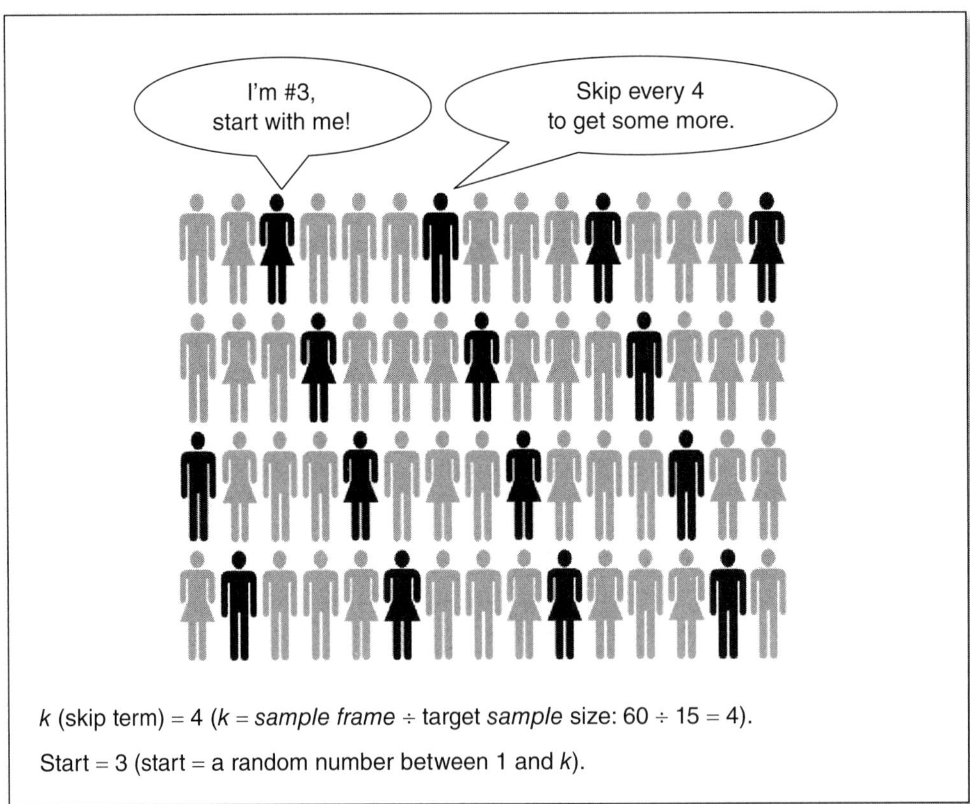
I'm #3,
start with me!
Skip every 4
to get some more.
k (skip term) = 4 (*k* = *sample frame* ÷ target *sample* size: 60 ÷ 15 = 4).
Start = 3 (start = a random number between 1 and *k*).

sample. In this case, the following 15 participants would be selected: 3, 7, 11, 15, 19, 23, 27, 31, 35, 39, 43, 47, 51, 55, and 59 (Figure 2.6).

Area Sampling

Area sampling, also referred to as *cluster sampling* or *multistage cluster sampling,* is typically used when it comes to gathering samples from a geographical region or when a sample frame is not available. Since the characteristics of neighborhoods and their residents can vary substantially from block to block, it is unwise to gather data from only one region. Area sampling enables you to gather a more representative sample that spans the entire geographical region specified.

This multistage process begins with acquiring a *sample frame* containing a list of the domestic addresses within a given geographical domain. For example, Smalltown consists of a population of 2,000 people spanning 20 residential blocks. Your target sample size is to conduct 40 surveys. Based on these figures, calculate the number of samples that will be drawn from each block using the following formula: **Samples per block = Target sample size ÷ Blocks:**

Area Sampling

Samples per block = Target sample size ÷ Blocks

Samples per block = 40 ÷ 20

Samples per block = 2

In this case, two samples will be randomly selected from each of the 20 blocks. Next build the *block strata* (Block 1, Block 2, Block 3, . . . Block 20). Each block stratum contains the addresses of every dwelling on that block. Finally, randomly select two addresses from each of the 20 blocks (strata) (20 blocks × 2 households per block = target *sample* size of 40) (Figure 2.7).

Area sampling is similar to *systemic sampling,* in that both are designed to help draw the *sample* more evenly from the *sample frame* as opposed to taking the chance that *simple random sampling* may draw too many (or too few) from any one area.

For simplicity, this example presumed uniform population density across the 20 blocks of Smalltown—that each block contains about the same number of dwellings and about the same number of people living in each dwelling. Naturally, prior to selecting the sample, it would be wise to statistically check this assumption and consider adjusting the sampling proportions to best represent the residents of Smalltown. For example, if it is found that 10% of the residents of Smalltown live on one block, then it would be appropriate to draw 10% of the overall sample from that single block.

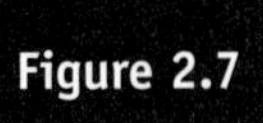

Figure 2.7 Area sampling. Surveying two households (indicated by dots) from each of the 20 *blocks* produces a target *sample* of 40.

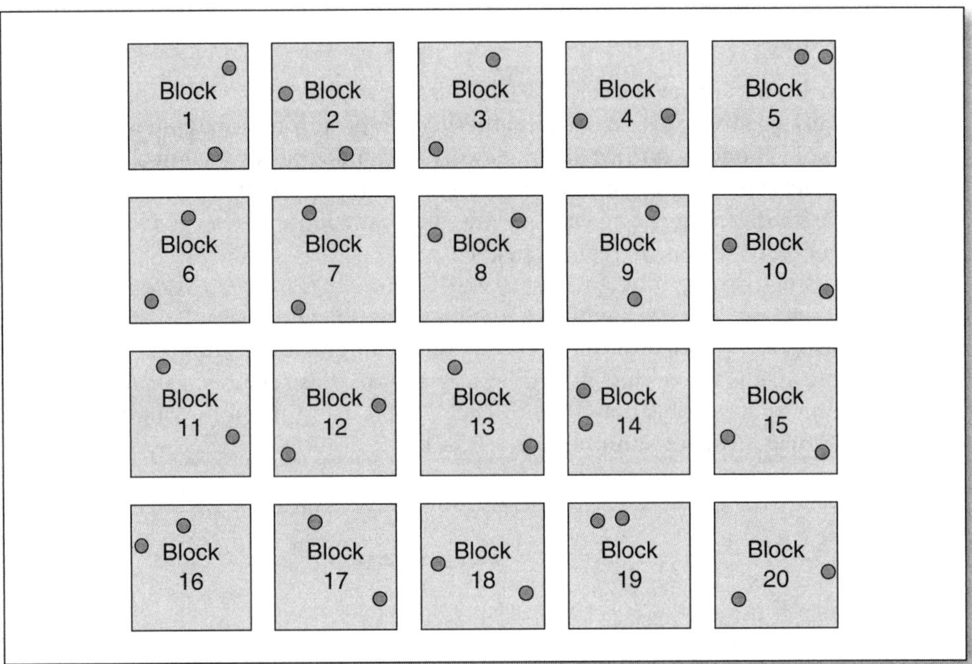

NONPROBABILITY SAMPLING

In *probability sampling,* each item in the *sample frame* has an equal chance of being selected when it comes to being included in the sample. In *nonprobability sampling,* either the *sample frame* does not exist or the researcher does not consider it relevant to the investigation at hand.

In nonprobability sampling, the elements that will constitute the *sample* will not be drawn randomly from a *sample frame;* rather, they will have some special characteristic(s), which is not proportionally representative of the overall *population.* As such, *external validity,* the ability to viably generalize the findings from your *sample* to the overall *population,* is the first casualty of *nonprobability sampling.* Still, much can be learned from *nonprobability sampling.*

Convenience Sampling

Convenience sampling, sometimes referred to as *availability sampling,* is exactly what it sounds like; the researcher recruits whoever is relevant to the line of investigation and readily accessible. For example, suppose you wanted to conduct a survey detailing people's exercise routines (e.g., How many days a week do you exercise? What exercise(s) do you do? How long is each exercise session?). You have noticed that a line at a neighborhood walk-in clinic forms starting at about 7:00 a.m. daily (the clinic opens at 8:00 a.m.). For 1 week, during the 1 hour before the clinic opens, you recruit volunteer participants who are waiting in that line to partake in your exercise survey (Figure 2.8).

In terms of *external validity*, clearly this survey was not designed to characterize the overall *population* of this city; instead, it was designed to provide the clinicians at this facility some clues as to the exercise propensity of their patients.

Figure 2.8 Convenience/availability sampling: surveying those who are standing in a line.

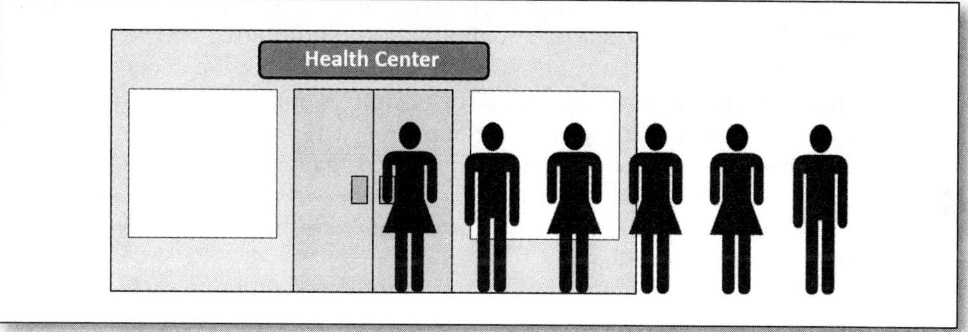

Purposive Sampling

Purposive sampling is used when the characteristics that the researcher is interested in are presumed to be of low prevalence in the population; in other words, since most of the people in the *population* would not meet the (multiple) criteria of interest, *probability sampling* would be an inefficient recruitment method. For example, suppose a researcher is interested in the effects that a particular drug has on patients undergoing radiation therapy. To be a viable participant in this study, each individual must meet *all* of the following criteria:

Participant Eligibility Criteria

- ☑ Between 18 and 65 years old
- ☑ Diagnosed with cancer
- ☑ Set to begin radiation therapy
- ☑ The prescribed course of radiation therapy consists of three to five treatments
- ☑ Willing to take an experimental drug or placebo
- ☑ Not using any nonprescribed medications

Purposive sampling may involve one or several criteria for participant selection. In this case, all six criteria must be met in order for an individual to be a potential participant. Clearly, it would be virtually impossible to encounter a sufficient number of individuals who meet all of these criteria simply by chance, as would be used in *probability sampling*. As you have likely surmised by now, each time an additional criterion is added in *purposive sampling,* the potential participant pool shrinks.

Quota Sampling

Quota sampling is typically used when a prompt response is needed from the population. In quota sampling, one or several attributes are identified and quotas are set for each. For example, suppose you are interested in the number of sleep hours per night among those who smoke and those who do not smoke, and you set the following quotas: 20 smokers and 20 nonsmokers (Figure 2.9). Once the quota is met for a group, no further data will be collected for that group. Suppose after the first hour of gathering data in a public park, you have completed surveying 15 smokers and 20 nonsmokers; at this point, you would stop attempting to gather data from nonsmokers, even if they actively volunteered, since that quota has been satisfied. You would continue your efforts to gather data from an additional 5 smokers, at which point you could (immediately) process your data.

Figure 2.9 Quota sampling.

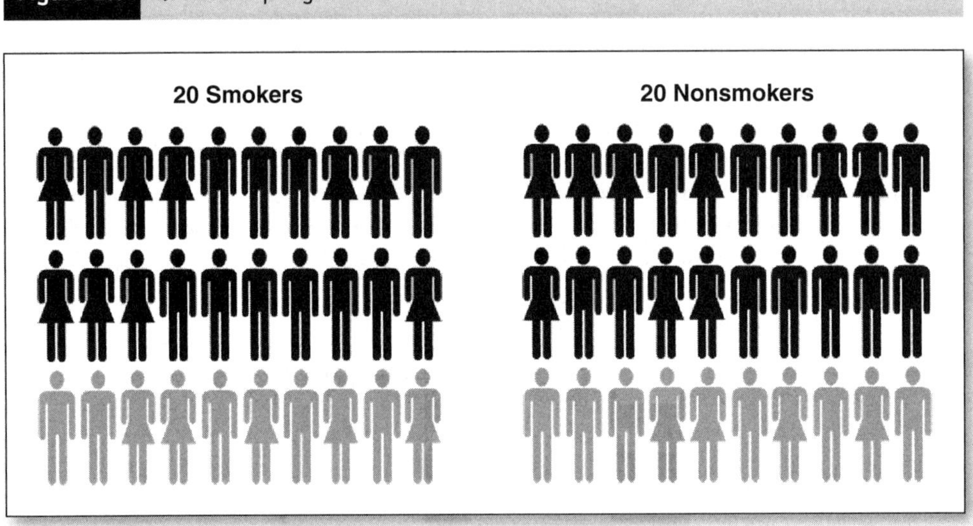

Snowball Sampling

The term *snowball sampling* comes from the (cartoon) notion that if you roll a small snowball downhill from the top of a snowy mountain, it will pick up more snow as it rolls along, ultimately amassing into a giant snowball. When it comes to *snowball sampling,* consider the proverb: *Birds of a feather flock together.*

Snowball sampling is useful when viable participants are scarce or difficult to readily identify. For example, suppose you are conducting a study of people who use a wheelchair, and by luck, you find someone in a wheelchair who is willing to participate in your study. After administering your survey/experiment, you courteously ask this person if he or she knows of anyone else who uses a wheelchair who might be interested in taking this survey. You would then follow up with these referrals and progressively ask each following participant for his or her list of referrals and so on—hence, the sample *snowballs up*. Referrals may lead to direct sources (e.g., their friends, family, colleagues, etc.) or indirect sources (e.g., wheelchair repair shop, wheelchair accessory website, rehab center, etc.). Figure 2.10 depicts an example of *snowball sampling,* wherein the first suitable participant refers you to the second participant, the second person refers you to the third, the third directs you to two more people, and so on.

Figure 2.10 Snowball sampling is based on referrals from the participant.

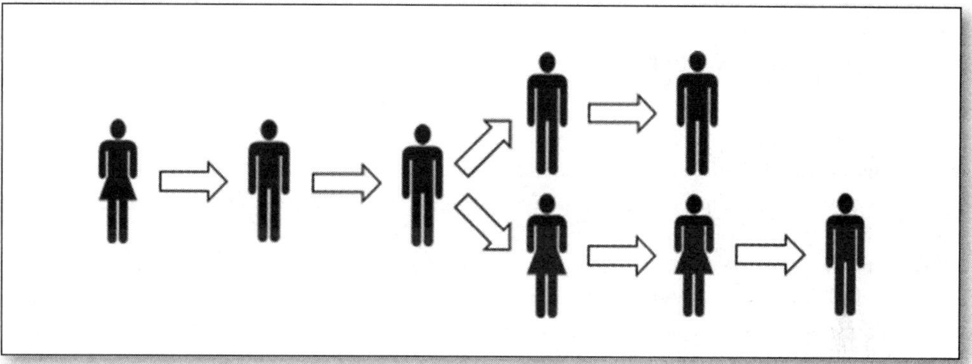

Unlike the wheelchair example, the sample that you are interested in may need to be drawn from an *invisible* or *hidden population*. This does not mean that these individuals are literally invisible or in hiding; it merely means that the feature(s) that you are interested in is not readily observable. For instance, such individuals may be invisible in that upon casual observation, they simply possess no identifying characteristics that would suggest that they meet your research criteria (e.g., single parent, bisexual, dyslexic, diabetic, etc.). Alternatively, some individuals deliberately hide the fact that they would meet the criteria for your research because revealing such information could have legal consequences (e.g., undocumented immigrants, involvement in criminal activities, etc.) or be embarrassing (e.g., peculiar obsessions, fetishes, unpopular belief systems, stigmatized disease/disorder, uncommon interests, etc.).

In any case, if you are fortunate enough to find one such person and are able to establish a professional rapport with a genuine nonthreatening and nonjudgmental demeanor, *snowball sampling* may lead you to other suitable subjects.

SAMPLING BIAS

Sampling bias occurs, perhaps unintentionally, when participants with certain characteristics are more (or less) likely to be selected. Such bias can corrupt the external validity of the findings. Depending on the methods used to identify potential participants or gather the sample, sampling bias can be a concern. For example, while it may seem reasonable to administer a survey via the Internet, this method would preclude individuals who are not computer savvy or do not have access to the Internet.

Recruitment location can also introduce survey bias; imagine the bias your data would be subject to if you were to post recruitment flyers (only) in a women's locker room, a sports bar, the lobby of a technology company, a liquor store in an impoverished neighborhood, and so forth. Such strategies would clearly be inappropriate unless you are deliberately seeking to sample and comprehend individuals endemic to those domains.

It may not be possible to completely control for sample bias in every situation, but awareness of this potential confound can be helpful when considering the credibility of the research of others and in designing and implementing your own investigations.

OPTIMAL SAMPLE SIZE

When it comes to determining the optimal sample size, there are disadvantages to samples that are too small or too large. Samples that are too small can produce unstable statistical findings, wherein a slight change in one or several scores could radically alter the statistical outcome. On the other hand, sample sizes that are too large involve spending more time, money, and effort to gather the data, as well as unnecessarily placing additional subjects at potential risk. The process of determining an optimal sample size is managed by *power calculations*. Each statistical test has its own set of power calculation equations. Although this text does not formally cover such calculations, the **Pretest Checklists** included in future chapters specify the minimum sample size necessary to produce robust statistical results. As a rule of thumb, when it comes to sample sizes, it is better to have too many than too few.

GOOD COMMON SENSE

When it comes to sampling, keep in mind that the quality of your statistical findings is dependent on the quality of the data gathered and from whom it was gathered. Methodical errors in sampling can produce misleading findings. For example, consider the relative ease of assembling and deploying a web-based survey; without careful consideration and control, your survey may attract inappropriate responders who may offer less-than-genuine responses, possibly more than once. Make it a point to best target a sample that suits the desired characteristics of your study. Additionally, anything you can do to administer your data collection in an environment that has the fewest distractions will help to enhance the quality of your findings.

Key Concepts

- Rationale for sampling
  - Time
  - Cost
  - Feasibility
  - Extrapolation
- Population
- Sample frame
- Sample
- Representative sample
- External validity
- Probability sampling
  - Simple random sampling
  - Stratified sampling
  - Systematic sampling
  - Area sampling
- Nonprobability sampling
  - Availability sampling
  - Purposive sampling
  - Quota sampling
  - Snowball sampling
- Sampling bias
- Optimal sample size

Practice Exercises

Exercise 2.1

1. Explain the rationale for sampling in terms of
   a. Time
   b. Cost
   c. Feasibility
   d. Extrapolation
2. Define the following terms and provide an example for each:
   a. Population
   b. Sample frame
   c. Sample
   d. Representative sample
3. Acme Community Clinic is interested in knowing how far their patients commute (from their home). To date, 20,000 unique patients have received care at this facility; the clinic operates Monday through Friday and sees about 200 patients per day. You have been commissioned to conduct a survey of their patients to gather home addresses, mode of transportation, and round-trip commute time. Your goal is to gather data on 10% of the patients who enter the clinic for a week. You will use simple random sampling.
   a. Define the population.
   b. Define the sample frame.
   c. Explain how you would select the sample.
   d. Explain how you would gather the data.

4. Acme Dialysis Center, which serves 250 patients, has commissioned you to conduct a patient satisfaction survey, providing you with a list of 120 patients who consented to being contacted; the target sample size is 20. The list contains their names and phone numbers. You will use systemic sampling.
    a. Define the population.
    b. Define the sample frame.
    c. Explain how you would select the sample.
    d. Explain how you would gather the data.
5. A team of public health nurses is deployed to a local high school for one day to gather body mass index (BMI) data from students; they will also record age and gender. There are 2,500 enrolled and 100 are absent on this day. Their goal is to sample as many students as possible on that day.
    a. Define the population.
    b. Define the sample frame.
    c. Explain how you would select the sample.
    d. Explain how you would gather the data.
6. Prior to building a fitness center in Cityville, Acme Corporation wants to conduct a survey of the residents. They provide you with a list of the 6,000 residential addresses covering the 300 blocks of Cityville. You will use area sampling to gather data from 900 households.
    a. Define the population.
    b. Explain how you would select the sample.
    c. Explain how you would gather the data.
7. A health science researcher has hired you to help determine the prevalence of smoking in a community. You will use availability sampling.
    a. Explain how you would select the sample.
    b. Explain how you would gather the data.
8. A learning lab has commissioned you to administer a survey of people with dyslexia. You will use snowball sampling.
    a. Explain how you would begin the snowball sampling process.
    b. Explain how you would gather data on additional respondents.
9. Acme Exercise Center has selected you to conduct a survey of their clients. They want data on 25 minors (younger than 18 years) and 50 adults (18 years or older). You will use quota sampling.
    a. Explain how you would select the sample.
    b. Explain how you would gather the data.
10. Acme Community Recreation Center has implemented a nutritional cooking class program for local youths. Before and after the 4-week session, each child's height, weight, and BMI data will be gathered. Participants must be between 10 and 14 years old, be available 3 days a week from 3:30 to 5:00 p.m., and have written parental consent to participate. You will use purposive sampling.
    a. Explain how you would select the sample.
    b. Explain how you would gather the data.

CHAPTER 3

Working in SPSS

*Welcome to **SPSS**.*

- Data View
- Variable View
- Codebook
- Saving Data Files

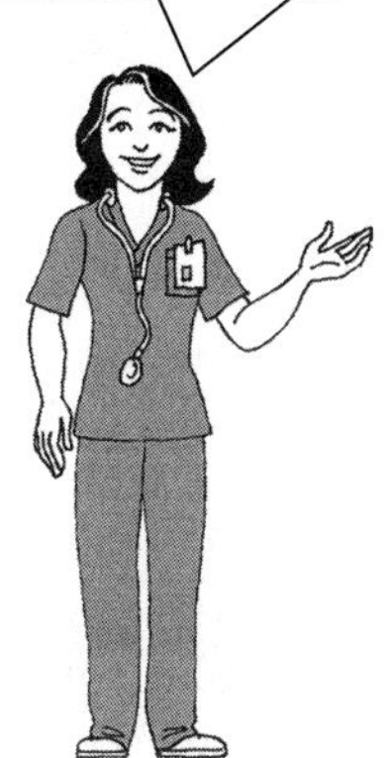

Computers are useless. They can only give you answers.

—Pablo Picasso

LEARNING OBJECTIVES

Upon completing this chapter, you will be able to:

- Operate in the two primary views in SPSS: Variable View and Data View
- Establish or modify variable definitions on the Variable View screen: name, type, width, decimals, label, values, missing, columns, align, measure, and role
- Use the value label icon to alternate between numeric and label (text) displays
- Interpret and use a codebook to configure variables in SPSS
- Enter data into SPSS
- Save and identify SPSS data files

VIDEO

The video for this chapter is **Ch 03 – Working in SPSS.mp4.** This video provides guidance on setting up an SPSS database, entering data, and saving SPSS files.

OVERVIEW – SPSS

Based on what you have read thus far, you have probably figured out that when it comes to statistics, larger sample sizes facilitate more robust statistical findings. Appropriately large sample sizes are also important when it comes to gathering a *representative sample,* which helps when it comes to generalizing the findings from your sample to the overall population from which it was drawn (*external validity*). Processing large samples can involve hundreds or even thousands of calculations. For most statistical formulas, the mathematical complexity does not go beyond simple algebra, however; such formulas typically involve multiple mathematical operations on each record. Attempting to process such data by hand would be inefficient in two ways: (1) It would be very time-consuming, and (2) accuracy would be compromised. Performing multiple calculations on a lengthy data set is bound to produce some errors along the way. Even if each mathematical operation was correct, the data would be vulnerable to cumulative rounding error. With the advent of affordable, powerful computers and menu-driven statistical programs, it is now possible to accurately perform a variety of statistical analyses in a matter of seconds. This chapter will provide you with what you need to know to get started using SPSS. SPSS, which originally stood for "Statistical Program for the Social Sciences," has gone through some substantial evolution over time; some versions are referred to as PASW—"Predictive Analytics Software." For the remainder of the text, the term *SPSS* will be used. Regardless of the name, the SPSS functionality of the statistics covered in this text has remained relatively stable across the evolution of the software.

TWO VIEWS: VARIABLE VIEW AND DATA VIEW

SPSS is laid out as two main screens: the *Variable View,* which is used for establishing or modifying the characteristics of each variable, and the *Data View,* which contains the gathered data. We will begin with the Variable View.

Variable View

The Variable View provides a screen for you to systematically set up the variables that will contain your data. This is where you will assign the name and characteristics of each variable that you will be including in the data set. To access the Variable View screen, click on the tab at the bottom of the screen that says *Variable View,* as shown in Figure 3.1.

Basically, for each variable, you are telling SPSS the name of the variable and the kind of data it will contain (e.g., regular numbers, dates, text, etc.), along with some other properties (parameters). Once you have established each variable in the Variable View screen, you can proceed to enter the data that you have gathered on the Data View screen, which resembles a traditional spreadsheet. The Variable View screen has 11 properties that you can set for each variable. Some versions of SPSS may have a different amount of properties; you should be able to proceed nonetheless. Naturally, you will use care when establishing variables on the Variable View screen, but there is no need to be nervous; even after you have entered data on the Data View screen, you can always return to the Variable View screen and make changes (e.g., include more variables, delete variables, rename variables, and modify the properties of existing variables).

The cursor is initially positioned in the *Name* column for the first variable; this is where the data definition process begins.

Figure 3.1 SPSS Variable View screen.

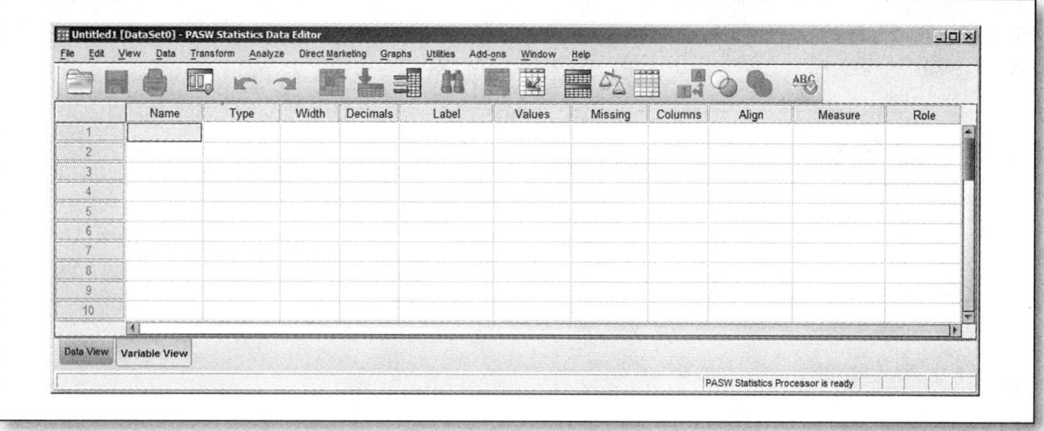

Name

Each variable needs a unique name. The name can contain up to 64 letters and numbers; the first character must be a letter. Some older versions of SPSS allow only eight characters for variable names, so you may need to be imaginative when it comes to assigning briefer variable names. Spaces are not allowed in the variable name, but you can use the underscore (_) character instead. For your own convenience, try to assign meaningful names (e.g., age, date_of_birth, first_name, last_name, gender, test01, question01, question02, question03, etc.). It is okay if you are unable to assign a perfect variable name; this will be discussed in more detail when we look at the *Label* property. The cursor is positioned in the first cell for the first variable. We will build a database containing two variables: *Gender* (a categorical variable) and *Age* (a continuous variable). Begin by entering *Gender* (in row 1 under *Name*). When you press Enter, notice that SPSS automatically enters default values for all of the remaining properties except for label. Each of these properties can be changed, but we will accept the automatic defaults for some.

Type

The system needs to know what *type* of data the variable will contain. The system assigns the default type as a numeric variable with a width of eight integer digits and two decimal digits (which you can change), meaning that this variable will accommodate a number such as 12345678.12 (Figure 3.2).

To access the menu shown in Figure 3.2, click on the *Type* cell for that variable. The options for variable type are fairly self-explanatory except for *String;* a *string* variable contains alphanumeric (letters and numbers) data (e.g., name, note, comment, memo, etc.). A string variable is useful for data that contain information that will not be processed mathematically consisting of letters, numbers, punctuation, or a mixture of letters and numbers, such as an ID code, an address, or a name (e.g., APB-373, 852 S. Bedford Street, Dusty Jones, etc.); if your data are not a date or a numeric value, then consider it alphanumeric and select *String* type. While string variables may contain valuable information, it is not possible to perform statistical operations on such variables.

Figure 3.2 SPSS Variable Type window.

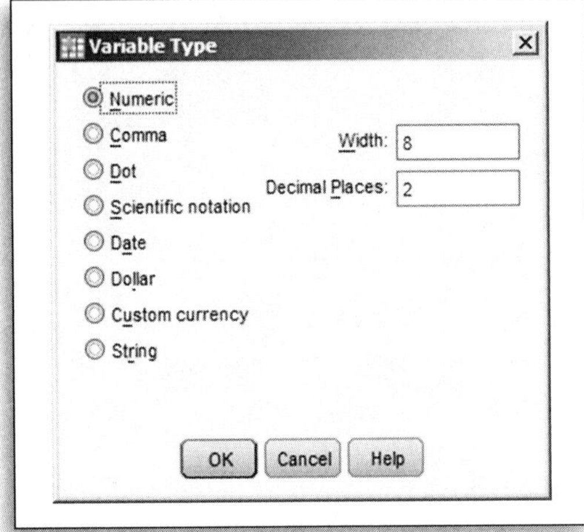

Width

The *Width* refers to the number of characters SPSS will allow you to enter for the variable. If it is a numerical value with decimals, the total *Width* has to include the decimal point and each digit (Figure 3.2). For example, if you were entering data for income (including dollars and cents) and the largest value expected was 123456.78, you would want to be sure to set the *Width* to at least 9.

Decimals

The *Decimals* property refers to the number of decimals that you want to display in your output (Figure 3.2). The default is 2 decimal places. When assigning this value, consider whether the variable is likely to need to be expressed with decimals. For example, a cash amount should have 2 decimal places (for the cents), whereas for categorical variables (e.g., Gender: Female = 1, Male = 2), a decimal is not needed, so the value should be set to 0.

Label

If the *Label* property is left blank, SPSS will use the variable *Name* in all output reports; otherwise, it will use whatever you specify as the label. For example, suppose the name of the variable is *DOB,* but in your reports, you want it to display as *Date of Birth;* in that case, simply enter *Date of Birth* in the *Label* property. Notice that the *Label* can contain spaces, but the *Name* cannot.

Values

The *Values* property provides a powerful instrument for assigning meaningful names to the values (numbers) contained in categorical variables. For example, *Gender* is a nominal variable consisting of two categories (1 = Female, 2 = Male). When it comes to nominal variables, SPSS handles categories as numbers (1, 2) as opposed to the textual names (Female, Male). The *Values* property allows you to assign the textual name to each category number, so even though you will code *Gender* using 1s and 2s, the output reports will exhibit these 1s and 2s as *Female* and *Male*.

Here is how it works:

1. In the *Name* column, create a variable called *Gender;* accept all the default values, except change the *Decimals* property to *0*.
2. Click on the *Values* cell for *Gender;* this will bring up the *Value Labels* menu (Figure 3.3).
3. Assign the values one at a time; begin by entering *1* in *Value* and *Female* in *Label,* then click *Add*.
4. Do the same for the second category: Enter *2* in *Value* and *Male* in *Label,* then click *Add*.
5. To finalize these designations, click *OK*.

You will see the utility of this labeling system when you enter data on the Data View screen and when you run your first report.

Missing

Sometimes, when the source data are either erroneous or missing, the cell is simply left blank, in which case, the *Missing* property can remain blank as well. Other times, the erroneous or missing data are represented by special numeric codes; a common convention is to code erroneous data as 888, and missing data are represented as 999—this conveys that a blank cell is not an oversight. Consider the variable *Age;* if the data contained an erroneous entry (e.g., "I'm a kid"), or if

Figure 3.3 SPSS Variable Labels window.

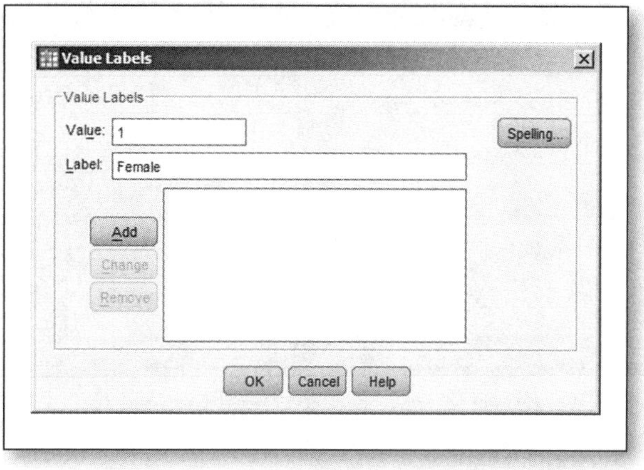

the entry were left blank, the corresponding 888 or 999 codes would radically throw off the statistical (age) calculations. The *Missing* property enables us to specify such codes (888 and 999) that we want SPSS to ignore so that they will not be processed in the statistical calculations.

Here is how it works:

1. Create a variable with the name *Age;* accept all the default values, except change the *Decimals* property to *0.*
2. Click on the Select *Discrete missing values* and enter *888* and *999* (Figure 3.4).
3. If you need to indicate more than three such values, you may opt for the *Range plus one optional discrete missing value* function, which would enable you to specify a range of values (e.g., *Low: 888, High: 999*—meaning that all values from 888 through 999 inclusive will be omitted from all statistical analysis for that variable). In addition, you can specify one additional value (e.g., *Discrete value: −1*).
4. To finalize these designations, click *OK.*

The numbers 888 and 999 have been generally adopted as special values since they are visually easy to recognize in a data set. Also, if these special values are not properly designated as erroneous/missing values, statistical clues will begin to emerge, such as a report indicating an average age of 347 or a maximum height of 999 inches or centimeters. Such extreme results alert you to check that the missing/erroneous designations have been properly specified for a variable.

Figure 3.4 SPSS Missing Values window.

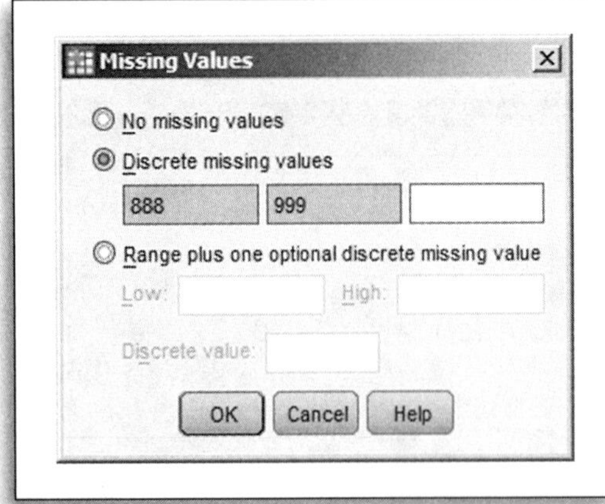

Columns

The *Columns* property allows you to change the column width on the Data View screen and in the reports; you can specify how many characters wide you want that column to be.

Align

The *Align* property lets you specify how you want the variable to be presented on the Data View screen and in the output reports. Typically, *Right* alignment (justification) is used for numeric data and *Left* alignment is used for text such as string data or categorical variables with data labels assigned to them. *Center* is also an option.

Measure

The *Measure* property pertains to the four levels of measures (*nominal, ordinal, interval,* and *ratio*) covered in the level of measure section in Chapter 1. For variables that contain *continuous* (interval or ratio) variables, select *Scale.* For *categorical* (nominal or ordinal) variables, which may contain value labels, select either *Nominal or Ordinal, depending on the variable type.*

Role

Some versions of SPSS have the *Role* property; do not panic if the version that you are using does not include this property—it will not be used in this text. Role enables you to define how the variable will be used in the statistical processes. If your version of the software includes the *Role* property, just use the default setting: *Input.*

Use SPSS to set up the Variable View screen to establish the *Gender* and *Age* variables as shown in Figure 3.5.

Figure 3.5 SPSS Variable View screen.

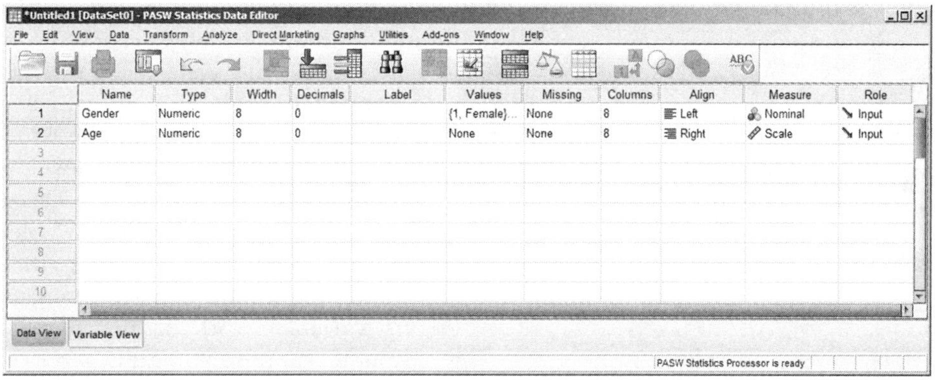

	Name	Type	Width	Decimals	Label	Values	Missing	Columns	Align	Measure	Role
1	Gender	Numeric	8	0		{1, Female}...	None	8	Left	Nominal	Input
2	Age	Numeric	8	0		None	None	8	Right	Scale	Input

Data View

Now that the properties for each variable have been established on the Variable View screen, the next step is to enter the actual data. To switch to the data entry mode, click on the *Data View* tab at the bottom of the screen. As you enter the data in Table 3.1 into the Data View screen, notice that for the *Gender* variable, you can access the pull-down menu in each cell to select *Female* or *Male.* Alternatively, you can enter the corresponding numbers that you defined: 1 for *Female* or 2 for *Male.* Notice that SPSS will not allow

Table 3.1 Gender and Age Source Data.

	Gender	Age
1	Male	24
2	Female	25
3	Male	31
4	Male	19
5	Female	27

NOTE: You do not need to enter the data in the leftmost column (1, 2, 3, 4, 5); this column pertains to the row (record) numbers that SPSS provides automatically.

you to type the words *Female* or *Male* directly in the *Gender* field; you will need to enter a number (in this case, 1 or 2) or use the pull-down menu feature to select *Female* or *Male* for this variable. The Data View screen should resemble Figure 3.6.

Value Labels Icon

When it comes to viewing your data, there will be times when you will want to see the value labels (e.g., *Female, Male*) and other times when you will want to see the source numbers (e.g., 1, 2). To toggle this display back and forth, from numbers to text (and back), click on the *Value Labels* icon (with the *1 A* on it), as shown in Figure 3.7.

Codebook

For learning purposes, the two-variable data set used in this chapter is admittedly simple. Even so, without being told that for the variable *Gender,* 1 stands for *Female* and 2 stands for *Male*, this coding scheme would lead to confusion. Designations such as 1 = *Female* and 2 = *Male* and other characteristics of each variable in a data set are traditionally contained in the *codebook,* which is the companion to the data set. The codebook is written by the person who develops the experiment or survey; it provides a list and a description of each variable contained in a data set. This is particularly valuable in data sets that contain numerous variables with arcane names. For example, suppose you came across a variable named *Q105 (Question 105)* and it appeared to contain dates. Without the codebook, we would have no idea what any of this means; we would not know how this variable was gathered or be able to assign any meaning to these dates (e.g., birth date, graduation date, anniversaries, date of arrest, date admitted to a hospital, etc.); if you do not know the story of a variable, that variable is virtually useless. Although there is no standard form for codebooks, a quality codebook should

Figure 3.6 Data View screen with data entered.

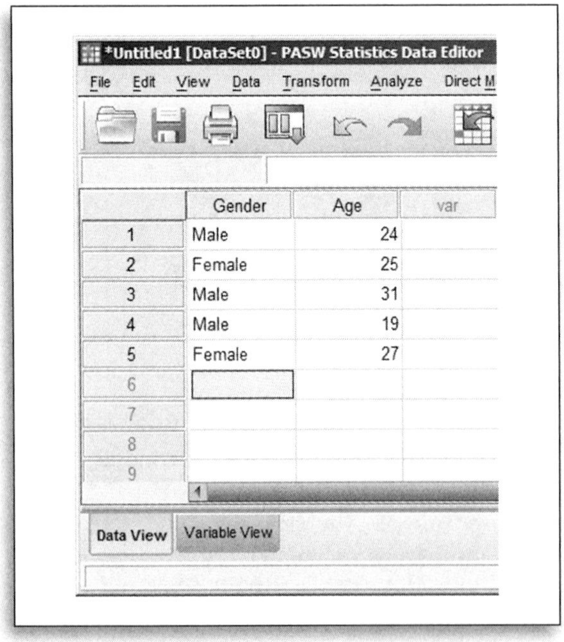

*Untitled1 [DataSet0] - PASW Statistics Data Editor
File Edit View Data Transform Analyze Direct M

	Gender	Age	var
1	Male	24	
2	Female	25	
3	Male	31	
4	Male	19	
5	Female	27	
6			
7			
8			
9			

Data View | Variable View

Figure 3.7 The *Value Labels* icon alternates the display of categorical variables from text to numeric display (and back).

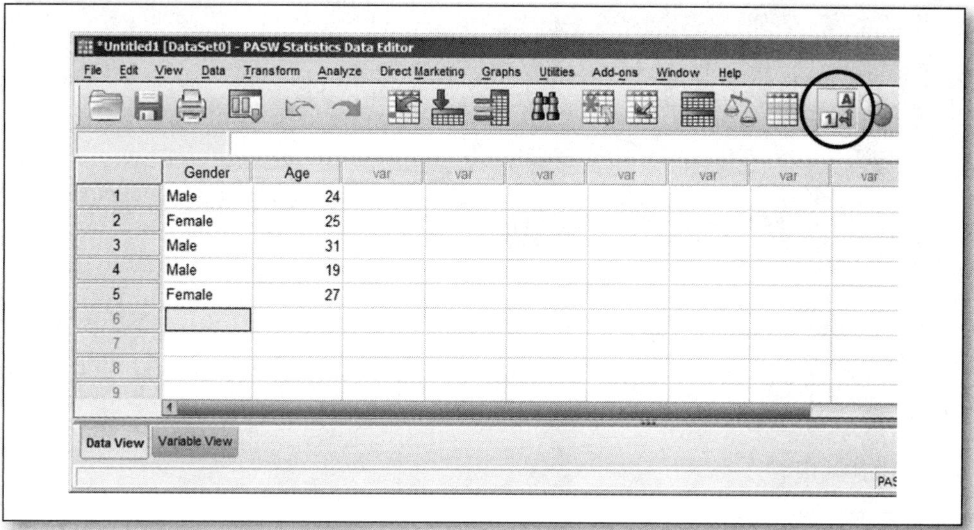

indicate the information essential to understanding each variable in the data set. Continuing with the *Q105* example, a reasonable codebook entry for this variable might look like this:

Codebook:

Variable:	Q105
Definition:	High school graduation date (Question #105)
Type:	Date (MM/DD/YYYY)

For our simple two-variable database detailed in Table 3.1, the codebook would look like this:

Codebook:

Variable:	Gender
Definition:	Gender of respondent
Type:	Categorical (1 = Female, 2 = Male)
Variable:	Age
Definition:	Age of respondent
Type:	Continuous

Figure 3.8 The *Save this document* icon.

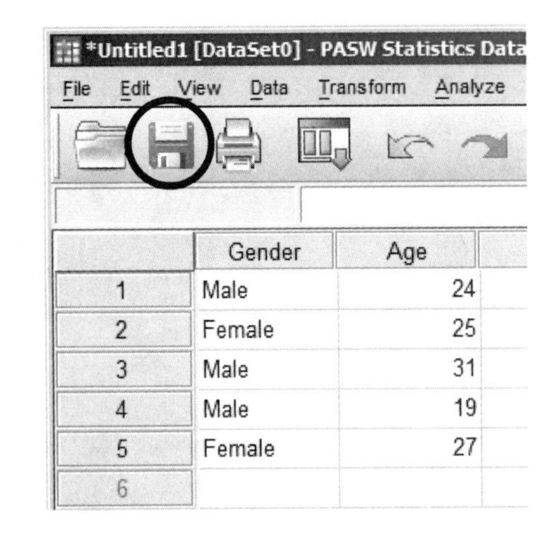

Saving Data Files

To save the file, click on the *Save this document* icon as shown in Figure 3.8. Use the file name *First Data Set;* SPSS automatically appends the *.sav* extension (suffix) to the *File name.* The file on your system will be listed as *First Data Set.sav.*

GOOD COMMON SENSE

The acronym GIGO (pronounced *gig-oh*) comes from the early days of computing; it stands for *Garbage In, Garbage Out,* and it is just as valid today. Basically, it means that if you input junk data into a program, the output will be junk too. *Junk data* can consist of missing or erroneous responses, responses to misconstrued questions, data entry errors, or other anomalies that may have allowed imprecise data to be entered into the database. Skillful statisticians will inspect and assess the data for such errors prior to embarking on analyses; this process is referred to as *cleaning the data*.

For example, a survey question may ask for the participant's *Age* (e.g., 25); however, the respondent enters a date (e.g., 9/18/1980). Clearly, data in date format will not fit into a variable that is configured to accept a three-digit numeric (*Age*) value. The statistician would then need to make a judgment call: The data could be coded as 888 (error), or one might presume that the date provided is the participant's birthdate, in which case, the *Age* could be calculated and entered into the specified field.

The accuracy of the statistical tests that you run will depend on the accuracy of the data definitions (on the *Variables View* screen) and the data entered (on the *Data View* screen). Considering that this book focuses on learning specific statistics, as opposed to coping with erroneous or missing data, the data sets that are provided contain *clean* data, which is ready for processing.

Key Concepts

- Variable View
  - Name
  - Type
  - Width
  - Decimals
  - Label

- Values
- Missing
- Columns
- Align
- Measure
- Role

- Data View
    - *Value Labels* icon
    - Codebook
    - Saving data files
        - *Save this document* icon
        - .sav files

Practice Exercises

TEST RUN

Use the provided codebook in each exercise to create the variables on the *Variable View* screen, and then enter the five records of data provided on the *Data View* screen. To check your work, produce a variable list; click on *Analyze, Reports, Codebook,* as shown in Figure 3.9.

Next, select all the variables that you want to include in the codebook report; move the variables from the left *Variables* window to the right *Codebook Variables* window (using double-click, drag & drop, or the arrow button), then click *OK*, as shown in Figure 3.10.

This will generate a report showing the properties of all variables, as shown in Table 3.2.

After each exercise, clear out the data; click on *File, New, Data,* as shown in Figure 3.11.

Figure 3.9 Ordering a list of all variables; click on *Analyze, Reports, Codebook.*

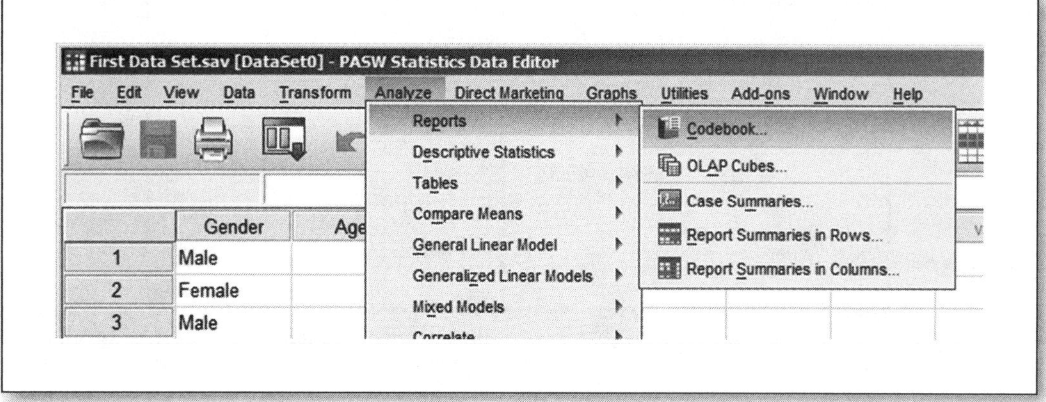

Figure 3.10 Codebook report order screen; move variables of interest to right (Codebook Variables) window.

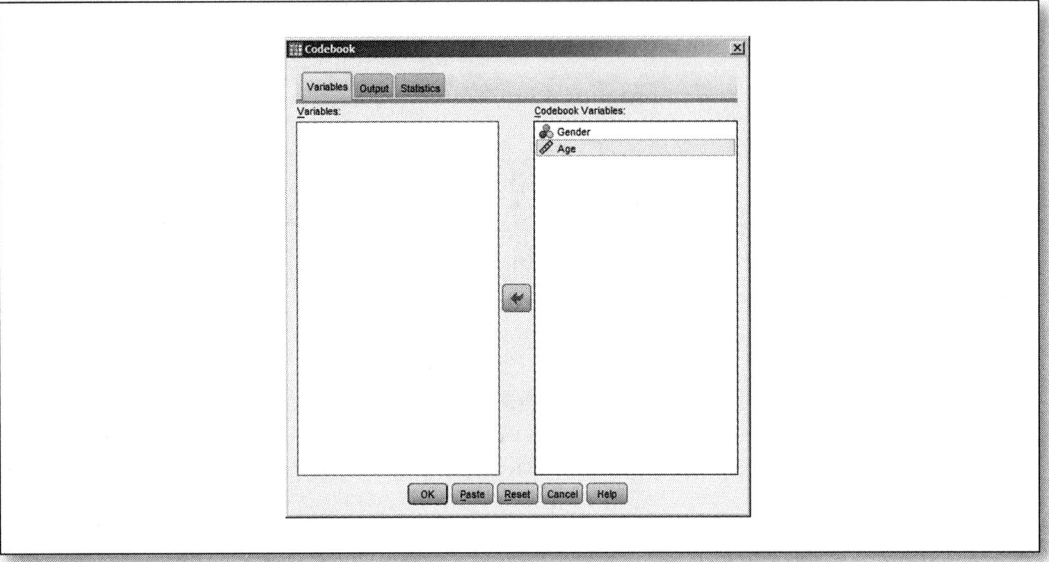

Table 3.2 Codebook Report Displaying the Variable Properties.

Gender

		Value	Count	Percent
Standard Attributes	Position	1		
	Label	<none>		
	Type	Numeric		
	Format	F8		
	Measurement	Nominal		
	Role	Input		
Valid Values	1	Female	2	40.0%
	2	Male	3	60.0%

Age

		Value
Standard Attributes	Position	2
	Label	<none>
	Type	Numeric
	Format	F8
	Measurement	Scale
	Role	Input
N	Valid	5
	Missing	0
Central Tendency and Dispersion	Mean	25.20
	Standard Deviation	4.382
	Percentile 25	24.00
	Percentile 50	25.00
	Percentile 75	27.00

Figure 3.11 To clear the data, click on: *File, New, Data.*

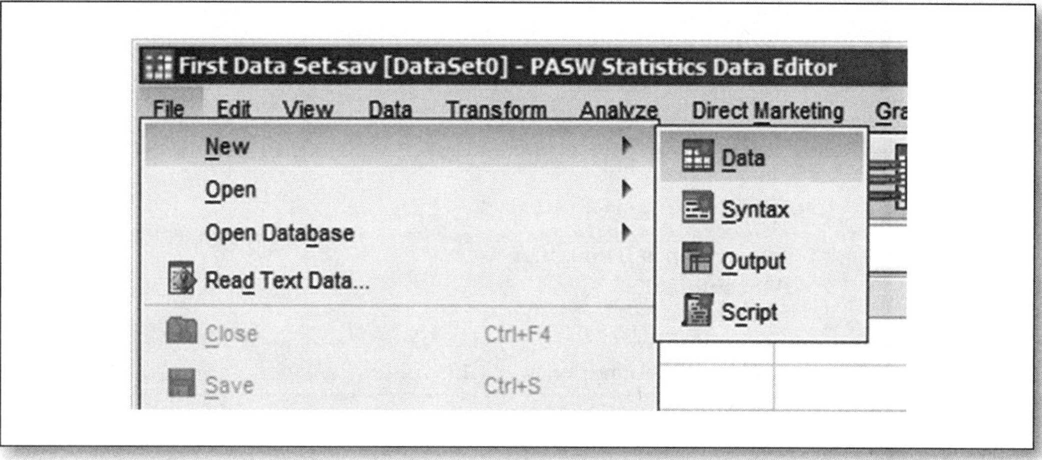

Exercise 3.1

Codebook

Variable: Enrolled
Definition: Enrollment status (Is the respondent currently enrolled?)
Type: Categorical (1 = Yes, 2 = No)

Variable: Courses
Definition: Total number of courses the student is currently enrolled in
Type: Continuous

Variable: Hours
Definition: Total number of hours per week are allocated for academic work
Type: Continuous

REMINDER: You do not need to enter the data in the leftmost column (1, 2, 3, 4, 5 . . .); this column pertains to the record numbers that SPSS provides automatically for each row.

Data set:

	Enrolled	Courses	Hours
1	Yes	3	16
2	Yes	3	10
3	No	0	0
4	Yes	4	19
5	Yes	2	7

Exercise 3.2

Codebook

Variable: ID
Definition: Respondent's ID number
Type: Alphanumeric

Variable: Volhours
Definition: Number of hours per week the volunteer is willing to provide
Type: Continuous

Data set:

	ID	Volhours
1	QF732	2.00
2	AL331	1.50
3	JW105	3.00
4	RK122	0.50
5	DD987	4.00

Exercise 3.3

Codebook

Variable: Gender
Definition: Gender
Type: Categorical (1 = Female, 2 = Male)

Variable: Height
Definition: Height (in inches)
Type: Continuous

Variable: Weight
Definition: Body weight (in pounds)
Type: Continuous

Variable: Age
Definition: Age
Type: Continuous

Data set:

	Gender	Height	Weight	Age
1	Male	71	212	24
2	Female	60	127	37
3	Female	68	160	52
4	Male	72	235	44
5	Female	65	136	68

Exercise 3.4

Codebook

Variable: Employ
Definition: Employment status
Type: Categorical (1 = Unemployed, 2 = Temporary, 3 = Part-time, 4 = Full-time)

Variable: Work
Definition: Number of hours worked in an average week
Type: Continuous

Variable: Sleep
Definition: Number of hours of sleep in an average night
Type: Continuous

Data set:

	Employ	Work	Sleep
1	Unemployed	0	10.00
2	Temporary	16	9.00
3	Full-time	40	7.50
4	Full-time	45	8.00
5	Part-time	20	7.00

Exercise 3.5

Codebook

Variable: Finitial
Definition: First initial of first name
Type: Alphanumeric

Variable: Lname
Definition: Last name
Type: Alphanumeric

Variable: Siblings
Definition: Total number of brothers and sisters
Type Continuous

Variable: Adopted
Definition: Adoption status (Is the respondent adopted?)
Type: Categorical (1 = Yes, 2 = No)

Data set:

	Finitial	Lname	Siblings	Adopted
1	J	Gower	0	No
2	D	Freeman	2	No
3	T	Rexx	3	No
4	P	Smith	2	Yes
5	V	Jones	1	No

Exercise 3.6

Codebook

Variable: Pt_ID
Definition: Patient ID number
Type: Continuous

Variable: Age
Definition: Age
Type: Continuous

Variable: Temp
Definition: Body temperature (in Fahrenheit)
Type: Continuous

Variable: Flu_shot
Definition: Flu shot status (Has the respondent had a flu shot this season?)
Type: Categorical (1 = Yes; 2 = No, and I don't want one; 3 = Not yet, but I'd like one)

Variable: Rx
Definition: Current medications
Type: Alphanumeric

Data set:

	Pt_ID	Age	Temp	Flu_shot	Rx
1	2136578099	22	98.6	Yes	
2	8189873094	24	99.0	No, and I don't want one	Multivitamin
3	2144538086	53	101.5	Not yet, but I want one	
4	8046628739	81	98.8	Yes	
5	5832986812	38	100.9	Yes	Xamine, Tutsocol

NOTE: Drug names are fictitious.

HINT: For variables that contain data that exceed eight digits (e.g., Pt_ID, Flu_shot, Rx), consider increasing the *Width* and *Columns* properties accordingly when establishing the variables.

Exercise 3.7

Codebook

Variable: ER
Definition: Have you ever been treated in an emergency room?
Type: Categorical (1 = Yes, 2 = No, 3 = Decline to answer)

Variable: DOB
Definition: Date of birth
Type: Date (MM/DD/YYYY)

Data set:

	ER	DOB
1	No	1/23/1936
2	Yes	8/18/1928
3	Yes	3/1/1987
4	Decline to answer	2/1/1993
5	No	3/11/1998

Exercise 3.8

Codebook

Variable: Dog
Definition: Dog allergy
Type: Categorical (1 = Allergic, 2 = Not allergic)

Variable: Cat
Definition: Cat allergy
Type: Categorical (1 = Allergic, 2 = Not allergic)

Variable: Pets
Definition: Number of pets at home that patient is allergic to
Type: Continuous

Data set:

	Dog	Cat	Pets
1	Not allergic	Not allergic	0
2	Not allergic	Allergic	0
3	Not allergic	Not allergic	0
4	Not allergic	Allergic	1
5	Not allergic	Not allergic	0

Exercise 3.9

Codebook

Variable: Blood_type
Definition: Blood type
Type: Categorical (1 = A−, 2 = A+, 3 = B−, 4 = B+, 5 = AB−, 6 = AB+, 7 = O−, 8 = O+)

Variable: Gender
Definition: Gender
Type: Categorical (1 = Female, 2 = Male)

Variable: Prior_donor
Definition: Prior blood donations
Type: Categorical (1 = Yes, 2 = No)

Data set:

	Blood_type	Gender	Prior_donor
1	B+	Female	Yes
2	A+	Female	No
3	A−	Male	No
4	AB+	Male	No
5	0−	Male	Yes

Exercise 3.10

Codebook

Variable: Send_labs
Definition: Method for sending laboratory results
Type: Categorical (1 = Phone call, 2 = Text message)

Variable: Phone
Definition: Phone number
Type: Alphanumeric

Data set:

	Send_labs	Phone
1	Text message	(555) 555-5150
2	Phone call	(555) 555-3536
3	Phone call	(555) 555-6753
4	Text message	(555) 555-5080
5	Text message	(555) 555-2749

PART II

Summarizing Variables

This chapter explains how to explore variables on an individual basis.

Chapter 4: Descriptive Statistics provides guidance on comprehending the values contained in continuous and categorical variables.

CHAPTER 4

Descriptive Statistics

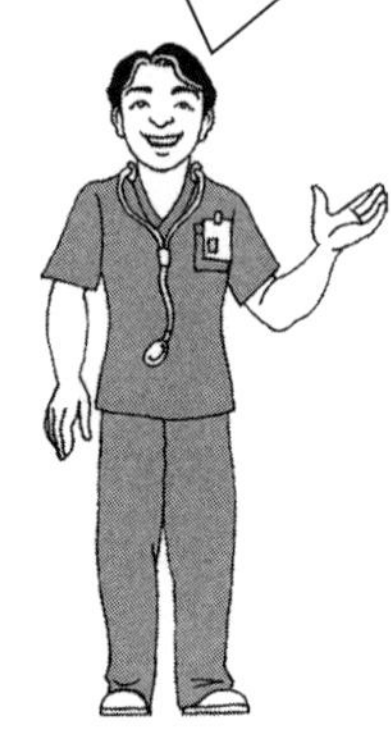
To summarize a variable, run descriptive statistics.

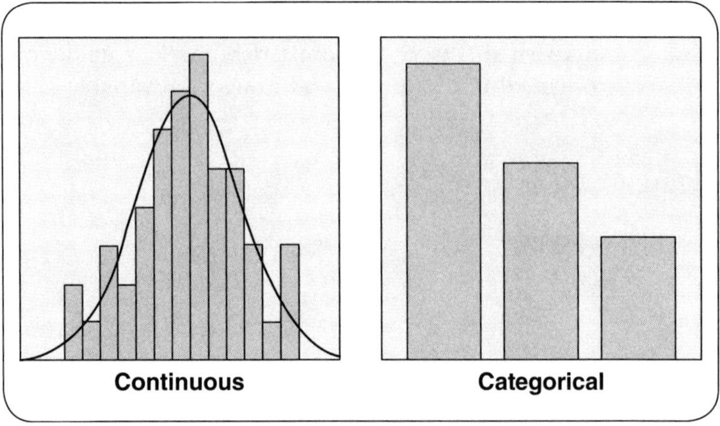
Continuous
Categorical

Whenever you can, count.

—Sir Francis Galton

LEARNING OBJECTIVES

Upon completing this chapter, you will be able to:

- Comprehend the meaning of each descriptive statistic: number (*n*), mean, median, mode, standard deviation, variance, minimum, maximum, and range
- Load an SPSS data file
- Order and interpret descriptive statistics for continuous variables: frequency statistics table, histogram with normal curve, and skewed distribution
- Order and interpret descriptive statistics for categorical variables: frequency statistics table, bar chart, and pie chart
- Select records to process/rule out
- Select all records to process

VIDEO

The videos for this chapter are **Ch 04 – Descriptive Statistics**, **Continuous.mp4** and **Ch 04 – Descriptive Statistics**, **Categorical.mp4.** These videos provide guidance on setting up, processing and interpreting descriptive (summary) statistics for continuous and categorical variables using the data set: **Ch 04 – Example 01 – Descriptive Statistics.sav**.

OVERVIEW – DESCRIPTIVE STATISTICS

Statistics is about understanding data, which could consist of one or many groups and involve data sets of virtually any size. Take a look at the data set in Table 4.1; if someone were to ask you to describe this data set, you might say, "It looks like a list of about half women and half men, mostly in their 20s," which would not be wrong, but we can be more precise than that. This list consists of (only) 50 records and 100 data items, but how would you make a viable summary statement if the list consisted of 100, 1,000, or even 100,000 records? Such data would span multiple pages and defy cursory visual inspection.

Table 4.1 Data Set Containing 50 Records With Two Variables per Record: Gender and Age.

Male	24	Male	30	Female	22	Male	26	Female	25
Male	25	Male	25	Male	25	Male	25	Female	25
Male	31	Female	26	Male	25	Female	24	Female	22
Female	19	Male	27	Female	24	Male	29	Male	22
Female	27	Male	24	Female	23	Male	23	Female	20
Male	20	Female	25	Male	25	Female	21	Female	22
Male	28	Male	24	Female	19	Female	22	Male	18
Female	23	Female	26	Female	23	Female	21	Female	18
Male	26	Female	23	Female	28	Female	24	Female	23
Male	24	Male	22	Female	24	Male	26	Female	27

To better comprehend and communicate the nature of a data set, we use *descriptive statistics,* sometimes referred to as *summary statistics*. Descriptive statistics enable us to concisely understand a data set of any size using a handful of figures and simple graphs that serve to concisely describe the contents of a variable.

Continuous variables can be summarized using the nine descriptive statistics: number (n), mean, median, mode, maximum, minimum, range, standard deviation, and variance. Graphically, continuous variables can be depicted using a histogram (a kind of bar chart) with a normal curve.

Categorical variables can be summarized using number (n) and percent. Graphically, categorical variables are depicted using a simple bar chart or pie chart. You can see examples of a histogram with a normal curve for a continuous variable and a bar chart for a categorical variable on the first page of this chapter and on the cover of this book.

We will begin with an explanation of the nine summary statistics used to analyze continuous variables. For simplicity, we will work with a small data set—the first 10 ages drawn from the second column of Table 4.1: 24, 25, 31, 19, 27, 20, 28, 23, 26, and 24.

DESCRIPTIVE STATISTICS

Number (n)

The most basic descriptive statistic is the *number,* represented by the letter n. To compute the n, simply count the number of elements (numbers) in the sample; in this case, there are 10 elements: 24 is the first, 25 is the second, 31 is the third, . . . 24 (at the end) is the tenth, so $n = 10$.

The lowercase n is the number of elements in a *sample,* whereas the uppercase N is the number of elements in the (whole) *population*. SPSS output reports always use the capital N. Since it is rare to be processing a data set consisting of an entire population, it is considered good practice to use the lowercase n in your documentation, as such: n(Age) = 10.

Mean (μ)

In statistical language, the *average* is referred to as the *mean*. The calculation for the mean is the same as the average: Add up all the numbers and then divide that amount by the total number of numbers ($n = 10$):

$$\text{Mean(Age)} = (24 + 25 + 31 + 19 + 27 + 20 + 28 + 23 + 26 + 24) \div 10$$

$$\text{Mean(Age)} = 247 \div 10$$

$$\text{Mean(Age)} = 24.7$$

The mean can be written using the lowercase Greek letter μ (pronounced *m-you*) or as the variable with a horizontal bar over it; hence, the mean may be documented as such:

$$\mu(\text{Age}) = 24.7$$

$$\overline{\text{Age}} = 24.7$$

For consistency throughout the rest of this text, the mean will be documented using the more common μ(Age) style.

Median

The median is the middle value of a variable. Think of the term *median* in terms of a street—the median is in the middle; it splits the street in half. To find the median, arrange the data in the variable from lowest to highest and then select the middle value(s). In smaller data sets, the mean can be altered substantially by outlier scores—scores that are unexpectedly high or low. In such instances, the median can provide a more stable indicator of the central value than the mean.

When the n is even, as in the data set below ($n = 10$), there are two middle numbers: 24 and 25. The median is the mean of these two middle numbers:

19, 20, 23, 24, (24, 25), 26, 27, 28, 31

Median(Age) = (24 + 25) ÷ 2

Median(Age) = (49) ÷ 2

Median(Age) = 24.5

When the n is odd, as in this small data set below ($n = 5$), there is (only) one middle number—hence, the median is simply the (one) middle number: 86.

6, 24, (86), 91, 99

Mode

The mode is the most common number in the data set. Notice that ***mode*** and ***most*** share the first two letters. In this case, we see that each number in this data set is present only once, except for 24, which occurs twice, and hence the mode is 24.

19, 20, 23, (24, 24), 25, 26, 27, 28, 31

It is possible for a data set to have more than one mode; the example below has two modes: 24 and 31 since both have the most (there are two 24s and two 31s; all the other numbers appear just once). Such a variable would be referred to as *bimodal*—meaning two modes.

19, 20, 23, (24, 24), 25, 26, 27, 28, (31, 31)

Although it is relatively rare, a variable may have more than two modes, which would be referred to as *multimodal*.

When SPSS detects more than one mode within a variable, it only reports the lowest one and provides a footnote indicating that there is more than one mode.

The mean, median, and mode are referred to as *measures of central tendency*, as they suggest the center point of the variable.

Standard Deviation (*SD*)

The standard deviation (*SD*) indicates the dispersion of the numbers within a variable. If a variable contains numbers that are fairly similar to each other, this produces a low(er) standard deviation; conversely, if there is more variety in the numbers, this renders a high(er) standard deviation.

Take a look at Figure 4.1. First, notice that the three people in Group A are all around the same height (67", 68", and 67"); their heights are just slightly above or below the mean ($\mu = 67.33$). Statistically speaking, their heights do not *deviate* much from the mean; hence, this group produces a low(er) standard deviation ($SD = .577$).

Now, focus on the three people in Group B; notice that they have very diverse heights (86", 45", and 71"); their heights are fairly far apart from each other—substantially above or below the mean ($\mu = 67.33$). Statistically speaking, their heights *deviate* much more from the mean, producing a high(er) standard deviation (*SD* = 20.744)—more than 35 times the standard deviation for Group A (*SD* = .577).

For clarity, the heights for Groups A and B have been set to produce the same means ($\mu = 67.33$). The point is, if all we had was the mean for each group, we might get the (wrong) impression that the heights in Group A are just like the heights in Group B. The standard deviation statistic tells us if the numbers contained within a variable *deviate* a little from the mean, as in Group A, wherein the heights are fairly similar to the mean (and each other), or if the numbers *deviate* more from the mean (and each other), as in Group B, wherein the heights are more spread out.

In statistical reporting, the standard deviation is often presented with the mean (e.g., $\mu = 67.33$ [*SD* = .577]).

Figure 4.1 Standard deviation (*SD*) illustrated: Low(er) diversity (Group A) renders lower standard deviation; higher diversity (Group B) renders high(er) standard deviation.

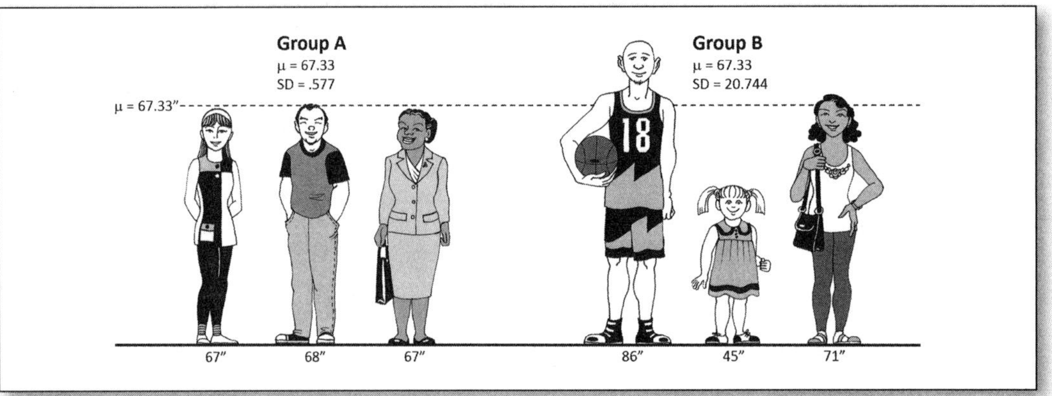

Variance

The variance is simply the standard deviation squared. For example, we will calculate the variance of Group B in the height example, where *SD* = 20.774.

$$\text{Variance(Height)} = [\text{Standard deviation(Height)}]^2$$

$$\text{Variance(Height)} = 20.774^2$$

$$\text{Variance(Height)} = 20.774 \times 20.774$$

$$\text{Variance(Height)} = 431.559$$

The variance is seldom included in statistical reports; it is primarily used as a term within other statistical formulas.

Minimum

The minimum is the smallest number in a variable. In the data set below, the minimum is 19.

(19), 20, 23, 24, 24, 25, 26, 27, 28, 31

Maximum

The maximum is the largest number in a variable. In the data set below, the maximum is 31.

19, 20, 23, 24, 24, 25, 26, 27, 28, (31)

Identifying the minimum and maximum values has some utility, but try not to bring inappropriate suppositions to your interpretation of such figures—bigger is not necessarily better. The meaning of the minimum and maximum values depends on the nature of the variable. For example, high IQ scores are considered good, while low BMI (body mass index) is considered good, and high (or low) patient ID numbers are considered neither good nor bad.

Range

The range is the span of the data set; the formula for the range is **maximum – minimum**. In the data set below, we would calculate: 31 – 19 = 12; the range is 12 (years).

(19), 20, 23, 24, 24, 25, 26, 27, 28, (31)

SPSS—LOADING AN SPSS DATA FILE

For clarity, the examples used thus far have involved only 10 data items (n = 10). Now it is time to use SPSS to process descriptive statistics using the entire data set consisting of 50 records and both variables (*Gender* and *Age*).

Run SPSS

DATA SET

Figure 4.2 *Open Data Document* icon.

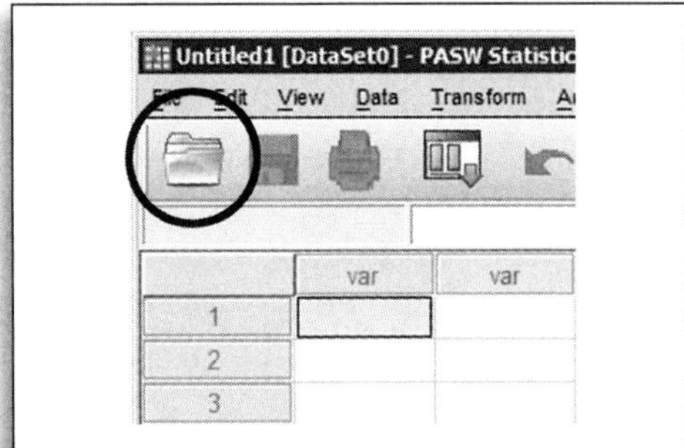

Use the *Open Data Document* icon (Figure 4.2) to load the SPSS data file: **Ch 04 – Example 01 – Descriptive Statistics.sav.**

Codebook

Variable:	Gender
Definition:	Gender of participant
Type:	Categorical (1 = Female, 2 = Male)
Variable:	Age
Definition:	Age of participant
Type:	Continuous

TEST RUN

SPSS—DESCRIPTIVE STATISTICS: CONTINUOUS VARIABLES (AGE)

There are two types of variables in this SPSS file: *Age* is a continuous variable, and *Gender* is a categorical variable. In this section, we will process descriptive statistics for the continuous variable (*Age*); later in this chapter, we will process the categorical variable (*Gender*).

1. After loading the data, click on *Analyze, Descriptive Statistics, Frequencies* (Figure 4.3).

Figure 4.3 Running descriptive statistics report; click on *Analyze, Descriptive Statistics, Frequencies*

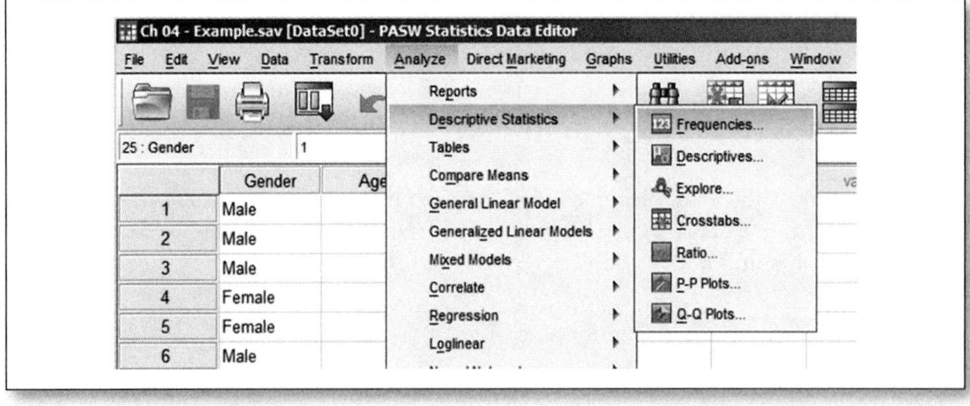

2. SPSS will then prompt you to select the variable(s) that you would like to process. Move the *Age* variable to the *Variable(s)* window (Figure 4.4).

Figure 4.4 Move the variable(s) to be analyzed (*Age*) from the left window to the right *Variable(s)* window.

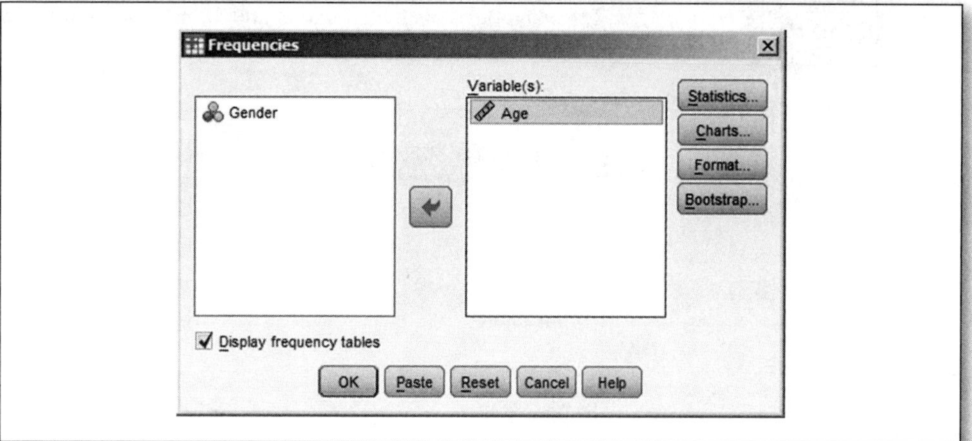

3. Click on the *Statistics* button.

Figure 4.5 *Frequencies: Statistics* menu.

Frequencies: Statistics
Percentile Values
Quartiles
Cut points for: 10 equal groups
Percentile(s):
Add
Change
Remove
Central Tendency
Mean
Median
Mode
Sum
Values are group midpoints
Dispersion
Std. deviation
Minimum
Variance
Maximum
Range
S.E. mean
Distribution
Skewness
Kurtosis
Continue
Cancel
Help

4. Select the descriptive statistics indicated by the checkboxes (Figure 4.5): *Mean, Median, Mode, Std. deviation, Variance, Range, Minimum,* and *Maximum.*

5. Click on the *Continue* button. This will take you back to the *Frequencies* menu (Figure 4.4).

Figure 4.6 *Frequencies: Charts* menu; select *Histograms* and *Show normal curve on histogram.*

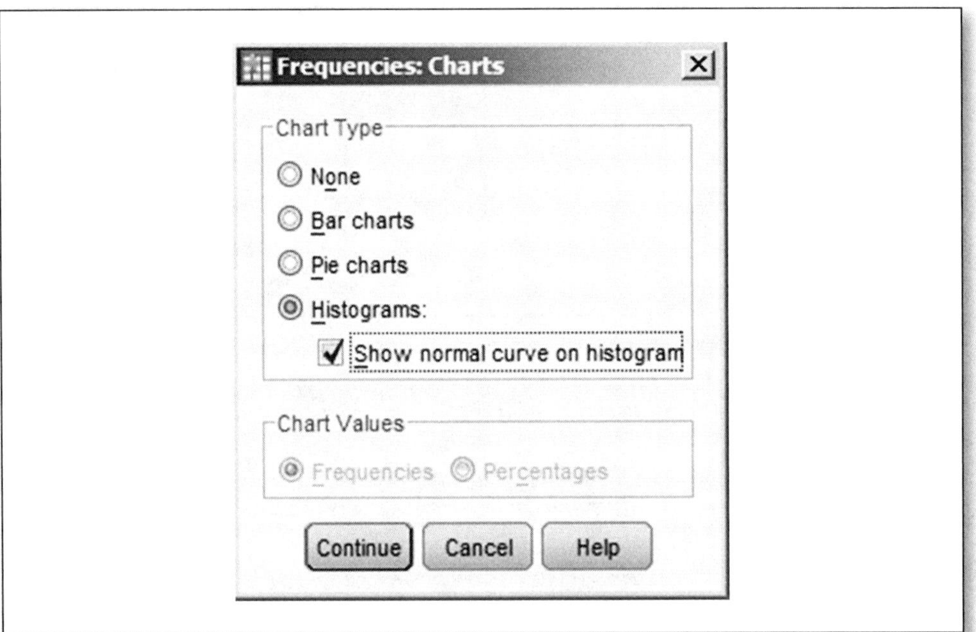

6. On the *Frequencies* menu (Figure 4.4), click on the *Charts* button.

7. Select *Histograms* and *Show normal curve on histogram* (Figure 4.6).

8. Click on the *Continue* button. This will take you back to the *Frequencies* menu (Figure 4.4).

9. Click on the *OK* button on the *Frequencies* menu; this tells SPSS to process the Frequencies report based on the parameters that you just specified. SPSS should produce this report in under a minute.

Frequency Statistics Tables

The first part of the report is the *Frequency Statistics* table (Table 4.2), which shows the summary statistical results as discussed earlier.

The second part of the report shows the frequency of each value in the *Age* variable (Table 4.3). Focus on columns 1 and 2 of this table, which show that the numbers 18, 19, 20, and 21 each occur twice in the data set; 22 and 23 each occur six times; 24 occurs eight times; 25 occurs nine times; and so on.

Table 4.2 *Frequency Statistics* Table Showing Summary Statistics for *Age*.

Statistics

Age

N	Valid	50
	Missing	0
Mean		24.00
Median		24.00
Mode		25
Std. Deviation		2.857
Variance		8.163
Range		13
Minimum		18
Maximum		31

Histogram With Normal Curve

The next part of this report is the histogram of the *Age* variable. The histogram is simply a graphical representation of the frequency statistics. Basically, Figure 4.7 is a picture of the data in Table 4.3. Notice that the first four bars are each two units tall; this is because the first four numbers in the table (18, 19, 20, and 21) each occur two times in the data set. Notice that

Figure 4.7 *Histogram* of the *Age* variable.

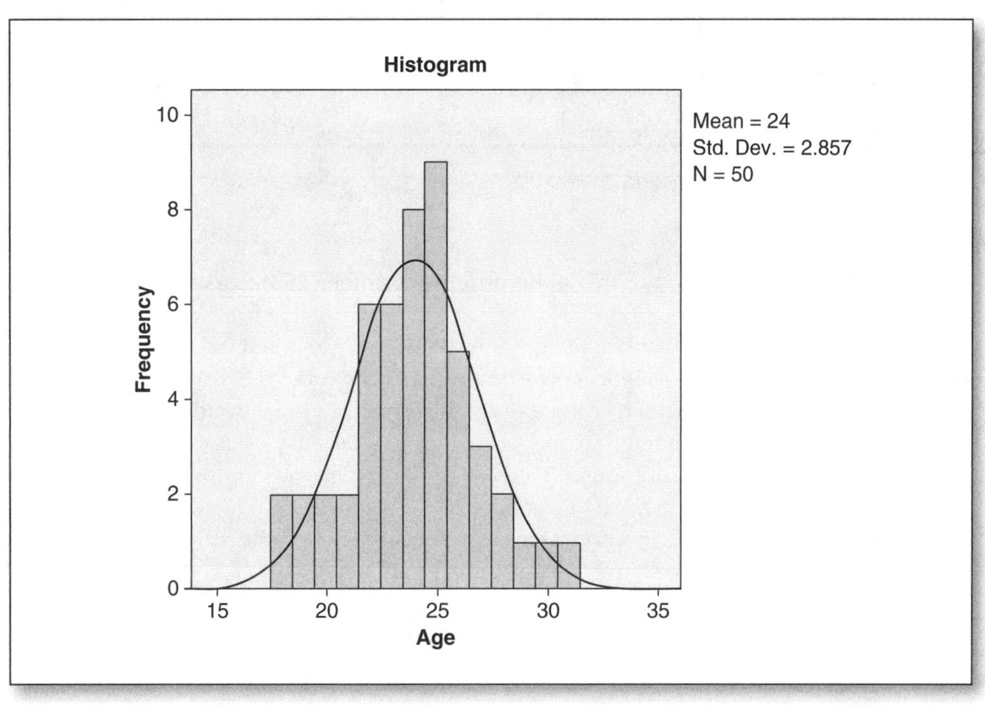

Table 4.3 Frequency Statistics Table Showing the Frequency of Each Value in the *Age* Variable.

Age

		Frequency	Percent	Valid Percent	Cumulative Percent
Valid	18	2	4.0	4.0	4.0
	19	2	4.0	4.0	8.0
	20	2	4.0	4.0	12.0
	21	2	4.0	4.0	16.0
	22	6	12.0	12.0	28.0
	23	6	12.0	12.0	40.0
	24	8	16.0	16.0	56.0
	25	9	18.0	18.0	74.0
	26	5	10.0	10.0	84.0
	27	3	6.0	6.0	90.0
	28	2	4.0	4.0	94.0
	29	1	2.0	2.0	96.0
	30	1	2.0	2.0	98.0
	31	1	2.0	2.0	100.0
	Total	50	100.0	100.0	

the tallest bar is nine units tall; this is because the number 25 occurs nine times in the data set.

The histogram provides further insight into the (descriptive) characteristics of a continuous variable—a picture is indeed worth a thousand words.

In addition to the bars, which constitute the histogram, it is also traditional to include a normal curve—sometimes referred to as a "bell curve" because of its shape. The normal curve is derived from the same source data as the bar chart; you can think of this normal curve as the smoothed-out version of the bar chart. More often than not, we see this sort of symmetrical distribution in continuous variables—most of the values are gathered toward the middle, with the frequencies progressively dropping off as the values depart above or below the mean.

For example, if we were to measure the height of 100 randomly selected people, we would expect to find that most people are moderate height (which would constitute the tallness in the middle of the normal curve). We would also expect to find a few exceptionally short people and about the same amount of exceptionally tall people, which would account for the tapering off seen on the left and right tails of the normal curve. This phenomenon of the bell-shaped distribution is so common that it is referred to as a *normal distribution,* as represented by the normal curve. When inspecting a histogram for normality, it is expected that the bars may have some jagged steps from bar to bar; however, to properly assess a variable for normality, our focus is on the symmetry of the normal curve more so than the bars. If we were to slice a proper normal curve vertically down the middle, the left half of the normal curve should resemble a mirror image of the right half.

Skewed Distribution

As with any rule, there are exceptions; not all histograms produce normally shaped curves. Depending on the distribution of the data within the variable, the histogram may be skewed, meaning that the distribution is shifted to one side or the other, as shown in Figures 4.8 and 4.9.

In Figure 4.8, we see that most of the data are on the right, between about 150 and 300, but there is a small scattering of lower values (under 100), forcing the left tail of the curve to be extended out. These few low values that substantially depart from the majority of the data are referred to as *outliers*. Typically, outliers become apparent when graphing the data. We would say that the histogram in Figure 4.8 has outliers to the left—hence, it is *skewed left,* or *negatively skewed.*

Outliers are not always negative. Figure 4.9, which is a virtual mirror image of Figure 4.8, shows outliers scattered to the right; this distribution would be referred to as being

Figure 4.8 Negative (left) skew.

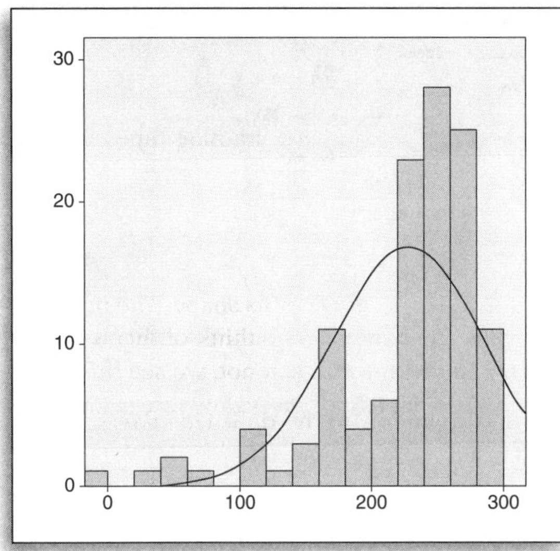

Figure 4.9 Positive (right) skew.

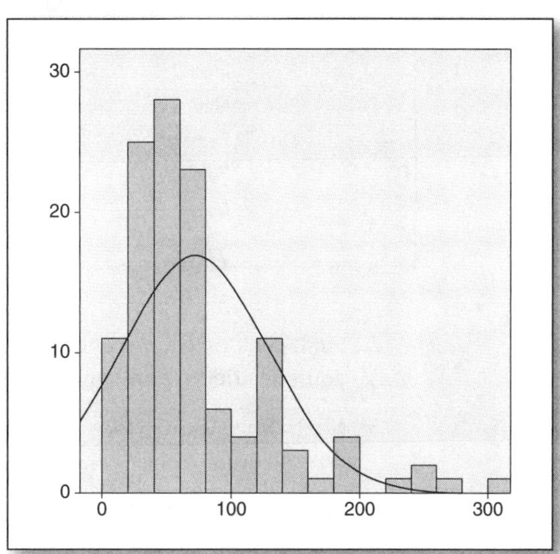

skewed right, or *positively skewed.* The notion of normality of the data distribution will be discussed further in future chapters.

SPSS—DESCRIPTIVE STATISTICS: CATEGORICAL VARIABLES (GENDER)

Descriptive statistics for categorical variables are derived using the same ordering menus as for continuous variables, except you will be specifying different options. Although it is plausible to compute the mode for a categorical variable to determine which is the largest category, it would be inappropriate to compute statistics such as mean, median, maximum, minimum, range, standard deviation, and variance. For example, in this data set, the *Gender* variable is coded as 1 for *Female* and 2 for *Male;* if we ordered the mean for *Gender,* the result would be 1.46, which is essentially meaningless.

1. Click on *Analyze, Descriptive Statistics, Frequencies.* (Figure 4.10).

Figure 4.10 Running descriptive statistics report; click on *Analyze, Descriptive Statistics, Frequencies.*

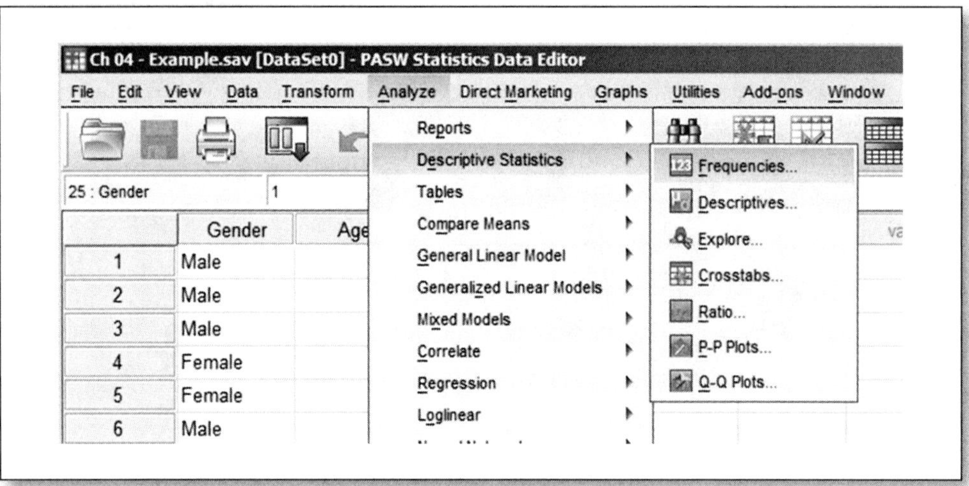

2. First, click on the *Reset* button; this will clear the parameters on the submenus that you specified when running the summary statistics for *Age.*
3. Next, move the *Gender* variable from the left window to the right *Variable(s)* window (Figure 4.11).
4. Click on the *Charts* button.

Figure 4.11 Click on the *Reset* button to clear prior options, then move the variable(s) to be analyzed (*Gender*) from the left window to the right *Variable(s)* window.

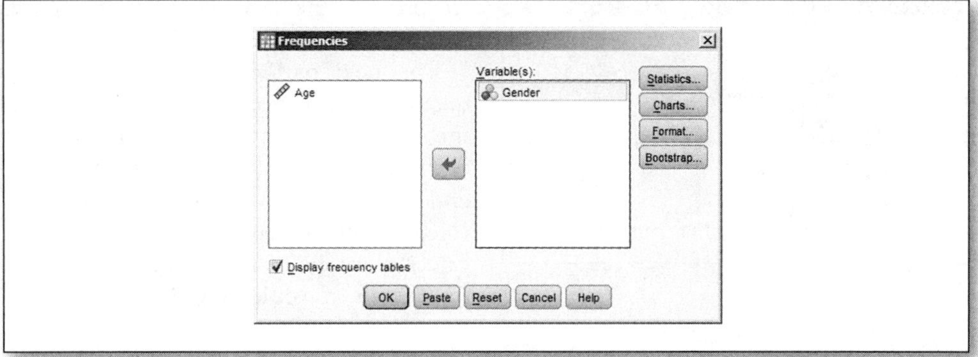

5. On the *Frequencies: Charts* menu, there are two viable options for categorical variables: *Bar charts* or *Pie charts* (Figure 4.12). In statistics, bar charts are used more often than pie charts. You can also choose to represent the numbers as frequencies (the actual counts) or percentages. For this example, select *Frequencies.*

Figure 4.12 *Frequencies: Charts* menu; select *Bar charts* and *Frequencies.* After running this analysis as specified, feel free to return to this menu to rerun this analysis using different settings (e.g., *Bar charts* with *Percentages, Pie charts*).

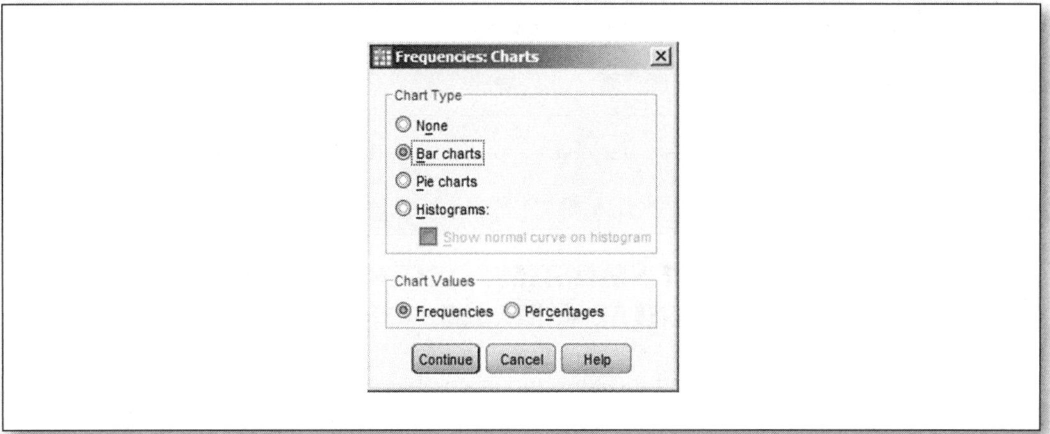

6. Click on the *Continue* button; this will return you to the *Frequencies* menu.

7. Click on the *OK* button on the *Frequencies* menu; this tells SPSS to process the *Frequencies* report based on the parameters that you just specified.

Frequency Statistics Tables

Table 4.4 Descriptive Statistics for *Gender*: *N* Valid and Missing.

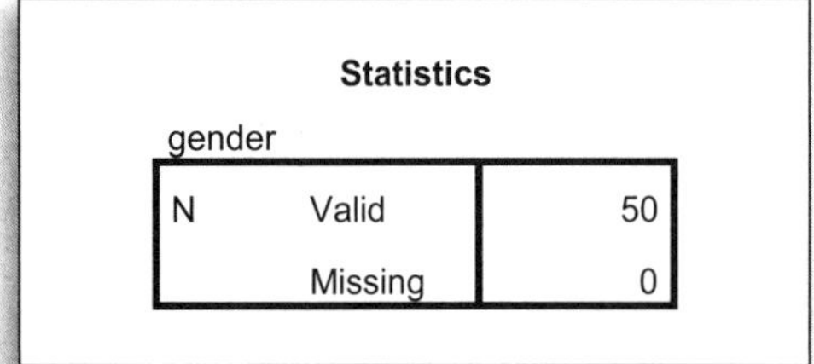

Statistics

gender

N	Valid	50
	Missing	0

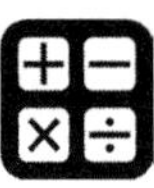

The first part of this frequency report shows the overall *N* (*n*)—the total number of entries (records) in the variable: 50 valid records and 0 missing as shown (Table 4.4).

The next part of the report provides more detailed information regarding the *N*, indicating the frequency (actual number) and percent for each category within the *Gender* variable (*Female* and *Male*), as shown in Table 4.5. Incidentally, to calculate the percent, divide the frequency for the category by the (valid) *n* and multiply by 100, so for *Female*, it would be (27 ÷ 50) × 100 = 54%.

Table 4.5 Descriptive Statistics for Gender: *Frequency* and *Percent*.

Gender

		Frequency	Percent	Valid Percent	Cumulative Percent
Valid	Female	27	54.0	54.0	54.0
	Male	23	46.0	46.0	100.0
	Total	50	100.0	100.0	

Bar Chart

Last, the report provides a bar chart representing the two *Gender* categories (*Female* and *Male*) (Figure 4.13).

SPSS—DESCRIPTIVE STATISTICS: CONTINUOUS VARIABLE (AGE) SELECT BY CATEGORICAL VARIABLE (GENDER)—FEMALES ONLY

So far, we have processed the continuous variable, *Age*, with both genders combined, but it is also possible to produce separate reports for *Females* only and *Males* only, showing the summary statistics and histograms for each. This technique not only satisfies curiosity about what is going on in each category but it will also be essential for running the *pretest checklist* reports that will be covered in future chapters.

We will begin with processing the *Age* summary statistics for *Females* only, and then we will repeat the process selecting data for *Males* only. The *Select Cases* option allows

Figure 4.13 *Bar chart* of the *Gender* variable.

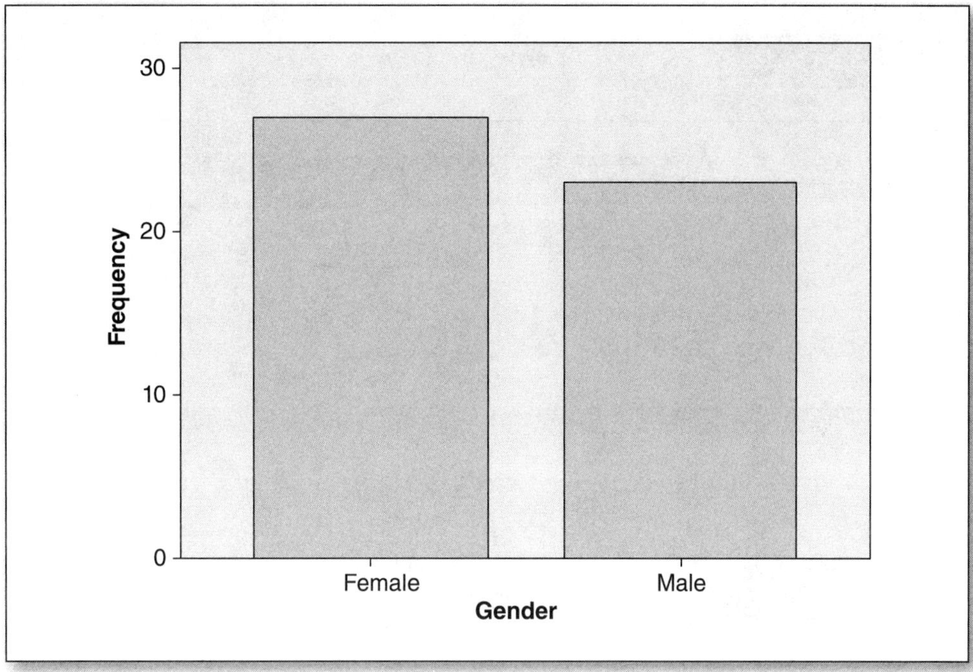

you to efficiently specify which cases (rows of data, also known as *records*) you would like to process; SPSS will temporarily ignore all other cases—they will not be included in any statistical computations until you choose to reselect them.

The following procedure will select only the cases where *Gender* = 1 (*Female*).

1. Click on the *Select Cases* icon (Figure 4.14).

Figure 4.14 The *Select Cases* icon.

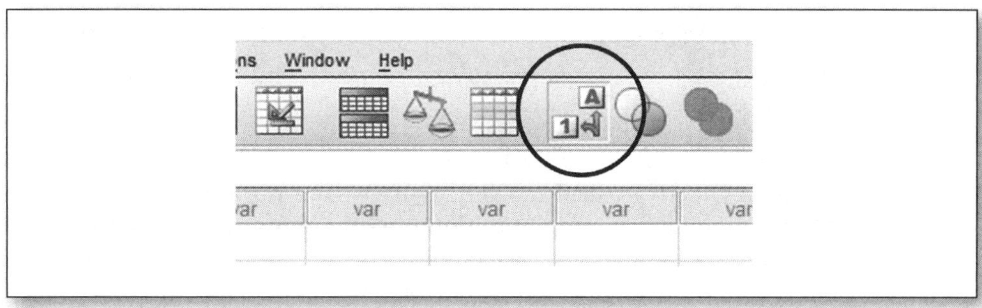

2. On the *Select Cases* menu (Figure 4.15), the default Selection is *All* cases. Click on *If condition is satisfied,* then click on the *If* button.

Figure 4.15 The *Select Cases* menu (top only).

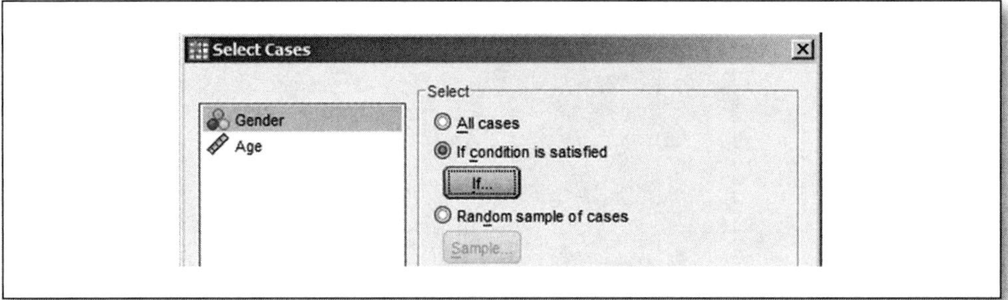

3. This will bring you to the *Select Cases*: *If* menu (Figure 4.16).

Figure 4.16 The *Select Cases: If* menu (top only).

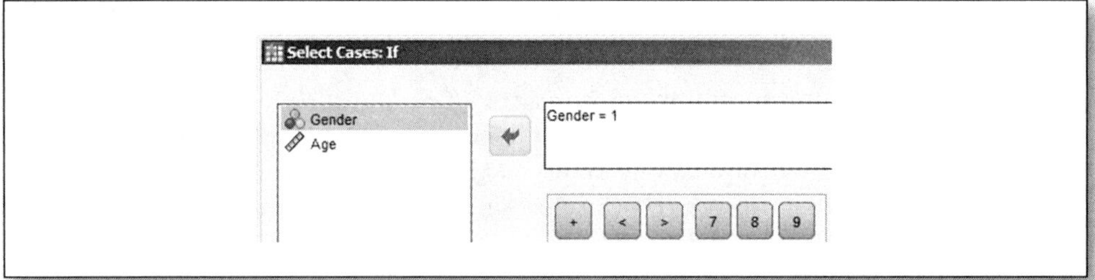

4. Remember: SPSS handles categorical variables as numbers; earlier, we had established that for the categorical variable *Gender,* 1 = *Female* and 2 = *Male*. Since we want statistical reports on *Females* only, we enter the inclusion criteria, *Gender* = *1,* in the big box at the top of the menu. Then click on the *Continue* button.

5. This will return you to the *Select Cases* menu. Click on the *OK* button, and the system will process your selection criteria.

6. Switch back to the *Data View* screen. First, notice that the record (row) numbers for each *Male* is slashed out (Figure 4.17). You can think of all the data in the slashed-out rows as being in a sort of penalty box—they are still part of the data set, but they cannot play. Slashed-out data will not be included in any statistical processing until they are reselected; however, you can still edit such data.

Figure 4.17 The *Data View* screen after *Select Cases (Gender = 1)* has been executed (section only).

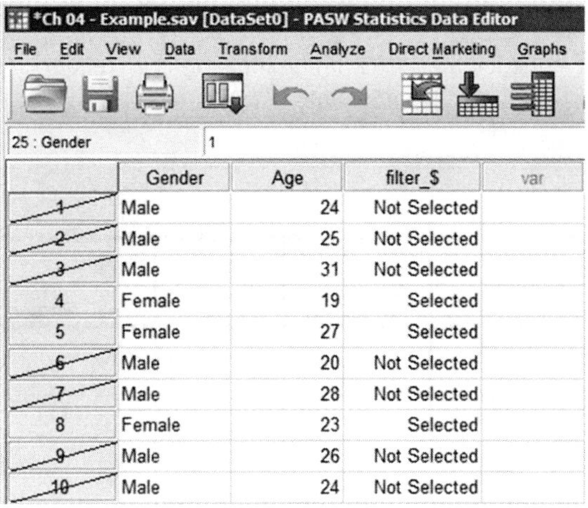

*Ch 04 - Example.sav [DataSet0] - PASW Statistics Data Editor

File Edit View Data Transform Analyze Direct Marketing Graphs

25 : Gender 1

	Gender	Age	filter_$	var
1	Male	24	Not Selected	
2	Male	25	Not Selected	
3	Male	31	Not Selected	
4	Female	19	Selected	
5	Female	27	Selected	
6	Male	20	Not Selected	
7	Male	28	Not Selected	
8	Female	23	Selected	
9	Male	26	Not Selected	
10	Male	24	Not Selected	

Notice that SPSS has created the temporary variable *filter_$* in the last column, which corresponds to the slashes in each row. If you click on the *Value Labels* icon or go to the *Variable View* screen, you will see that the *filter_$* variable contains two categories: *0 = Not Selected* and *1 = Selected.*

Since we selected only cases where *Gender* = *1,* this means that if we were to (re)run the descriptive statistics, the summary statistics and histogram would reflect *Females* only, as opposed to the earlier report that combined *Females* and *Males.*

7. Rerun the analysis for the *Age* variable using the procedure (go to the ★ icon on page **58**). The resulting statistical report should resemble the data shown in Table 4.6.

Table 4.6 *Frequency Statistics* Table Showing Summary Statistics for *Age* for Females Only.

Statistics

Age

N	Valid	27
	Missing	0
Mean		23.19
Median		23.00
Mode		23
Std. Deviation		2.543
Variance		6.464
Range		10
Minimum		18
Maximum		28

8. Notice that the *N* has changed from 50, which included both *Females* and *Males,* to 27, which is *Females* only. Compared to the first report, all other statistics have changed as well. Continuing our analysis of the *Females* only, observe the frequency statistics (Table 4.7) and corresponding histogram (Figure 4.18).

Table 4.7 Frequency Statistics Table Showing the Frequency of Each Value in the *Age* Variable for *Females* Only.

Age

		Frequency	Percent	Valid Percent	Cumulative Percent
Valid	18	1	3.7	3.7	3.7
	19	2	7.4	7.4	11.1
	20	1	3.7	3.7	14.8
	21	2	7.4	7.4	22.2
	22	4	14.8	14.8	37.0
	23	5	18.5	18.5	55.6
	24	4	14.8	14.8	70.4
	25	3	11.1	11.1	81.5
	26	2	7.4	7.4	88.9
	27	2	7.4	7.4	96.3
	28	1	3.7	3.7	100.0

9. As you can see, there is a lot to be learned by selecting the data and examining statistics pertaining to *Females* only. The next step is to run the same reports for *Males* only.

10. Begin the *Males only* analysis by selecting only the cases that pertain to males only; go to the ★ icon on page **66**, except when you get to **Step 4,** instead of specifying *Gender* = *1,* change that to *Gender* = *2* (remember, we established *Gender* as 1 for *Female* and 2 for *Male*).

11. Upon rerunning the data for *Males,* notice that the slashes, *filter_$,* and output reports have all changed to reflect *Males* only (see Table 4.8, Table 4.9, and Figure 4.19).

Figure 4.18 Histogram of the *Age* variable for *Females* only.

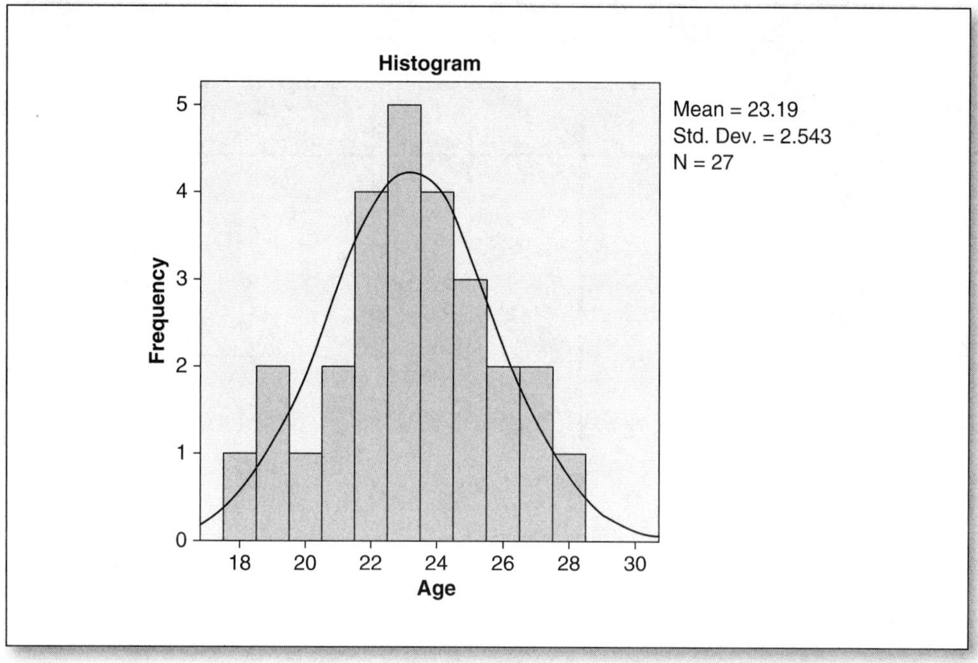

Table 4.8 *Frequency Statistics* Table Showing Summary Statistics for *Age* for *Males* Only.

Statistics

Age

N	Valid	23
	Missing	0
Mean		24.96
Median		25.00
Mode		25
Std. Deviation		2.962
Variance		8.771
Range		13
Minimum		18
Maximum		31

Table 4.9 Frequency Statistics Table Showing the Frequency of Each Value in the *Age* Variable for *Males* Only.

Age

		Frequency	Percent	Valid Percent	Cumulative Percent
Valid	18	1	4.3	4.3	4.3
	20	1	4.3	4.3	8.7
	22	2	8.7	8.7	17.4
	23	1	4.3	4.3	21.7
	24	4	17.4	17.4	39.1
	25	6	26.1	26.1	65.2
	26	3	13.0	13.0	78.3
	27	1	4.3	4.3	82.6
	28	1	4.3	4.3	87.0
	29	1	4.3	4.3	91.3
	30	1	4.3	4.3	95.7
	31	1	4.3	4.3	100.0
	Total	23	100.0	100.0	

Figure 4.19 Histogram of the *Age* variable for *Males* only.

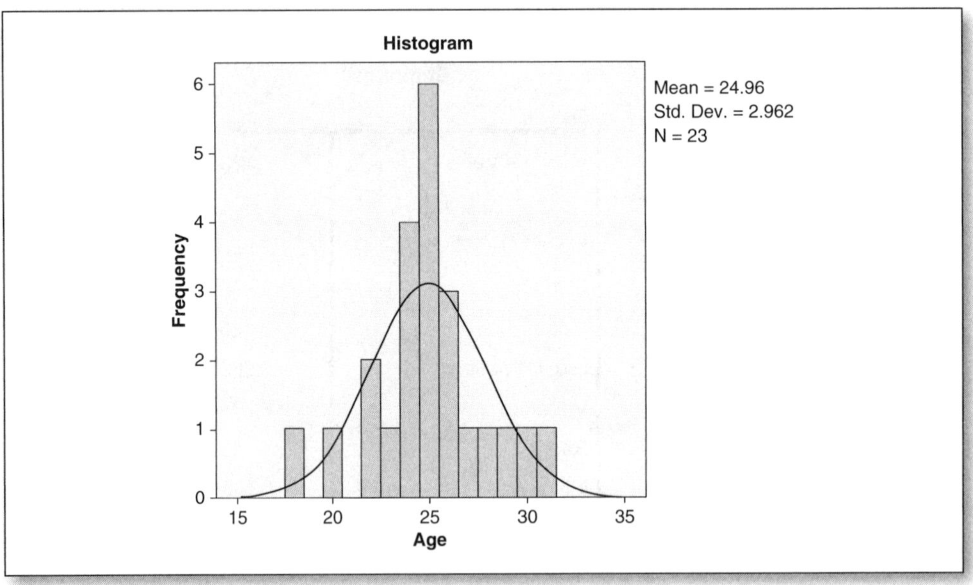

SPSS—(RE)SELECTING ALL VARIABLES

At this point, we have run three sets of descriptive statistics on *Age:* (1) all records, (2) *Females* only, and (3) *Males* only. Now, suppose we want to perform further analyses using the *entire* data set again; there are several ways to reactivate all of the slashed-out records:

- On the *Data View* screen, click on the column header *filter_$* (which will highlight the whole column) and press the *Delete* key.
- On the *Variable View* screen, click on the corresponding row number—in this case, row 3 (which will highlight the whole row)—and press the *Delete* key.
- Click on the *Select Cases* icon, then click on the *All Cases* button. Finally, click on the *OK* button.

GOOD COMMON SENSE

Although SPSS is proficient at processing statistical data, keep in mind that the program has no real intelligence per se—it just pushes the numbers through the functions using the parameters that you specify. As such, it is up to you to enter the data accurately and make intelligent processing selections.

In the examples detailed in this chapter, we ordered a variety of statistical analyses on the *Age* variable, which makes sense; knowing the mean age can be useful. Larger databases are likely to contain other numeric variables such as patient ID numbers, street addresses, phone numbers, serial numbers, license numbers, and so on. Technically, you could order SPSS to compute descriptive statistics on such variables; SPSS is not bright enough to know that computing the mean for a series of phone numbers makes no sense; SPSS (or any other statistical processing software) would mindlessly process the variable and provide you with an average phone number, which would be useless. In summary, it is up to you to proceed mindfully when using any such software.

Key Concepts

Descriptive statistics

- Number (*n*)
- Mean (μ)
- Median
- Mode
- Standard deviation (*SD*)
- Variance
- Minimum
- Maximum
- Range

Loading SPSS data files

- Histogram
- Normal curve

- Skew
    - Negative (left) skew
    - Positive (right) skew
- Outlier
- Bar chart
- Pie chart
- Select cases
- Good common sense

Practice Exercises

Use the prepared SPSS data sets (download from **study.sagepub.com/statsfornursing**).

Load the specified data sets, then process and document your findings for each exercise.

Exercise 4.1

The administration provides you with data gathered from a recent student enrollment survey.

Data set: **Ch 04 – Exercise 01A.sav**

Codebook

Variable: Enrolled
Definition: Enrollment status (Is the respondent currently enrolled?)
Type: Categorical (1 = Yes, 2 = No)

Variable: Courses
Definition: Total number of courses the student is currently enrolled in
Type: Continuous

Variable: Hours
Definition: Total number of hours per week allocated for academic work
Type: Continuous

a. Run descriptive statistics and a bar chart for *Enrolled.*
b. Run descriptive statistics and a histogram with a normal curve for *Courses* but only for students who are *Enrolled* (*Enrolled* = *1*).
c. Run descriptive statistics and a histogram with a normal curve for *Hours* but only for students who are *Enrolled* (*Enrolled* = *1*).
d. Write an abstract under 200 words discussing the results of the study.

Repeat this exercise using data set: **Ch 04 – Exercise 01B.sav.**

Exercise 4.2

A local health clinic has asked their team of volunteers to indicate their weekly availability.

Data set: **Ch 04 – Exercise 02A.sav**

Codebook

Variable: ID
Definition: Respondent's ID number
Type: Alphanumeric

Variable: Volhours
Definition: Number of hours per week the volunteer is willing to provide
Type: Continuous

a. Run descriptive statistics and a histogram with a normal curve for *VolHours* (NOTE: On the *Analyze, Frequencies, Statistics* menu, along with the regular descriptive statistic selections, select ☑ ***Sum;*** this will produce the total number of weekly volunteer hours).
b. Write an abstract under 200 words discussing the results of the study.

Repeat this exercise using data set: **Ch 04 – Exercise 02B.sav.**

Exercise 4.3

The nurse in charge of a weight control program has gathered baseline data on the participants.

Data set: **Ch 04 – Exercise 03A.sav**

Codebook

Variable: Gender
Definition: Gender
Type: Categorical (1 = Female, 2 = Male)

Variable: Height
Definition: Height (in inches)
Type: Continuous

Variable: Weight
Definition: Body weight (in pounds)
Type: Continuous

Variable: Age
Definition: Age
Type: Continuous

a. Run descriptive statistics and a histogram with a normal curve for *Height, Weight,* and *Age* for females only (*Gender* = *1*).

NOTE: You can run three separate reports, or since these variables are all the same type (continuous), you can process all of them in one pass: On the *Analyze, Frequencies, Statistics* menu, move all three variables (*Height, Weight,* and *Age*) into the *Variable(s)* window.

b. Run descriptive statistics and a histogram with a normal curve for *Height, Weight,* and *Age* for males only (*Gender* = *2*).

c. Write an abstract under 200 words discussing the results of the study.

Repeat this exercise using data set: **Ch 04 – Exercise 03B.sav.**

Exercise 4.4

The rehabilitation department has conducted a survey of patients to comprehend their employment status and the amount of sleep for each patient.

Data set: **Ch 04 – Exercise 04A.sav**

Codebook

Variable: Employ
Definition: Employment status
Type: Categorical (1 = Unemployed, 2 = Temporary, 3 = Part-time, 4 = Full-time)

Variable: Work
Definition: Number of hours worked in an average week
Type: Continuous

Variable: Sleep
Definition: Number of hours of sleep in an average night
Type: Continuous

a. Run descriptive statistics and a bar chart for *Employ*.

b. Run descriptive statistics and a histogram with a normal curve for *Work* and *Sleep* for those who are unemployed (*Employ* = *1*).

NOTE: You can run two separate reports, or since these variables (*Work* and *Sleep*) are the same type (continuous), you can process both of them in one pass: On the *Analyze, Frequencies, Statistics* menu, move both variables (*Work* and *Sleep*) into the *Variable(s)* window.

c. Run descriptive statistics and a histogram with a normal curve for *Work* and *Sleep* for those with temporary employment (*Employ* = *2*).

d. Run descriptive statistics and a histogram with a normal curve for *Work* and *Sleep* for those with part-time employment (*Employ* = *3*).

e. Run descriptive statistics and a histogram with a normal curve for *Work* and *Sleep* for those with full-time employment (*Employ* = *4*).

f. Write an abstract under 200 words discussing the results of the study.

Repeat this exercise using data set: **Ch 04 – Exercise 04B.sav.**

Exercise 4.5

A genetics counselor has provided you with an excerpt from a patient database detailing the number of siblings and adoption status of each patient.

Data set: **Ch 04 – Exercise 05A.sav**

Codebook

Variable:	Finitial
Definition:	First initial of first name
Type:	Alphanumeric
Variable:	Lname
Definition:	Last name
Type:	Alphanumeric
Variable:	Siblings
Definition:	Total number of brothers and sisters
Type	Continuous
Variable:	Adopted
Definition:	Adoption status (Is the respondent adopted?)
Type:	Categorical (1 = Yes, 2 = No)

a. Run descriptive statistics and a bar chart for *Adopted*.

b. Run descriptive statistics and a histogram with a normal curve for *Siblings* for those who are not adopted (*Adopted = 2*).

c. Run descriptive statistics and a histogram with a normal curve for *Siblings* for those who are adopted (*Adopted = 1*).

d. Write an abstract under 200 words discussing the results of the study.

Repeat this exercise using data set: **Ch 04 – Exercise 05B.sav.**

Exercise 4.6

The administrator at a walk-in clinic has asked the triage nurse to gather patient information in order to help determine flu shot demand for the upcoming flu season.

Data set: **Ch 04 – Exercise 06A.sav**

Codebook

Variable:	Pt_ID
Definition:	Patient ID number
Type:	Continuous

Variable: Age
Definition: Age
Type: Continuous

Variable: Temp
Definition: Body temperature (in Fahrenheit)
Type: Continuous

Variable: Flu_shot
Definition: Flu shot status (Has the respondent had a flu shot this season?)
Type: Categorical (1 = Yes; 2 = No, and I don't want one; 3 = Not yet, but I'd like one)

Variable: Rx
Definition: Current medications
Type: Alphanumeric

a. Run descriptive statistics and a bar chart for *Flu_shot.*

b. Run descriptive statistics and a histogram with a normal curve for *Age* and *Temp.*

NOTE: You can run two separate reports, or since these variables are the same type (continuous), you can process both of them in one pass: On the *Analyze, Frequencies, Statistics* menu, move both variables (*Age* and *Temp*) into the *Variable(s)* window.

c. Write an abstract under 200 words discussing the results of the study.

Repeat this exercise using data set: **Ch 04 – Exercise 06B.sav.**

Exercise 4.7

The research team wants to determine how many patients in their clinic have ever been treated in an emergency room.

Data set: **Ch 04 – Exercise 07A.sav**

Codebook

Variable: ER
Definition: Have you ever been treated in an emergency room?
Type: Numeric (1 = Yes, 2 = No, 3 = Decline to answer)

Variable: DOB
Definition: Date of birth
Type: Date (MM/DD/YYYY)

a. Run descriptive statistics and a bar chart for *ER.*

b. Write an abstract under 200 words discussing the results of the study.

Repeat this exercise using data set: **Ch 04 – Exercise 07B.sav.**

Exercise 4.8

Providers at an immunology clinic want to better understand the prevalence of pet allergies among their patients.

Data set: **Ch 04 – Exercise 08A.sav**

Codebook

Variable: Cat
Definition: Cat allergy
Type: Categorical (1 = Allergic, 2 = Not allergic)

Variable: Dog
Definition: Dog allergy
Type: Categorical (1 = Allergic, 2 = Not allergic)

Variable: Pets
Definition: Number of pets at home that patient is allergic to
Type: Continuous

a. Run descriptive statistics and a bar chart for *Cat* and *Dog*.

NOTE: You can run two separate reports, or since these variables are the same type (categorical), you can process both of them in one pass: On the *Analyze, Frequencies, Statistics* menu, move both variables (*Cat* and *Dog*) into the *Variable(s)* window.

b. Run descriptive statistics and a histogram with a normal curve for *Pets*.
c. Write an abstract under 200 words discussing the results of the study.

Repeat this exercise using data set: **Ch 04 – Exercise 08B.sav.**

Exercise 4.9

A blood donor center wants to better comprehend the nature of their donors.

Data set: **Ch 04 – Exercise 09A.sav**

Codebook

Variable: Blood_type
Definition: Blood type
Type: Categorical (1 = A−, 2 = A+, 3 = B−, 4 = B+, 5 = AB−, 6 = AB+, 7 = O−, 8 = O+)

Variable: Gender
Definition: Gender
Type: Categorical (1 = Female, 2 = Male)

Variable: Prior_donor
Definition: Prior blood donations
Type: Categorical (1 = Yes, 2 = No)

a. Run descriptive statistics and a bar chart for *Blood_type, Gender,* and *Prior_donor.*

NOTE: You can run three separate reports, or since these variables are the same type (categorical), you can process all of them in one pass: On the *Analyze, Frequencies, Statistics* menu, move all three variables (*Blood_type, Gender,* and *Prior_donor*) into the *Variable(s)* window.

b. Write an abstract under 200 words discussing the results of the study.

Repeat this exercise using data set: **Ch 04 – Exercise 09B.sav.**

Exercise 4.10

Patients in the primary care clinic have the option to choose if they want to receive their laboratory results via a telephone call or a brief text message.

Data set: **Ch 04 – Exercise 10A.sav**

Codebook

Variable: Send_labs
Definition: Method for sending laboratory results
Type: Categorical (1 = Phone call, 2 = Text message)

Variable: Phone
Definition: Phone number
Type: Alphanumeric

a. Run descriptive statistics and a bar chart for *Send_labs.*
b. Write an abstract under 200 words discussing the results of the study.

Repeat this exercise using data set: **Ch 04 – Exercise 10B.sav.**

PART III

Measuring Differences Between Groups

These chapters provide tests for detecting differences between groups that involve continuous variables.

LAYERED LEARNING

Chapter 5: *t* Test and Mann-Whitney *U* Test: The ***t* test** is used in two-group designs (e.g., control vs. experimental) to detect if one group significantly outperformed the other. In the event that the data are not fully suitable to run a ***t* test,** the **Mann-Whitney *U* test** provides an alternative.

Chapter 6: ANOVA and Kruskal-Wallis Test: ANOVA is similar to the ***t* test,** but it is capable of processing *more than two groups*. In the event that the data are not fully suitable to run an **ANOVA,** the **Kruskal-Wallis test** provides an alternative.

Chapter 7: ANCOVA is similar to **ANOVA,** but it is capable of including a covariate, which adjusts the results to account for the potential influences of an identified confounding variable.

Chapter 8: MANOVA is similar to **ANOVA,** but it is capable of processing more than one outcome (dependent) variable.

CHAPTER 5

t Test and Mann-Whitney *U* Test

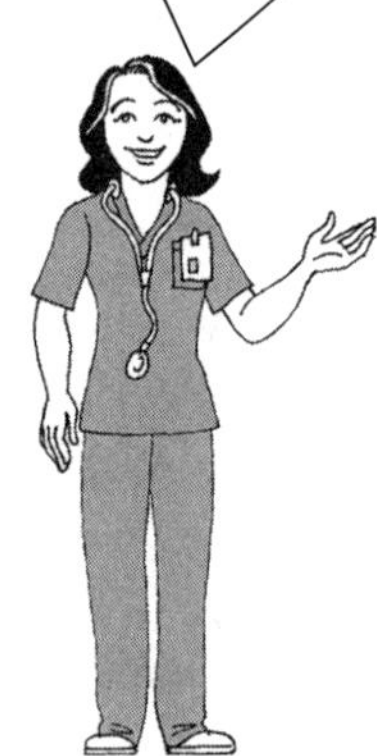

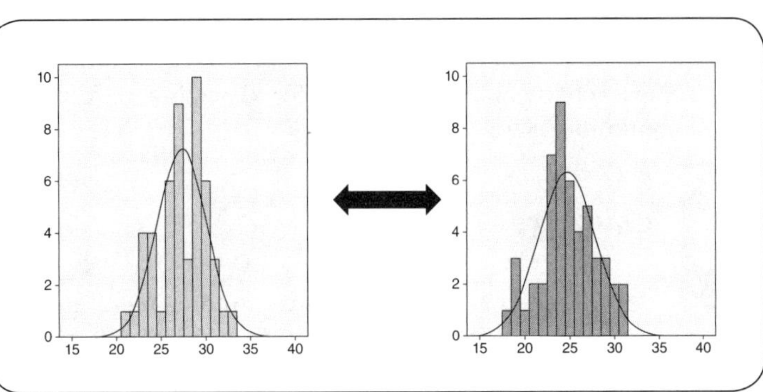

The difference between a violin and a viola is that a viola burns longer.

—Victor Borge

LEARNING OBJECTIVES

Upon completing this chapter, you will be able to:

- Determine when it is appropriate to run a *t* test
- Verify that the data meet the criteria for *t* test processing: normality, *n*, and homogeneity of variance
- Order a *t* test
- Interpret the test results
- Comprehend the α and *p* value
- Resolve the hypotheses

- Know when and how to run and interpret the Mann-Whitney *U* test
- Document the results in plain English
- Understand the implications of Type I and Type II errors
- Apply techniques for reducing the likelihood of committing Type I and Type II errors

NOTE: From here forward, the "μ" character will be used to symbolize the mean.

VIDEO

The videos for this chapter are **Ch 05 – t Test.mp4** and **Ch 05 – Mann-Whitney U Test.mp4**. These videos provide overviews of these tests, instructions for carrying out the pretest checklist, run, and interpreting the results of this test using the data set: **Ch 05 – Example 01 – t Test.sav**.

OVERVIEW—*t* TEST

The *t* test is one of the most common and versatile statistical tests in the realm of experimental research and survey methodology. The *t* test is used when there are two groups, wherein each group renders a continuous variable for the outcome (e.g., height, age, weight, number of teeth, bank account balance, IQ score, score on a depression assessment instrument, blood pressure, test score, typing speed, etc.).

In the most basic experimental setting, the design consists of two groups: a control group, which gets a placebo or treatment as usual, and a treatment group, which gets the innovative intervention that is the focus of the study.

We can compute the mean for each group, and we would not expect the two means to be identical; they would likely be different. The *t* test answers the question, *Is there a statistically significant difference between μ(Control) and μ(Treatment)?* In other words, the result of the *t* test helps us to determine if one group *substantially* outperformed the other or if the differences between the means are essentially *incidental*.

Example

The nurse manager is interested in identifying the most effective drug for managing patients with moderate hypertension (systolic between 130 mmHg and 140 mmHg).

Research Question

Drug A, which is the new drug, or Drug B, a commonly used drug?

Groups

The nurse manager recruits 60 volunteers who meet the criteria and consent to participate in this study. Each patient's name is written on slips of paper and placed in a hat. The nurse manager randomly draws 30 names from the hat; these patients will receive Drug A; the next 30 names drawn will get Drug B.

Procedure

Each participant is brought in to the clinic for a brief visit: Their blood pressure is taken to verify that they meet the criteria (systolic between 130 mmHg and 140 mmHg), and they are given a 30-day supply of the specified medication. After 30 days, each participant will return to the clinic and have his or her blood pressure taken. For purposes of this example, we will presume 100% dosage adherence.

Hypotheses

The null hypothesis (H_0) is phrased to anticipate that the experiment/intervention fails, indicating that *Drug A and Drug B perform the same in lowering blood pressure.* The alternative hypothesis (H_1) states that *Drug A will outperform Drug B in lowering blood pressure:*

H_0: Drug A and Drug B perform the same in lowering blood pressure.

H_1: Drug A outperforms Drug B in lowering blood pressure.

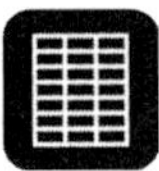

Data Set

Use the following data set: **Ch 05 – Example 01 – t Test.sav.**

Codebook

Variable: Group
Definition: Group number
Type: Categorical (1 = Drug A, 2 = Drug B)

Variable: SystolicBP
Definition: Systolic blood pressure (in mmHg)
Type: Continuous

NOTE: In this data set, records (rows) 1 through 30 are for Group 1 (Drug A), and records 31 through 60 are for Group 2 (Drug B). The data are arranged this way just for visual clarity; the order of the records has no bearing on the statistical results.

If you go to the *Variable View* and open the *Values* menu for the variable *Group,* you will see that the corresponding categorical labels have been assigned: 1 for Drug A and 2 for Drug B (Figure 5.1).

Figure 5.1 Value labels for a *t* test analysis.

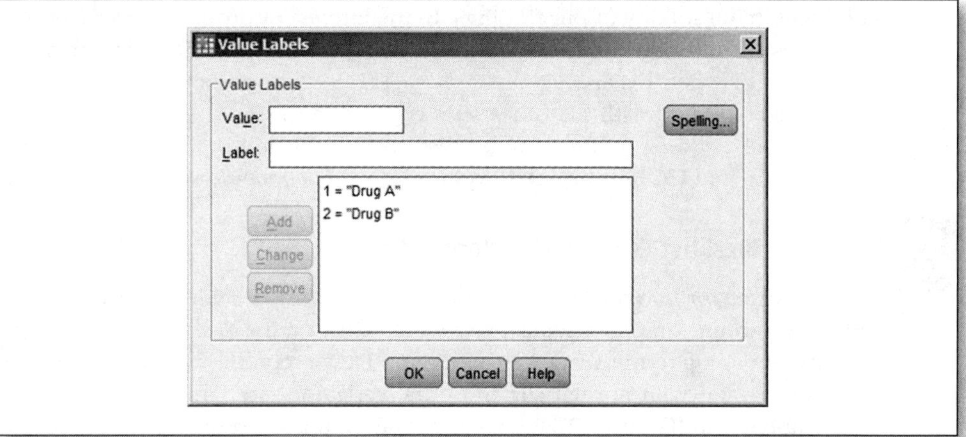

Pretest Checklist

t Test Pretest Checklist

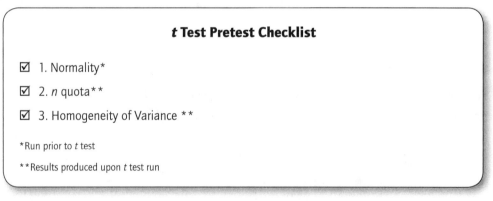

☑ 1. Normality*

☑ 2. *n* quota**

☑ 3. Homogeneity of Variance **

*Run prior to *t* test

**Results produced upon *t* test run

The statistical pretest checklist is akin to looking both ways before you cross the street; certainly you *could* cross the street without looking, but you would probably wind up in much better shape if you looked first. In terms of statistical tests, certainly you *could* run the statistical test without tending to the pretest checklist, but you may unknowingly generate misleading findings.

The formulas that compose each statistical test require that the source data meet a unique set of criteria in order for that test to operate properly. These criteria are referred to as *assumptions*—we *assume* that the data meet the criteria specified by the test at hand. Actually, we need to do more than just passively *assume* that the data are suitable for processing; we need to *actively* assess the source data before proceeding with the test.

When the tests on the pretest checklist (statistical assumptions) are satisfied, we can consider the statistical results relatively "robust." When one or more of the pretest checklist criteria are not satisfied, we still proceed with the analysis, but we would be a bit less confident in the solidity of our findings. In the interest of proper scientific ethics and the principles of full disclosure, it would be appropriate to mention any such (statistical) shortcomings when discussing the results. This notion pertains to the unique pretest checklists associated with the other tests covered in this text as well.

The pretest criteria for running a *t* test involve checking the data for **(1) normality**, **(2) *n* quota,** and **(3) homogeneity** (pronounced *hoe-moe-juh-nay-it-tee*) **of variance.**

Pretest Checklist Criterion 1—Normality

Checking for *normality* involves producing a histogram with a normal curve for each of the two groups. In this instance, you would click on the *Select Cases* icon to select the records pertaining to the Drug A group; the selection criteria would be Group = 1. Next, run a histogram (with normal curve) on the variable score. Then repeat the process for the Drug B group (Group = 2). For more details on this procedure, please refer to Chapter 4 ("SPSS—Descriptive Statistics: Continuous Variable (Age) Select by Categorical Variable (Gender)—Females Only"); see the star (★) icon on page **66**.

This will produce two histograms with normal curves—one for scores in the Drug A group and the other for the scores in the Drug B group. The histograms should resemble the graphs shown in Figures 5.2 and 5.3.

Figure 5.2 Histogram of score for Group 1: Drug A.

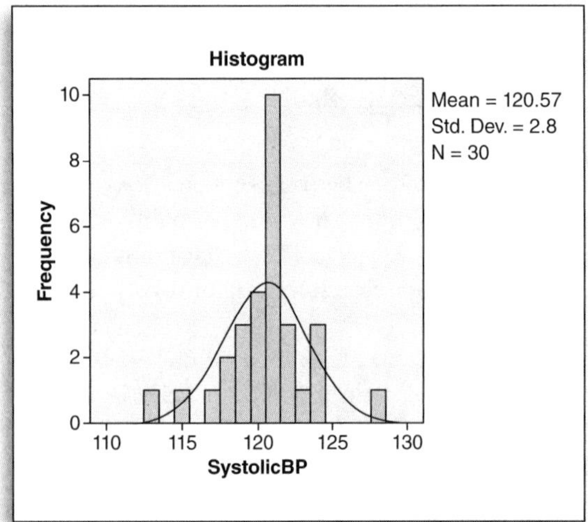

Figure 5.3 Histogram of score for Group 2: Drug B.

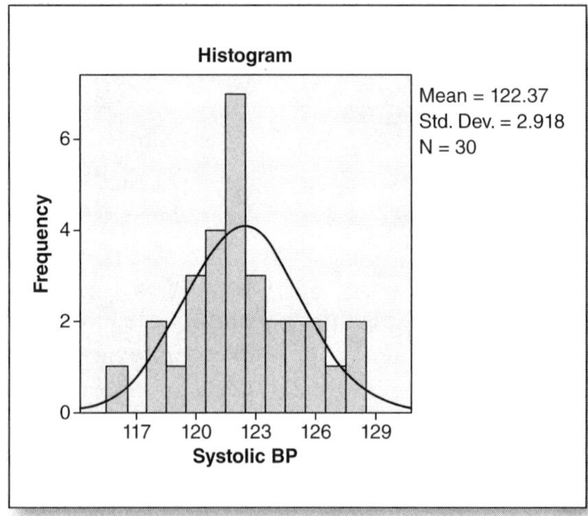

As we read these two histograms, set aside the X,Y scales and the possible irregularities among the bars; our attention is focused on the shape of the *normal curve* that is superimposed over the bars. We are looking for *normality* (symmetry) in these two curves. Although the normal curve in Figure 5.2 is shorter and fatter than the normal curve in Figure 5.3, in terms of normality, this is not an issue. The critical thing to observe is that both normal curves are sufficiently symmetrical—in other words, if you sliced this curve vertically down the middle, the left side would resemble a mirror image of the right side; sometimes this normal curve is aptly referred to by its characteristic shape as a "bell curve." In this example, we see that both curves are symmetrical; there is no notable *skew* in either curve. Hence, we would say that the criteria of normality are satisfied for both Drug A and Drug B.

Pretest Checklist Criterion 2—*n* Quota

Technically, you can process a *t* test with an *n* of any size in each group, but when the *n* is at least 30 in each group, the result of the *t* test is considered more robust. We will see the *n* reported for each group in the **Results** section, when we examine the findings produced by the *t* test.

Pretest Checklist Criterion 3—Homogeneity of Variance

Homogeneity pertains to *sameness;* the homogeneity of variance criteria involve checking that the variances of the two groups are not too different from each other. As a rule of thumb, homogeneity of variance is likely to be achieved if the variance from one group is not more than 2.2 times the variance of the other group. In this case, the variance ([standard deviation]^2) for SystolicBP in the Drug A group is 10.036 (3.168^2), and the variance for SystolicBP in the Drug B group is 8.515 (2.918^2). Since 10.036 is not more than twice 8.515, we would expect that the homogeneity of variance test would pass.

In SPSS, the homogeneity of variance test is an option selected during the actual run of the *t* test. If the homogeneity of variance test renders a significance (*p*) value that is greater than .05, then this suggests that there is no statistically significant difference between the variance from one group to the other group. This would mean that the data pass the homogeneity of variance test. The notion of the *p* value will be discussed in detail in the **Results** section in this chapter, when we examine the findings produced by the *t* test.

The remaining two pretest criteria, **(2) *n* quota** and **(3) homogeneity of variance,** will be processed during the **Test Run** and finalized in the **Results** section.

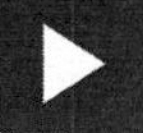

Test Run

You may have noticed a variety of *t* test options on the *Analyze, Compare Means* pull-down menu. We will be using the *One-Way ANOVA* menu to process the *t* tests; the reasoning for this option is threefold: (1) This is an easier menu to fill out, (2) it will produce the desired *t* test results, and (3) this will prepare you to efficiently run the ANOVA in the next chapter. NOTE: The *t* test is basically a two-group ANOVA.

1. On the main screen, click on *Analyze, Compare Means, One-Way ANOVA* (Figure 5.4).

Figure 5.4 Running a *t* test.

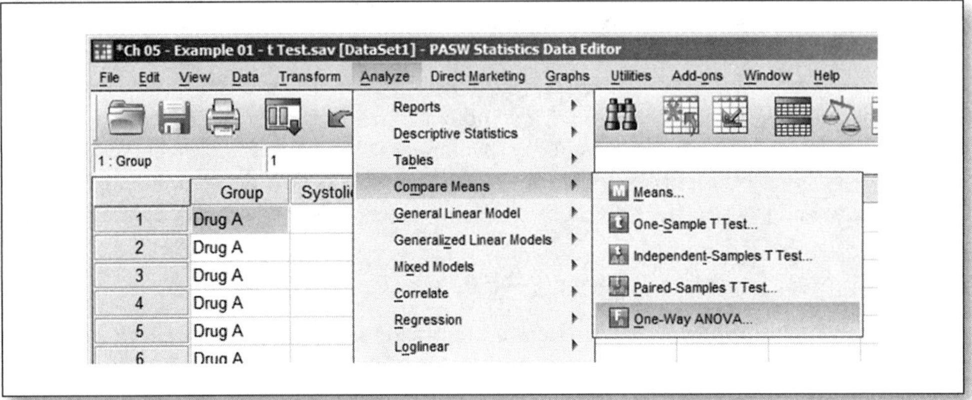

2. On the *One-Way ANOVA* menu, move the continuous variable that you wish to analyze (*SystolicBP*) into the *Dependent List* window, and move the variable that contains the categorical variable that specifies the group (*Group*) into the *Factor* window (Figure 5.5).

Figure 5.5 The one-way ANOVA menu.

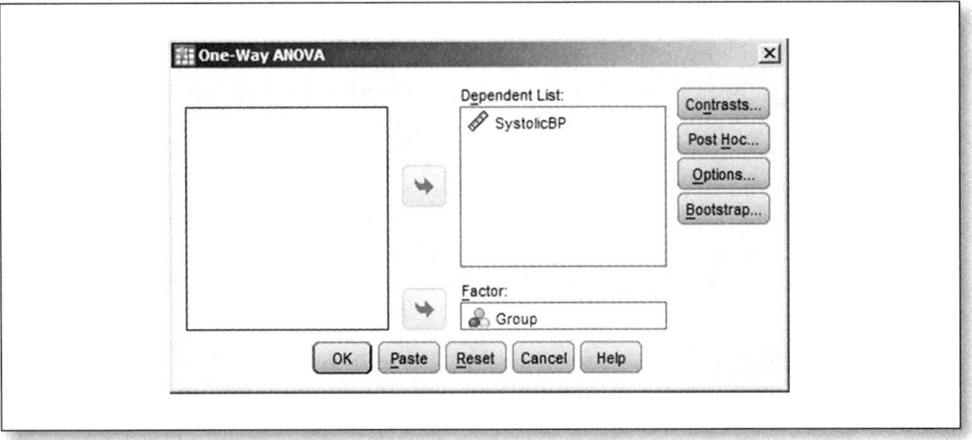

3. Click on the *Options* button. On the *One-Way ANOVA: Options* menu, check ☑ *Descriptive* and ☑ *Homogeneity of variance test,* then click on the *Continue* button (Figure 5.6). This will take you back to the *One-Way ANOVA* menu.

Figure 5.6 The one-way ANOVA: Options menu.

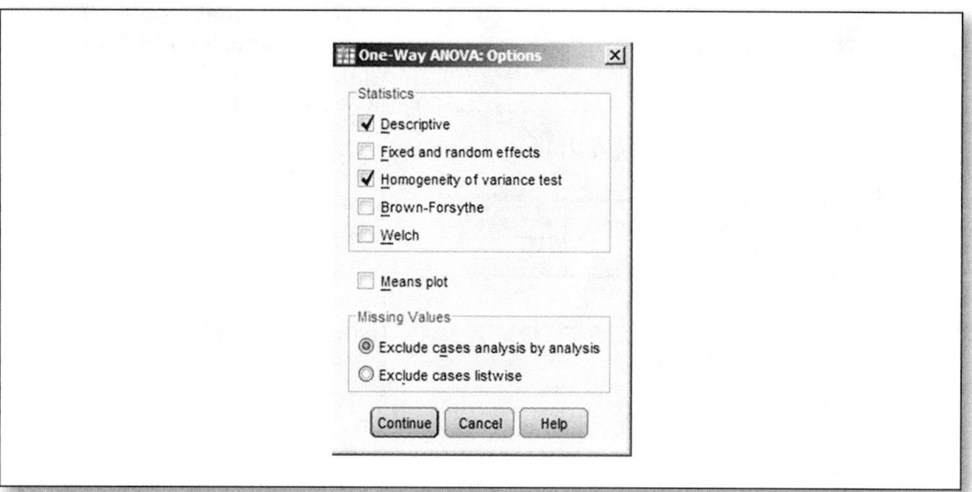

4. On the *One-Way ANOVA* menu (Figure 5.5), click on the *OK* button, and the test will process.

Results

Pretest Checklist Criterion 2—*n* Quota

The Descriptives table (Table 5.1) shows that each group has an *n* of 30. This satisfies the *n* assumption, indicating that the ANOVA test becomes more robust when the *n* for each group is at least 30.

Table 5.1 Descriptive Statistics Results.

Descriptives

SystolicBP

	N	Mean	Std. Deviation	Std. Error	95% Confidence Interval for Mean		Minimum	Maximum
					Lower Bound	Upper Bound		
Drug A	30	120.37	3.168	.578	119.18	121.55	112	128
Drug B	30	122.37	2.918	.533	121.28	123.46	116	128
Total	60	121.37	3.183	.411	120.54	122.19	112	128

Pretest Checklist Criterion 3—Homogeneity of Variance

Table 5.2 Homogeneity of Variance Test Results.

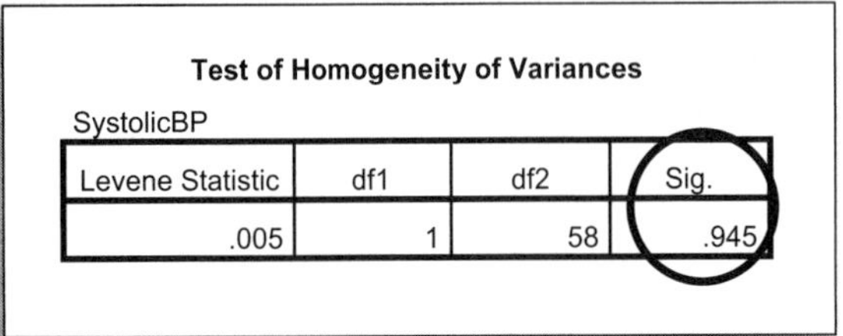

Test of Homogeneity of Variances

SystolicBP

Levene Statistic	df1	df2	Sig.
.005	1	58	.945

The last column of the homogeneity of variance table (Table 5.2) shows a Sig.(nificance) of .945; since this is greater than the α level of .05, this tells us that there is no statistically significant difference between the variances in the *SystolicBP* variable for the *Drug A* group compared with the *Drug B* group. We would conclude that the criteria of the homogeneity of variance have been satisfied. (NOTE: The Sig.(nificance) and α level are clarified in the following section.)

p Value

At this point, you have probably noticed column 3 in Table 5.1, which shows that the mean score for the Drug A group (120.37) is lower than the mean score for the Drug B group (122.37). On the basis of these means, you may hastily conclude that Drug A is the best since it performed better at lowering blood pressure than Drug B, but in statistics, the world is not so simple.

Statisticians recognize and actively acknowledge that we do not live in a perfect world; no matter how hard we try to conduct quality investigations, the scientific process can be a messy proposition littered with multiple confounding variables—conditions for which we cannot fully control or account for that can influence the outcome variable(s).

In our simple example, judging by the mean systolic blood pressure values of the two groups, it looks like the Drug A group outperformed the Drug B group, and this may in fact turn out to be the case, but other factors may have contributed to the differences observed between the (mean) scores of these two groups. For example, maybe the random distribution process unexpectedly routed more nonsmokers to the Drug A group; maybe the majority of dietary noncompliant patients were unknowingly routed to the Drug B group; maybe the members of the Drug B group had more stressful life circumstances than the patients who were issued Drug A; maybe the Drug A group had a more robust social support system that helped to promote better health practices than those in the Drug B group. Any number of these or other factors that we do not know about may have been occurring over the course of this study.

As you can see, there is virtually no limit to the variety of confounding variables that could potentially influence the outcome of a study. Since we cannot fully account for or compensate for such confounds, we know we do not have a perfect experimental setting. Hence, we do not speak of our statistical findings with *absolute certainty;* rather, we speak of how much *confidence* we have in our findings.

The key question in this case is, *How certain can we be that the 2-point difference that we detected between the group means (μ(Drug A) = 120.37 and μ(Drug B) = 122.37) is actually due to the genuine superiority of Drug A and not due to chance alone?* In other words, we want a number that will tell us how likely we would detect this result (the

2-point difference in the means) if Drug A was actually no different from Drug B. This number is known as the significance level, represented by the letter *p*.

Here is how the significance (*p*) value works: Look at the last column of Table 5.3; the Sig.(nificance) score is .014; this is the *p* value. This tells us that we would expect to see the 2-point difference in the group scores about 1.4% of the time if it were occurring by (random) chance alone. In other words, based on the data gathered, if Drug A is exactly as effective as Drug B, we would see the Drug A group outperform the Drug B group by 2 points about 1.4% of the time.

Since the *p* value tells us how often we would be accepting the intervention as effective, when in fact it really is not, the lower the *p* value, the more significant the findings.

To exemplify the point further, suppose this experiment produced a *p* value of .01. This tells us that if Drug A were in fact clinically equivalent to Drug B, and we ran this experiment 100 times, 1 of those iterations would, through random chance, produce results wherein Drug A outperforms Drug B. If the *p* value was .001, this indicates that we would have to run this experiment 1,000 times to see an instance where Drug A outperforms Drug B (merely due to random chance). Essentially, the lower the *p* value, the less likely it is that the findings (differences between the means of the groups) are occurring merely due to random chance, suggesting the stronger likelihood that the observed differences are due to the intervention—in this case, the effectiveness of Drug A.

In the next section, we will see how we use the *p* value to determine which hypothesis to reject and which to accept.

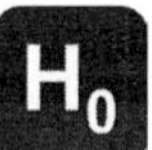

Hypothesis Resolution

We need to have a way of using the *p* value to guide us in making decisions about our pending hypotheses:

H_0: Drug A and Drug B perform the same in lowering blood pressure.

H_1: Drug A outperforms Drug B in lowering blood pressure.

Table 5.3 *t* Test Results Comparing *SystolicBP* of Drug A : Drug B.

ANOVA

SystolicBP

	Sum of Squares	df	Mean Square	F	Sig.
Between Groups	60.000	1	60.000	6.469	.014
Within Groups	537.933	58	9.275		
Total	597.933	59			

α Level

To do this, before we embark on our research process, we draw a somewhat arbitrary numerical line in the sand, known as the alpha (α) level. Typically the α level is set to .05. Think of the α level as a sort of statistical significance threshold—any p (Sig.) value that is .05 or less is considered statistically significant—hence, we reject H_0, which states that there is no significant difference between the groups. If the p value is over .05, then the differences between the means are not considered statistically significant—hence, we do not reject H_0. This will guide us in making our decisions regarding the hypotheses.

p Value Summary

- If $p \leq \alpha$, then there is a statistically significant difference; reject H_0.
- If $p > \alpha$, then there is no statistically significant difference; do not reject H_0.

NOTE: $\alpha = .05$ (.05 is the typical value used; some more stringent studies may use .01 or lower.)

Since the p is .014, which is less than or equal to α (.05), we would determine that there is a statistically significant difference between the scores—specifically, that 120.37 is statistically significantly less than 122.37. To finalize the hypotheses, we would reject H_0 and accept H_1:

REJECT: H_0: Drug A and Drug B perform the same in lowering blood pressure.

ACCEPT: H_1: Drug A outperforms Drug B in lowering blood pressure.

Documenting Results

Although it is essential to comprehend the meaning of the key values in the statistical reports, it would be inappropriate to simply present the figures in a results section without providing a concise narrative. While all figures below are technically correct, try to avoid documenting your findings as such:

Accurate but Inappropriate Numerical Statistical Abstract

Drug A: $n = 30$, $\mu = 120.37$ ($SD = 3.168$)

Drug B: $n = 30$, $\mu = 122.37$ ($SD = 2.918$)

$p = .014$, $\alpha = .05$, therefore, use Drug A

While the above data may be useful in assembling a table, it is important that you become proficient at translating your methodology and numerical findings into a brief textual abstract detailing the story of the study specifying the research question, along with an overview of how you got from the research question to the results.

Appropriate Verbose Statistical Abstract

A group of 60 patients with moderate hypertension (systolic between 130 mmHg and 140 mmHg) were recruited and randomly assigned to take an antihypertensive medication—either Drug A or Drug B.

After 30 days, patients in the Drug A group had a significantly lower mean systolic pressure reading (μ = 120.37, *SD* = 3.168) compared to those who took Drug B (μ = 122.37, *SD* = 2.918), *p* = .014, α = .05.

In addition to the full manuscript, scientific journals also require authors to submit an abstract that tells the overall story of the study and key findings; usually the limit for the abstract is about 200 words. While initially it can be a challenge to write technical information so concisely, this is a worthy skill to develop for journal publication and other forms of professional communication. The above abstract is under 100 words.

In the example processed in this chapter, we saw that the *t* test assessed the means of the two groups and revealed that the mean for the group that got Drug A was statistically significantly lower than the mean for the group that took Drug B, signifying that Drug A outperformed Drug B (in lowering blood pressure). As you will see in the exercises for this chapter, the *t* test is equally effective in detecting statistically significant differences when the mean from one group is *higher* than for the other group. For example, in an intervention designed to elevate the mood of depressed patients as measured by the Acme Mood Scale (1 = very depressed . . . 10 = very happy), success of the intervention would be signified by the treated group having a statistically significantly *higher* mean AMS score compared to the other group, as opposed to the antihypertension (Drug A : Drug B) example, wherein success was associated with *lowering* blood pressure. Remember: The *t* test is designed to simply detect statistically significant differences between the means of two groups; it does not matter which group mean is higher and which is lower.

Type I and Type II Errors

The world is imperfect; despite all best efforts, errors can occur in virtually any realm no matter how careful you are. Consider the two types of errors that can occur in a legal verdict:

Error 1: The court finds the defendant *guilty* when, in fact, he or she is actually *not guilty*.

Error 2: The court finds the defendant *not guilty* when, in fact, he or she actually *is guilty*.

These same two types of errors can happen in statistics. Consider this standard set of hypotheses:

H_0: There is no significant difference between the groups ($p > .05$; the treatment failed).

H_1: There is a statistically significant between the groups ($p \leq .05$; the treatment worked).

Type I Error

A Type I error (also known as alpha [α] error) occurs when the findings indicate that there is a statistically significant difference between two variables (or groups) ($p \leq .05$) when, in fact, on the whole, there actually is not, meaning that you would erroneously reject the null hypothesis. The consequence is that you would conclude that treatment was effective when, in fact, on the whole, it was not. This is connected with the p value; a p value of .05 means that there is a 5% chance that you have committed a Type I error—hence, the lower the p value, the less likely that you have committed a Type I error. A Type I error can be thought of as the court finding the defendant *guilty* when, in fact, he or she is actually *not guilty*.

Type II Error

A Type II error (also known as beta [β] error) occurs when the findings indicate that there is no statistically significant difference between two variables (or groups) ($p > .05$) when, in fact, on the whole, there actually is, meaning that you would erroneously accept the null hypothesis. The consequence is that you would conclude that the treatment was ineffective when, in fact, on the whole, it was. Sample size is inversely related to Type II errors—the higher the sample size, the lower the likelihood of committing a Type II error. A Type II error can be thought of as a court finding the defendant *not guilty* when, in fact, he or she actually *is guilty*.

There is no formal metric that you can run that will tell you if you have a Type I or Type II error on hand; they are just characteristics endemic in the realm of statistical testing. The point to keep in mind is that even if a statistical test produces a statistically significant p value (e.g., $p \leq .05$), this does not mean that you have solid evidentiary proof of anything; at best, you have reduced uncertainty. Essentially, a p value of .05 means that if the effect of the treatment group were the same as the control group (null intervention), we would see this (anomalous) statistical outcome, where the treatment group outperforms the control group, just by chance, about 5% of the time. Since p never goes to zero, there is always some level of uncertainty in statistical findings.

Occasionally, SPSS will produce results wherein the Sig. (p) value is *.000*. In such instances, the p value is so low that rounding it to three decimal digits produces the *.000* readout. In documenting such an occurrence, instead of writing $p = .000$ or $p = 0$, it is customarily documented as $p < .001$.

Remember: Statistics is not about proving or disproving anything; statistics is about reducing uncertainty—there is always some margin of error, no matter how small. The notion of Type I and Type II errors pertains to all other tests covered in the chapters that follow.

OVERVIEW—MANN-WHITNEY *U* TEST

One of the pretest criteria that must be met prior to running a *t* test states that the data from each group must be normally distributed (Figure 5.7); minor variations in the normal distribution are acceptable. Occasionally, you may encounter data that are substantially skewed (Figure 5.8), bimodal (Figure 5.9), flat (Figure 5.10), or may have some other atypical distribution. In such instances, the Mann-Whitney *U* statistic is an appropriate alternative to the *t* test.

Figure 5.7 Normal.

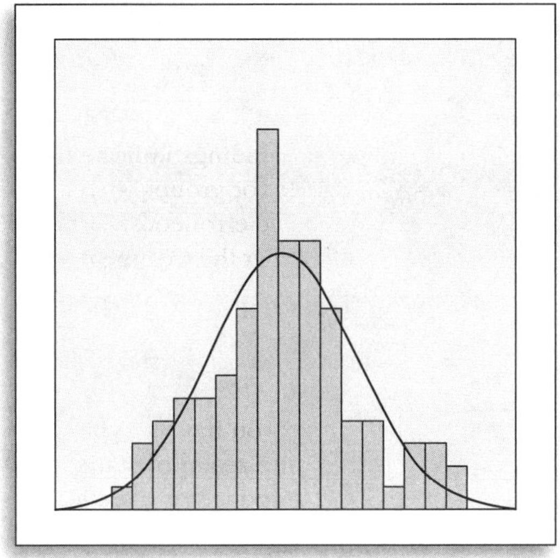

Figure 5.8 Skewed.

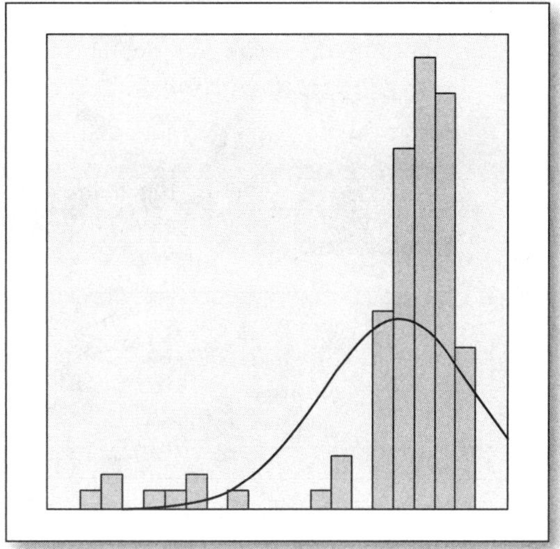

Test Run

For exemplary purposes, we will run the Mann-Whitney *U* test using the same data set (**Ch 05 – Example 01 – t Test.sav**) even though the data are normally distributed. This will enable us to compare the results of a *t* test to the results produced by the Mann-Whitney *U* test.

Figure 5.9 Bimodal.

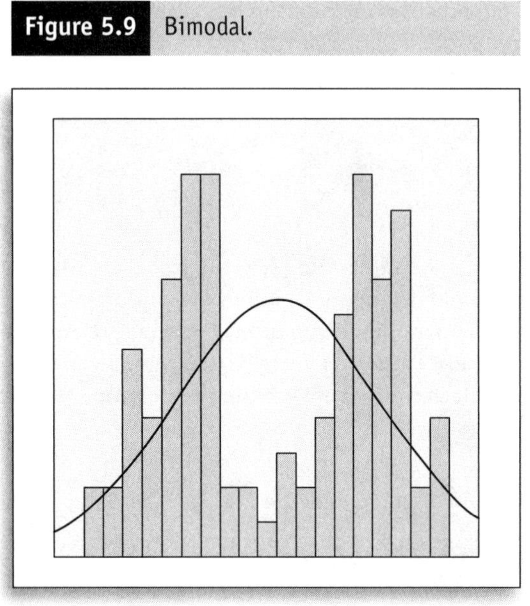

Figure 5.10 Flat.

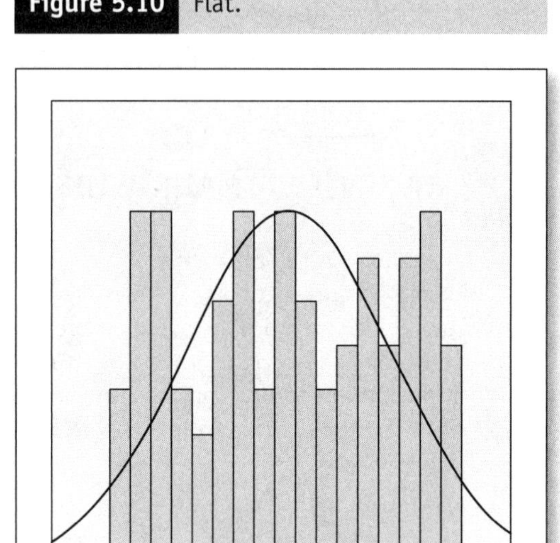

1. On the main screen, click on *Analyze, Nonparametric Tests, Legacy Dialogs, 2 Independent Samples* (Figure 5.11).

Figure 5.11 Ordering the Mann-Whitney *U* test: Click on *Analyze, Nonparametric Tests, Legacy Dialogs, 2 Independent Samples.*

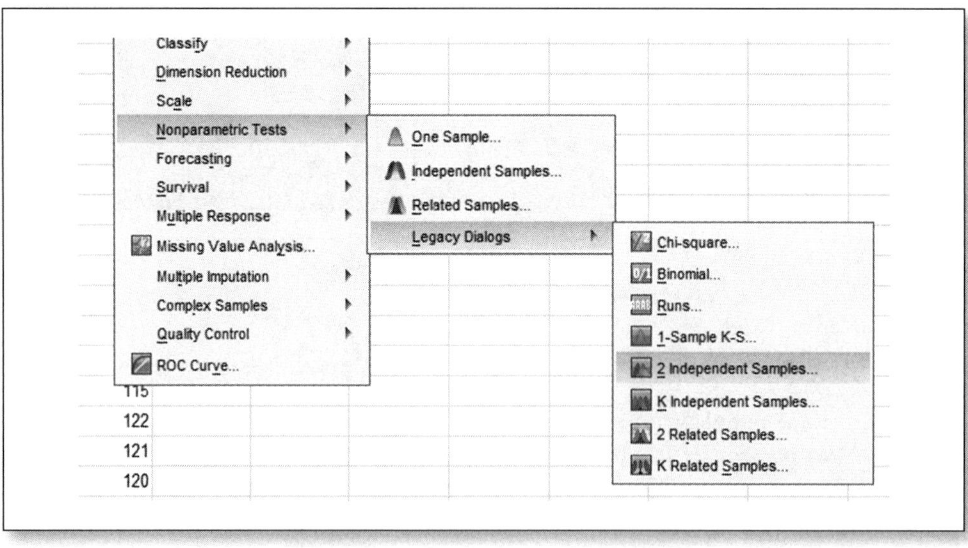

2. On the *Two-Independent-Samples Tests* menu, move *SystolicBP* to the *Test Variable List* window.

3. Move *Group* to the *Grouping Variable* box (Figure 5.12).

Figure 5.12 On the *Two-Independent-Samples Tests* menu, move SystolicBP to the *Test Variable List,* and move *Group* to the *Grouping Variable* box.

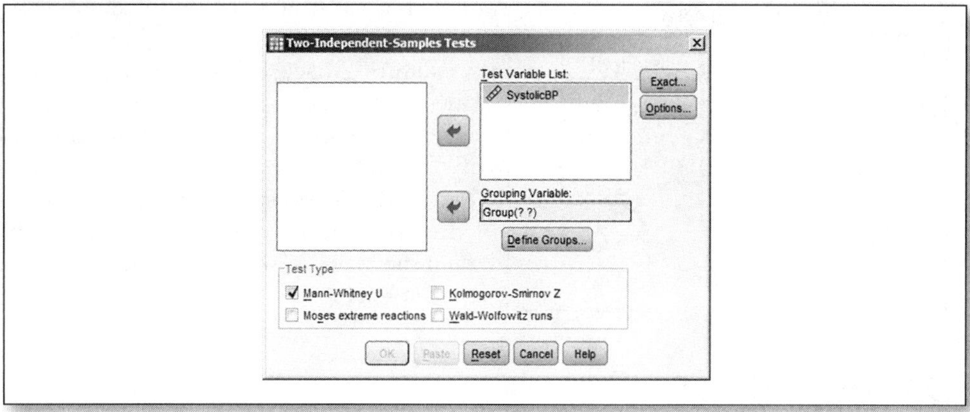

4. Click on *Group(? ?)*, then click on *Define Groups.*

5. On the *Two Independent Sample* submenu, for *Group 1,* enter *1;* for *Group 2,* enter *2* (this is because we defined Drug A as 1 and Drug B as 2) (Figure 5.13).

6. Click *Continue;* this will close this submenu.

Figure 5.13 On the *Two Independent Samples* submenu, for *Group 1,* enter *1;* for *Group 2,* enter *2.*

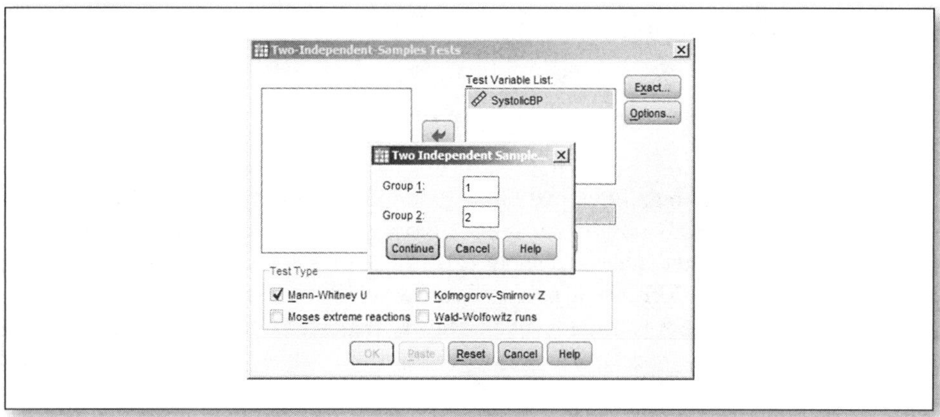

7. On the *Two-Independent-Samples Tests* menu, click on *OK*.

Results

Table 5.4 Mann-Whitney *p* Value = .011.

Test Statistics[a]

	SystolicBP
Mann-Whitney U	280.000
Wilcoxon W	745.000
Z	-2.533
Asymp. Sig. (2-tailed)	.011

a. Grouping Variable: Group

The Mann-Whitney U test result is found on the *Test Statistics* table (Table 5.4); the *Asymp. Sig. (2-tailed)* statistic rendered a *p* value of .011; since this is less than α (.05), we would conclude that there is a statistically significant difference between the performances of the two drugs.

Referring back, remember that the *t* test produced a *p* value of .014. The differences in these *p* values are due to the internal transformations that the Mann-Whitney *U* test conducts on the data. If one or more substantial violations are detected when running the pretest checklist for the *t* test, then the Mann-Whitney *U* test is considered a viable alternative.

GOOD COMMON SENSE

Clearly, it is essential that you comprehend key figures of the statistical reports that you order, but when it comes to using these findings to make decisions in the real world, other considerations must be taken into account.

Consider the results of the example processed in this chapter from the *t* test:

Systolic Blood Pressure Results

Drug A: $\mu = 120.37$

Drug B: $\mu = 122.37$

$p = .014$, $\alpha = .05$

Strictly speaking, the above findings identify that Drug A statistically significantly outperformed Drug B in reducing systolic blood pressure. Your first reaction might be to leap to the conclusion that Drug A should always be prescribed in substitution of Drug B. Before making such a decision, it may be worthy to take some real-world factors into account: (1) What if Drug A is not effective for every patient? (2) What if some patients are allergic to Drug A? (3) What if Drug A has the potential for serious side effects? (4) What if Drug A has adverse interactions with other drugs commonly prescribed?

(5) What if the dosage scheduling for Drug A is more complex (q4h) than Drug B (qd)? (6) What if Drug A is substantially more expensive than Drug B? (7) What if Drug A is injectable, and Drug B is oral? As you can see, in addition to the information that we gain from statistical analysis, there may be multiple viable considerations in making such decisions.

Another factor in assessing these results in the real world is to momentarily set aside the p value and look at the performance of each drug in terms of the means: The mean systolic blood pressure for Drug A is 120.37, and the mean for Drug B is 122.37; this is only a 2-point difference. Technically, this difference is statistically significant ($p = .014$), but one must ponder: *Does a 2-point reduction in blood pressure make any real difference in a patient's overall health profile?* The answer is essentially no.

Furthermore, suppose the goal of this study was to identify the drug(s) that would be most effective in controlling moderate hypertension (systolic between 130 mmHg and 140 mmHg), resulting in systolic blood pressure in the (normal) mid-120-mmHg range. If that was the goal, then one could plausibly conclude that Drug A and Drug B both successfully achieved that goal, so by these criteria, either drug could be considered a viable choice.

The lesson at hand is that when interpreting statistical findings, it is important that you not exclusively tend to the numbers but also mindfully comprehend that those numbers are only a part of the picture when it comes to making practical decisions in the real world.

Key Concepts

- *t* Test
- Pretest checklist
    - Normality
    - n
    - Homogeneity of variance
- α
- p
- Hypothesis resolution
- Documenting results
- Mann-Whitney *U* test
- Good common sense
- Type I (α) error
- Type II (β) error

Practice Exercises

Exercise 5.1

You want to determine if meditation can reduce resting pulse rate. Participants were recruited and randomly assigned to one of two groups: Members of Group 1 (the control group) will not meditate, and members of Group 2 (the treatment group) will meditate for 30 minutes per day on Mondays, Wednesdays, and Fridays over the course of 2 weeks. At the end, you gathered the resting pulse rates for each participant.

Data set: **Ch 05 – Exercise 01A.sav**

Codebook

Variable:	Group
Definition:	Group number
Type:	Categorical (1 = No meditation, 2 = Meditates 3 days)
Variable:	Pulse
Definition:	Pulse rate (beats per minute)
Type:	Continuous

a. Write the hypotheses.

b. Run each criterion of the pretest checklist (normality, homogeneity of variance, and n) and discuss your findings.

c. Run the t test and document your findings (ns, means, and Sig. [p value], hypotheses resolution).

d. Write an abstract under 200 words detailing a summary of the study, the t test results, hypothesis resolution, and implications of your findings.

Repeat this exercise using data set: **Ch 05 – Exercise 01B.sav.**

Exercise 5.2

You want to determine the optimal preceptor-to-nurse ratio. Nurses will be randomly assigned to one of two groups: Group 1 will involve each preceptor working with only one nurse, and in Group 2, each preceptor will work with two nurses. At the end of each shift, patients will be asked to complete the Acme Nursing Satisfaction Survey, which renders a score from 0 to 100.

Data set: **Ch 05 – Exercise 02A.sav**

Codebook

Variable:	Group
Definition:	Group number
Type:	Categorical (1 = One-to-one, 2 = Two-to-one)
Variable:	ANSS
Definition:	Acme Nursing Satisfaction Survey score (0–100)
Type:	Continuous

a. Write the hypotheses.

b. Run each criterion of the pretest checklist (normality, homogeneity of variance, and n) and discuss your findings.

c. Run the t test and document your findings (ns, means, and Sig. [p value], hypotheses resolution).

d. Write an abstract under 200 words detailing a summary of the study, the t test results, hypothesis resolution, and implications of your findings.

Repeat this exercise using **Ch 05 – Exercise 02B.sav.**

Exercise 5.3

Clinicians at a nursing home facility want to see if giving residents a plant to tend to will help lower depression. To test this idea, the residents are randomly assigned to one of two groups: Those assigned to Group 1 will serve as the control group and will not be given a plant. Members of Group 2 will be given a small bamboo plant along with a card detailing care instructions. After 90 days, all participants will complete the Acme Depression Scale, which renders a score between 1 and 100 (1 = Low depression . . . 100 = High depression).

Data set: **Ch 05 – Exercise 03A.sav**

Codebook

Variable:	Group
Definition:	Group number
Type:	Categorical (1 = No plant, 2 = Bamboo)

Variable:	Depress
Definition:	Acme Depression Scale (1 = Low depression . . . 100 = High depression)
Type:	Continuous

a. Write the hypotheses.

b. Run each criterion of the pretest checklist (normality, homogeneity of variance, and *n*) and discuss your findings.

c. Run the *t* test and document your findings (*n*s, means, and Sig. [*p* value], hypotheses resolution).

d. Write an abstract under 200 words detailing a summary of the study, the *t* test results, hypothesis resolution, and implications of your findings.

Repeat this exercise using **Ch 05 – Exercise 03B.sav.**

Exercise 5.4

You want to determine if chocolate enhances mood. Subjects will be recruited and randomly assigned to one of two groups: Those in Group 1 will be the control group and will eat their regular diet. Those in Group 2 will eat their usual meals and have a piece of chocolate at breakfast, lunch, and dinner over the course of a week. At the end of the week, all participants will complete the Acme Mood Scale (1 = Extremely bad mood . . . 100 = Extremely good mood).

Data set: **Ch 05 – Exercise 04A.sav**

Codebook

Variable:	Group
Definition:	Group number
Type:	Categorical (1 = No chocolate, 2 = Chocolate [1 per meal])

Variable: Mood
Definition: Acme Mood Scale score (1–100)
Type: Continuous

a. Write the hypotheses.
b. Run each criterion of the pretest checklist (normality, homogeneity of variance, and *n*) and discuss your findings.
c. Run the *t* test and document your findings (*n*s, means, and Sig. [*p* value], hypotheses resolution).
d. Write an abstract under 200 words detailing a summary of the study, the *t* test results, hypothesis resolution, and implications of your findings.

Repeat this exercise using **Ch 05 – Exercise 04B.sav.**

Exercise 5.5

During flu season, the administrators at a walk-in health clinic want to determine if providing patients with a pamphlet will increase their receptivity to flu shots. Each patient will be given a ticket at the check-in desk with a 1 or 2 on it; the tickets will be issued in (repeating) sequence (e.g., 1, 2, 1, 2, etc.). Once escorted to the exam room, patients with a number 1 ticket will serve as control participants and will not be offered any flu shot informational material. Patients with a number 2 ticket will be given a flu shot information pamphlet describing the rationale for the flu shot and flu prevention practices, emphasizing effective hand hygiene. At the end of the day, the charts were reviewed and two entries were made in the database: total number of flu shots given to patients in Group 1 and the total number of flu shots given to patients in Group 2.

Data set: **Ch 05 – Exercise 05A.sav**

Codebook

Variable: Group
Definition: Group number
Type: Categorical (1 = Nothing, 2 = Flu shot pamphlet)

Variable: Shots
Definition: Number of flu shots given in a day for each group
Type: Continuous

a. Write the hypotheses.
b. Run each criterion of the pretest checklist (normality, homogeneity of variance, and *n*) and discuss your findings.
c. Run the *t* test and document your findings (*n*s, means, and Sig. [*p* value], hypotheses resolution).
d. Write an abstract under 200 words detailing a summary of the study, the *t* test results, hypothesis resolution, and implications of your findings.

Repeat this exercise using **Ch 05 – Exercise 05B.sav.**

Exercise 5.6

You want to determine if introducing a video in the waiting area will help relax patients. This study will take place over 2 days: On the first day, Group 1 (the control group) will experience the waiting room as is—with the monitor off; on the second day, Group 2 will have a classic movie playing. The nurse will anonymously copy their pulse rate to a journal along with the day number (Group).

Data set: **Ch 05 – Exercise 06A.sav**

Codebook

Variable:	Group
Definition:	Group number
Type:	Categorical (1 = Control, 2 = Classic movie)

Variable:	Pulse
Definition:	Pulse rate (gathered by a pulse oximeter)
Type:	Continuous

a. Write the hypotheses.
b. Run each criterion of the pretest checklist (normality, homogeneity of variance, and *n*) and discuss your findings.
c. Run the *t* test and document your findings (*n*s, means, and Sig. [*p* value], hypotheses resolution).
d. Write an abstract under 200 words detailing a summary of the study, the *t* test results, hypothesis resolution, and implications of your findings.

Repeat this exercise using **Ch 05 – Exercise 06B.sav**.

Exercise 5.7

In an effort to determine the effectiveness of light therapy to alleviate depression, you recruit a group of subjects who have been diagnosed with depression. The subjects are randomly assigned to one of two groups: Group 1 will be the control group—members of this group will receive no light therapy. Members of Group 2 will get light therapy for 1 hour on even-numbered days over the course of 1 month. After 1 month, all participants will complete the Acme Mood Scale, consisting of 10 questions; this instrument renders a score between 1 and 100 (1 = Extremely bad mood . . . 100 = Extremely good mood).

Data set: **Ch 05 – Exercise 07A.sav**

Codebook

Variable:	Group
Definition:	Group number
Type:	Categorical (1 = No light therapy, 2 = Light therapy: even days)

Variable: Mood
Definition: Acme Mood Scale (1 = Extremely bad mood . . . 100 = Extremely good mood)
Type: Continuous

a. Write the hypotheses.
b. Run each criterion of the pretest checklist (normality, homogeneity of variance, and *n*) and discuss your findings.
c. Run the *t* test and document your findings (*n*s, means, and Sig. [*p* value], hypotheses resolution).
d. Write an abstract under 200 words detailing a summary of the study, the *t* test results, hypothesis resolution, and implications of your findings.

Repeat this exercise using **Ch 05 – Exercise 07B.sav.**

Exercise 5.8

It is thought that exercising early in the morning will provide better energy throughout the day. To test this idea, subjects are recruited and randomly assigned to one of two groups: Members of Group 1 will constitute the control group and not be assigned any walking. Members of Group 2 will walk from 7:00 to 7:30 a.m., Monday through Friday, over the course of 30 days. At the conclusion of the study, each participant will answer the 10 questions on the Acme End-of-the-Day Energy Scale. This instrument produces a score between 1 and 100 (1 = Extremely low energy . . . 100 = Extremely high energy).

Data set: **Ch 05 – Exercise 08A.sav**

Codebook

Variable: Group
Definition: Group number
Type: Categorical (1 = No walking, 2 = Walking: 30 minutes)

Variable: Mood
Definition: Acme End-of-the-Day Energy Scale (1 = Extremely low energy . . . 100 = Extremely high energy)
Type: Continuous

a. Write the hypotheses.
b. Run each criterion of the pretest checklist (normality, homogeneity of variance, and *n*) and discuss your findings.
c. Run the *t* test and document your findings (*n*s, means, and Sig. [*p* value], hypotheses resolution).
d. Write an abstract under 200 words detailing a summary of the study, the *t* test results, hypothesis resolution, and implications of your findings.

Repeat this exercise using **Ch 05 – Exercise 08B.sav.**

Exercise 5.9

In order to determine the best method for facilitating smoking cessation, patients who smoke two packs per day (40 cigarettes) are recruited and randomly assigned to one of two psychoeducational peer support groups with a qualified facilitator: Group 1 will meet once a week in an in-person setting, and Group 2 will meet once a week via Internet videoconferencing. After 10 weeks, each participant will be asked how many cigarettes he or she smokes per day.

Data set: **Ch 05 – Exercise 09A.sav**

Codebook

Variable: Group
Definition: Group number
Type: Categorical (1 = 1 meeting in-person, 2 = 1 meeting videoconference)

Variable: Smoking
Definition: Number of cigarettes each participant smokes per day after 10 weeks
Type: Continuous

a. Write the hypotheses.
b. Run each criterion of the pretest checklist (normality, homogeneity of variance, and *n*) and discuss your findings.
c. Run the *t* test and document your findings (*n*s, means, and Sig. [*p* value], hypotheses resolution).
d. Write an abstract under 200 words detailing a summary of the study, the *t* test results, hypothesis resolution, and implications of your findings.

Repeat this exercise using **Ch 05 – Exercise 09B.sav.**

Exercise 5.10

Due to numerous complications involving missed medication dosages, you implement a study to determine the best strategy for enhancing medication adherence. Patients who are on a daily medication regime will be recruited, receive a complimentary 1-month dosage of their regular medication(s), and be randomly assigned to one of two groups: Group 1 will serve as the control group (no treatment); Group 2 will participate in a 1-hour in-person nurse-administered medication adherence workshop. At the end of one month, participants will present their prescription bottle(s); the nurse will count the remaining pills and calculate the dosage adherence percentage (e.g., 0 pills remaining = 100% adherence).

Data set: **Ch 05 – Exercise 10A.sav**

Codebook

Variable: Group
Definition: Group number
Type: Categorical (1 = Control, 2 = Rx workshop)

Variable: RxAdhere
Definition: Percentage of medication adherence (0–100)
Type: Continuous

a. Write the hypotheses.
b. Run each criterion of the pretest checklist (normality, homogeneity of variance, and *n*) and discuss your findings.
c. Run the *t* test and document your findings (*n*s, means, and Sig. [*p* value], hypotheses resolution).
d. Write an abstract under 200 words detailing a summary of the study, the *t* test results, hypothesis resolution, and implications of your findings.

Repeat this exercise using **Ch 05 – Exercise 10B.sav.**

CHAPTER 6

ANOVA and Kruskal-Wallis Test

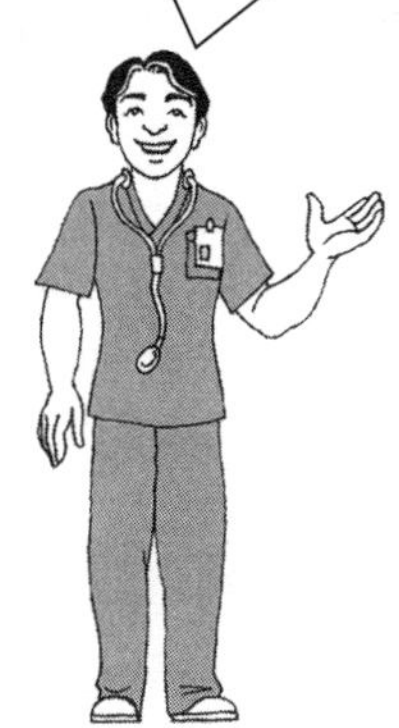
To compare more than 2 groups of continuous variables, run an **ANOVA**.

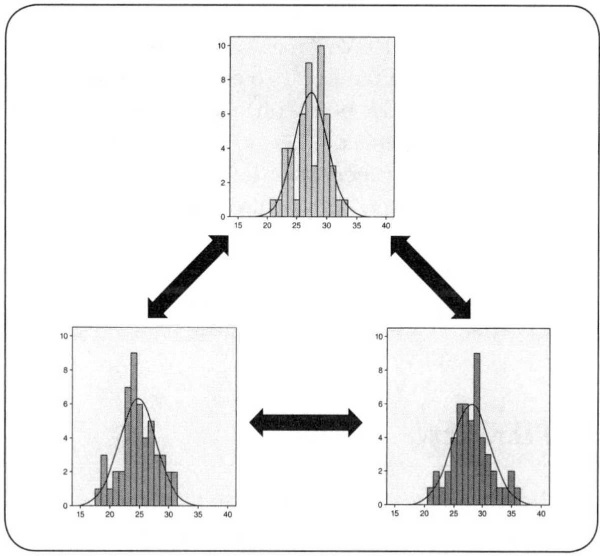

Three is a magic number.

—Bob Dorough

LEARNING OBJECTIVES

Upon completing this chapter, you will be able to:

- Determine when it is appropriate to run an ANOVA test
- Verify that the data meet the criteria for ANOVA processing: normality, *n*, and homogeneity of variance
- Order an ANOVA test with graphics
- Select an appropriate ANOVA post hoc test: Tukey or Sidak
- Derive results from the descriptives and multiple comparisons tables
- Calculate the unique pairs formula
- Resolve the hypotheses
- Know when and how to run and interpret the Kruskal-Wallis test
- Document the results in plain English

VIDEO

The videos for this chapter are **Ch 06 – ANOVA.mp4** and **Ch 06 – Kruskal-Wallis Test.mp4.** These videos provide overviews of these tests, instructions for carrying out the pretest checklist, run, and interpreting the results of this each test using the data set: **Ch 06 – Example 01 – ANOVA.sav**

LAYERED LEARNING

The *t* test and ANOVA (analysis of variance) are so similar that this chapter will use the same example and the same 10 exercises used in Chapter 5 (*t* Test); the only difference is that the data sets have been enhanced to include a third or fourth group. If you are proficient with the *t* test, you are already more than halfway there to comprehending ANOVA. The only real differences between the *t* test and ANOVA are in ordering the test run and interpreting the test results; several other minor differences will be pointed out along the way.

That being said, let us go into the expanded example, drawn from Chapter 5, which involved Group 1 (Drug A), Group 2 (Drug B), and now a third group: Group 3 (Drug C). The ANOVA test will reveal which (if any) of these drugs statistically significantly outperforms the others in effectively controlling hypertension.

OVERVIEW—ANOVA

The ANOVA test is similar to the *t* test, except whereas the *t* test compares two groups of continuous variables to each other, the ANOVA test can compare three or more groups to each other.

Example

The nurse manager is interested in identifying the most effective drug for managing patients with moderate hypertension (systolic between 130 mmHg and 140 mmHg).

Research Question

Which is the best drug for lowering moderate hypertension: Drug A, Drug B, or Drug C?

Groups

The nurse manager recruits 90 volunteers who meet the criteria and consent to participate in this study. Each patient's name is written on slips of paper and placed in a hat. The nurse manager randomly draws 30 names from the hat; these patients will receive Drug A, the next 30 names drawn will get Drug B, and the remaining 30 will be given Drug C.

Procedure

Each participant is brought in to the clinic for a brief visit: Their blood pressure is taken to verify that they meet the criteria (systolic between 130 mmHg and 140 mmHg), and they are given a 30-day supply of the specified medication. After 30 days, each participant will return to the clinic and have his or her blood pressure taken. For purposes of this example, we will presume 100% dosage adherence.

Hypotheses

The null hypothesis (H_0) is phrased to anticipate that the experiment/intervention fails, indicating that *no drug outperformed any of the others*. The alternative hypothesis (H_1) states that *at least one drug did outperform another:*

H_0: There is no statistically significant difference in the performance of the three drugs.

H_1: At least one drug (group) outperformed another.

Admittedly, H_1 is phrased fairly broadly. The Post Hoc Multiple Comparisons table, which is covered in the Results section, will identify which drug(s), if any, outperformed which.

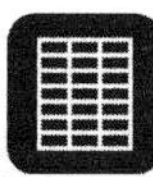

Data Set

Use the following data set: **Ch 06 – Example 01 – ANOVA.sav.**

Notice that this data set has 90 records; the first 60 records (rows) are the same as the *t* test example data set used in Chapter 5 (records 61 through 90 are new):

Codebook

Variable:	Group
Definition:	Group number
Type:	Categorical (1 = Drug A, 2 = Drug B, 3 = Drug C)
Variable:	SystolicBP
Definition:	Systolic blood pressure (in mmHg)
Type:	Continuous

NOTE: In this data set, records (rows) 1 through 30 are for Group 1 (Drug A), records 31 through 60 are for Group 2 (Drug B), and records 61 through 90 are for Group 3 (Drug C). The data are arranged this way just for visual clarity; the order of the records has no bearing on the statistical results.

If you go to the *Variable View* and open the *Values* menu for the variable *Group,* you will see that the label *Drug C* for the third group has been assigned to the value 3 (Figure 6.1).

Figure 6.1 Value labels for a three-group ANOVA analysis.

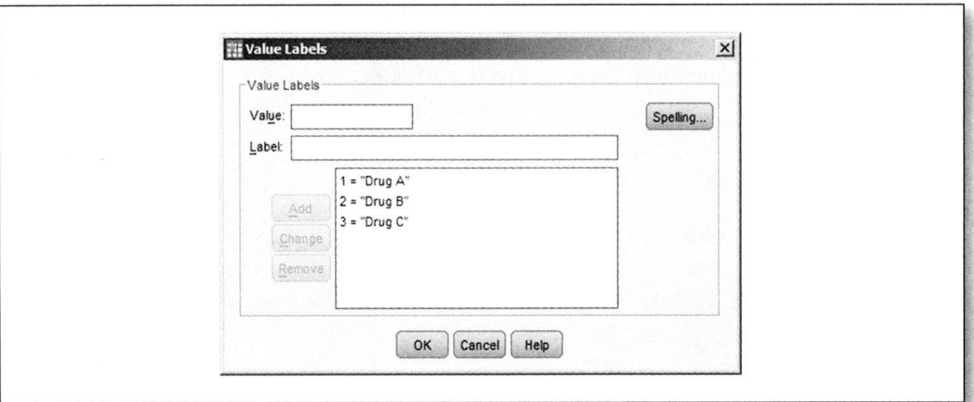

Pretest Checklist

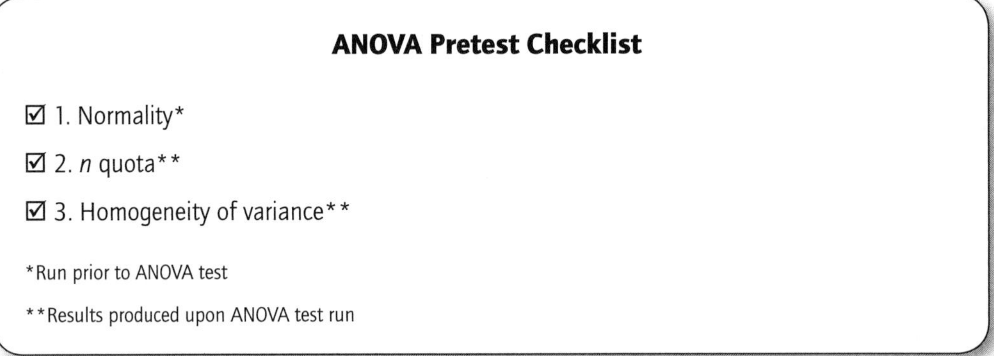

ANOVA Pretest Checklist

☑ 1. Normality*

☑ 2. *n* quota**

☑ 3. Homogeneity of variance**

*Run prior to ANOVA test

**Results produced upon ANOVA test run

The statistical pretest checklist for the ANOVA is similar to the *t* test: **(1) normality, (2) *n*,** and **(3) homogeneity of variance,** except that you will assess the data for more than two groups.

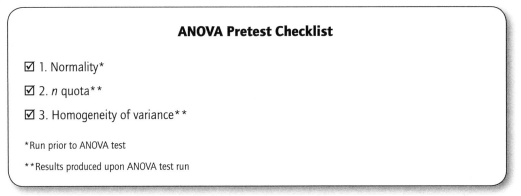

Pretest Checklist Criterion 1—Normality

Check for normality by inspecting the histogram with a normal curve for each of the three groups. Begin by using the *Select Cases* icon to select the records pertaining to the Drug A group (*Group* = 1); the selection criteria would be *Group* = *1*. Next, run a histogram (with normal curve) on the variable *Score*. For more details on this procedure, refer to Chapter 4 ("SPSS—Descriptive Statistics: Continuous Variable (Age) Select by Categorical Variable (Gender)—Females Only"); see the star (★) icon on page **66**.

Then repeat the process for the Drug B group (*Group* = 2), and finally, repeat the process a third time for the Drug C group (*Group* = 3).

This will produce three histograms with normal curves—one for the scores in the Drug A group, a second for the scores in the Drug B group, and a third for the Drug C group. The histograms should resemble the graphs shown in Figures 6.2, 6.3, and 6.4.

As we read these three histograms, our focus is on the *normality of the curve,* as opposed to the characteristics of the individual bars. Although the height and width of each curve are unique, we see that each is bell shaped and shows good symmetry with no substantial *skewing*. On the basis of the inspection of these three figures, we would conclude that the criteria of *normality* are satisfied for all three groups.

Next, (re)activate all records for further analysis; you can either delete the temporary variable *filter_$* or click on the *Select Cases* icon and select the *All cases* button. For more details on this procedure, please refer to Chapter 4 ("SPSS—(Re)Selecting All Variables"); see the star (★) icon on page **73**.

Pretest Checklist Criterion 2—*n* Quota

Again, as with the *t* test, technically, you can run an ANOVA test with an *n* of any size in each group, but when the *n* is at least 30 in each group, the ANOVA is considered

Figure 6.2 Histogram of score for Group 1: Drug A.

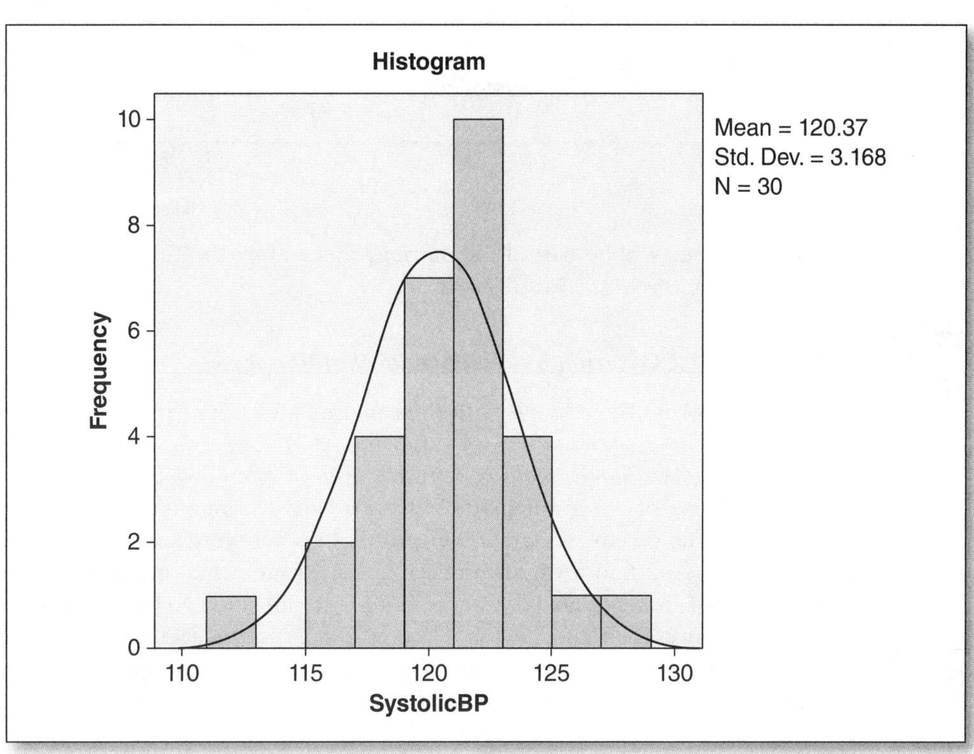

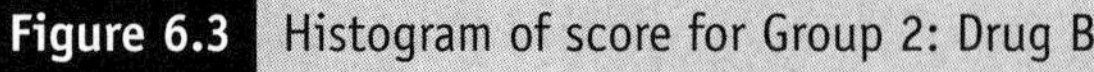

Figure 6.3 Histogram of score for Group 2: Drug B.

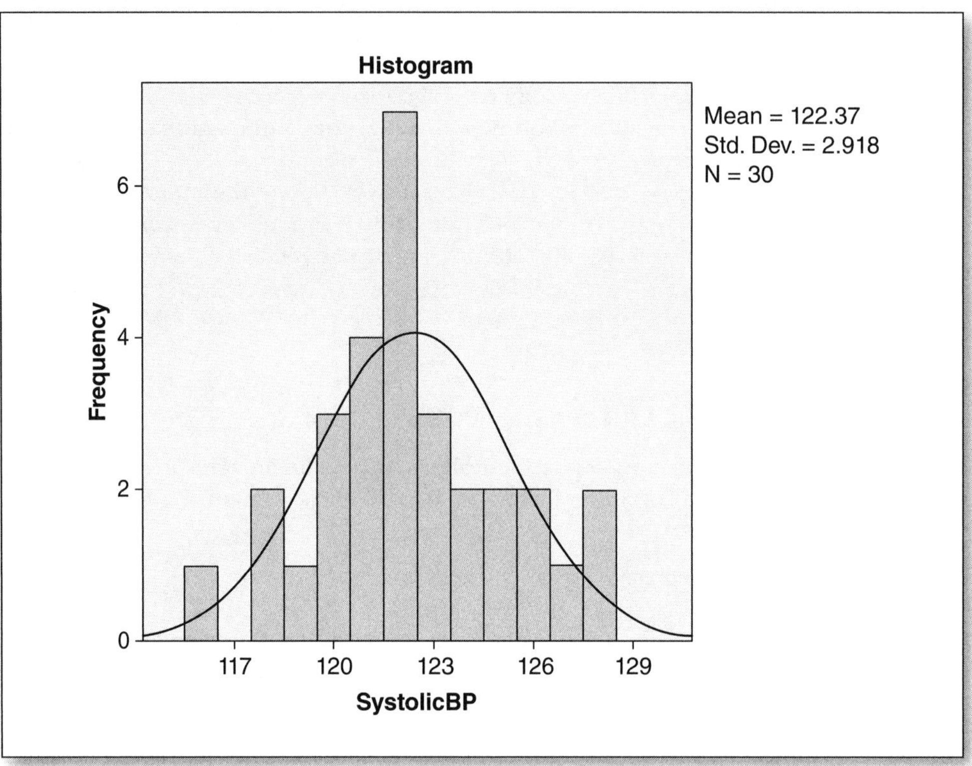

more robust. The *n*s will be part of the output produced by the Test Run procedure; we will revisit this criteria in the Results section.

Pretest Checklist Criterion 3—Homogeneity of Variance

Since we process the ANOVA with the same menu as the *t* test, we will select the *homogeneity of variance test* when we order the ANOVA test and read the findings as part of the results. The *homogeneity of variance* rule of thumb for the ANOVA test is just like the *t* test: None of the groups should have a variance (standard deviation^2) that is more than twice the variance of any other group. In other words, if Group 1 had a variance of 20.1, Group 2 had a variance of 24.7, and Group 3 had a variance of 90.6, we would expect the homogeneity of variance criteria to fail since 90.6 is clearly more than twice as large as 20.1 or 24.7.

The remaining two pretest criteria, **(2) *n* quota** and **(3) homogeneity of variance,** are processed during the **Test Run** and finalized in the **Results** section.

Figure 6.4 Histogram of score for Group 3: Drug C.

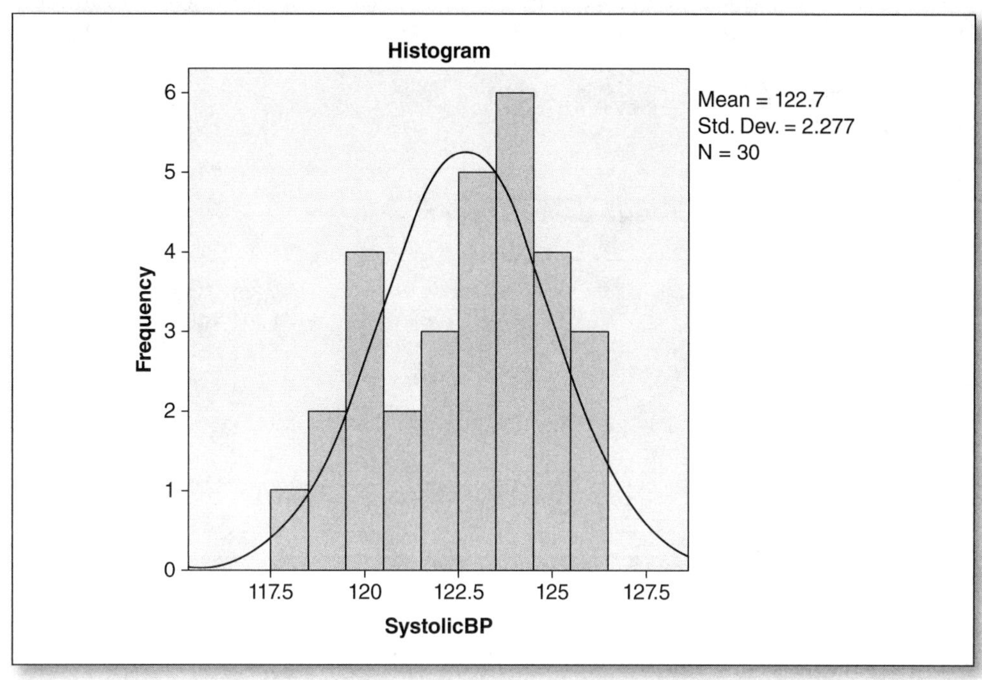

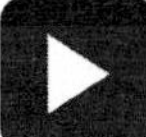

Test Run

1. On the main screen, click on *Analyze, Compare Means, One-Way ANOVA* (Figure 6.5).

Figure 6.5 Running an ANOVA test.

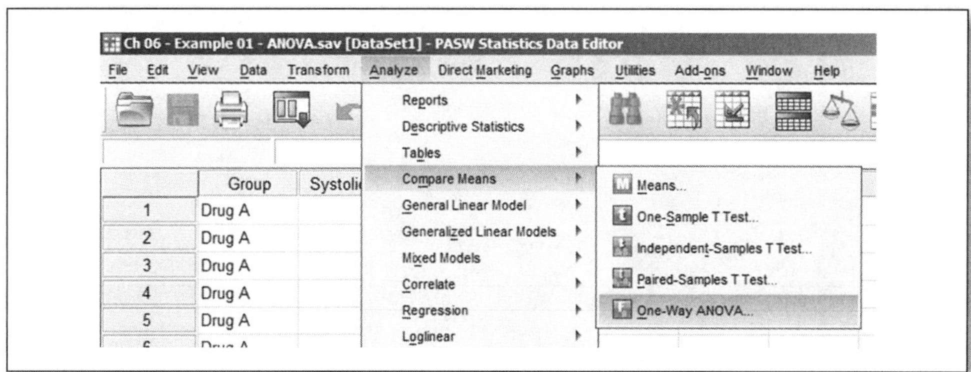

2. On the *One-Way ANOVA* menu, move the continuous variable that you wish to analyze (*SystolicBP*) into the *Dependent List* window, and move the variable that contains the categorical variable that specifies the group (*Group*) into the *Factor* window (Figure 6.6).

Figure 6.6 The one-way ANOVA menu.

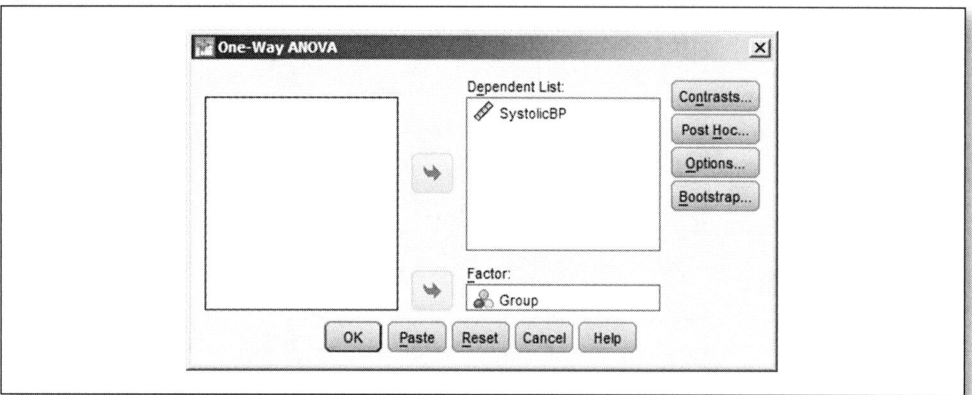

3. Click on the *Options* button. On the *One-Way ANOVA: Options* menu, check *Descriptive* and *Homogeneity of variance test,* then click on the *Continue* button (Figure 6.7). This will take you back to the *One-Way ANOVA* menu.

Figure 6.7 The one-way ANOVA: Options menu.

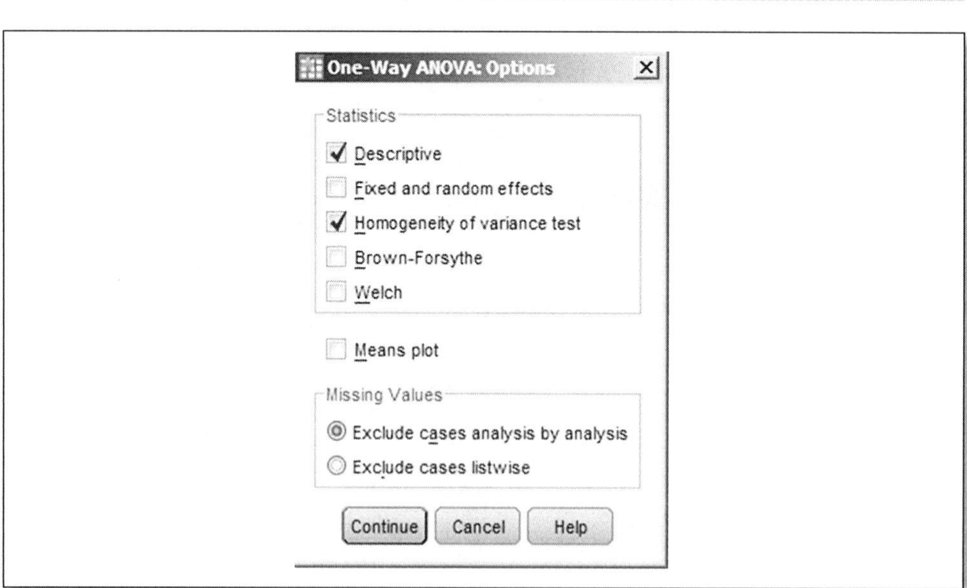

4. Click on the *Post Hoc* button.
5. This will take you to the *One-Way ANOVA: Post Hoc Multiple Comparisons* menu (Figure 6.8).

Figure 6.8 The *One-Way ANOVA: Options* menu.

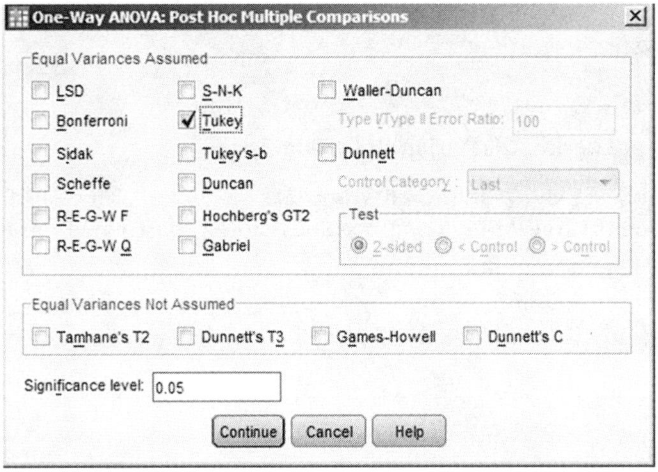

One-Way ANOVA: Post Hoc Multiple Comparisons

Equal Variances Assumed

LSD | S-N-K | Waller-Duncan
Bonferroni | Tukey | Type I/Type II Error Ratio: 100
Sidak | Tukey's-b | Dunnett
Scheffe | Duncan | Control Category: Last
R-E-G-W F | Hochberg's GT2 | Test
R-E-G-W Q | Gabriel | 2-sided, < Control, > Control

Equal Variances Not Assumed

Tamhane's T2 | Dunnett's T3 | Games-Howell | Dunnett's C

Significance level: 0.05

Continue | Cancel | Help

6. If you were to run the ANOVA test without selecting a post hoc test, then all it would return is a single p value; if that p is statistically significant, then that would tell you that somewhere among the groups processed, the mean for at least one group is statistically significantly different from the mean of at least one other group, but it would not tell you specifically *which* group is different from *which*. The post hoc test produces a table comparing the mean of each group with the mean of each other group, along with the p values for each pair of comparisons. This will become clearer in the *Results* section when we read the post hoc multiple comparisons table.

   As for which post hoc test to select, there are a lot of choices. We will focus on only two options: *Tukey* and *Sidak*. *Tukey* is appropriate when each group has the *same ns*; in this case, each group has an n of 30, so check the *Tukey* checkbox, then click on the *Continue* button (this will take you back to the *One-Way ANOVA* menu [Figure 6.6]). If the groups had *different ns* (e.g., n(Group 1) = 40, n(Group 2) = 55, n(Group 3) = 36), then the *Sidak* post hoc test would be appropriate. If you do not know the *ns* for each group in advance, then just select either *Tukey* or *Sidak* and observe the *ns* on the resulting report; if you chose wrong, then go back and rerun the analysis using the appropriate post hoc test.

ANOVA Post Hoc Summary

- If all groups have the same *n*s, then select *Tukey*.
- If the groups have different *n*s, then select *Sidak*.

7. On the *One-Way ANOVA* menu (Figure 6.6), click on the *OK* button, and the ANOVA test will process.

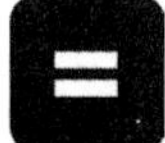

Results

Pretest Checklist Criterion 2—*n* Quota

Table 6.1 shows that each group has an *n* of 30. This satisfies the *n* assumption, indicating that the ANOVA test becomes more robust when the *n* for each group is at least 30.

Table 6.1 Descriptive Statistics (*n*) of Score for Drug A, Drug B, and Drug C.

Descriptives

SystolicBP

	N	Mean	Std. Deviation	Std. Error	95% Confidence Interval for Mean		Minimum	Maximum
					Lower Bound	Upper Bound		
Drug A	30	120.57	2.800	.511	119.52	121.61	113	128
Drug B	30	122.37	2.918	.533	121.28	123.46	116	128
Drug C	30	122.70	2.277	.416	121.85	123.55	118	126
Total	90	121.88	2.812	.296	121.29	122.47	113	128

Pretest Checklist Criterion 3—Homogeneity of Variance

As for the final item on the pretest checklist, Table 6.2 shows that the homogeneity of variance test produced a significance (p) value of .656; since this is greater than the α level of .05, this tells us that there are *no statistically significant differences among the variances of the SystolicBP variable for the three groups analyzed*. In other words, the variances for *SystolicBP* are similar enough among the three groups: Drug A, Drug B, and Drug C that we would conclude that the criteria of the homogeneity of variance has been satisfied.

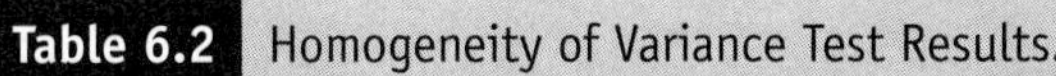

Table 6.2 Homogeneity of Variance Test Results.

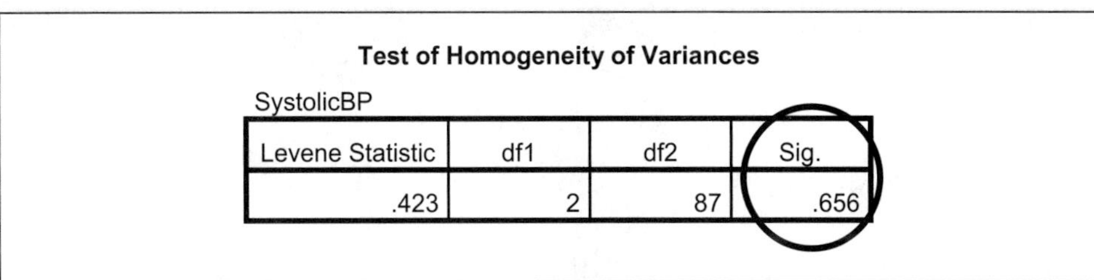

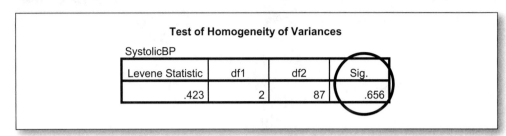

Test of Homogeneity of Variances

SystolicBP

Levene Statistic	df1	df2	Sig.
.423	2	87	.656

Next, we look at the ANOVA table (Table 6.3) and find a significance (p) value of .003; since this is less than the α level of .05, this tells us that there is a statistically significant difference between the (three) group means for *SystolicBP,* but unlike reading the results of the t test, we are not done yet.

Table 6.3 ANOVA Test Results Comparing Score of Drug A, Drug B, and Drug C.

ANOVA

SystolicBP

	Sum of Squares	df	Mean Square	F	Sig.
Between Groups	95.556	2	47.778	6.040	.003
Within Groups	688.233	87	7.911		
Total	783.789	89			

Remember that in the realm of the t test, there are only *two* groups involved, so interpreting the p value is fairly straightforward: If p is $\leq$ .05, there is no question as to which group is different from which—clearly, the mean from Group 1 is statistically significantly different from the mean of Group 2, but when there are *three or more groups,* we need more information to determine *which* group is different from which; that is what the post hoc test answers.

Consider this: Suppose you have *two* kids, Aaron and Blake; you are in the living room, and someone calls out from the den, *The kids are fighting again!* Since there are only two kids, you immediately know that the fight is between Aaron and Blake; this is akin to the t test, which involves comparing the means of two groups.

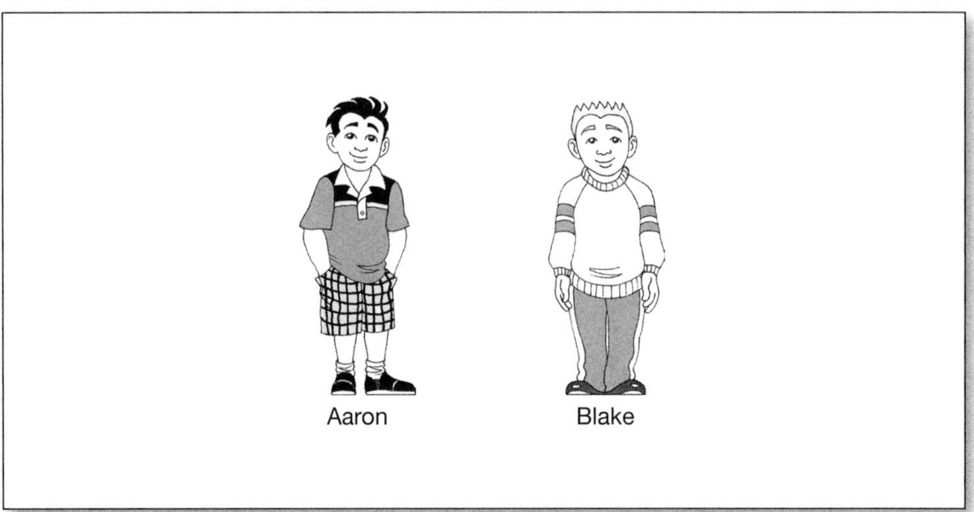

Now suppose you have *three* kids—Aaron, Blake, and Claire:

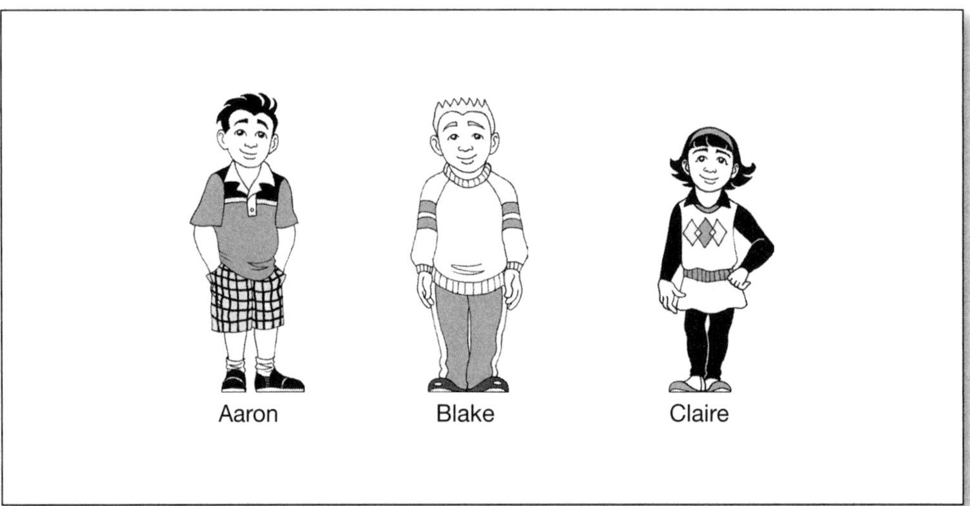

This time when the voice calls out, *The kids are fighting again!* you can no longer simply know that the fight is between Aaron and Blake; when there are *three* kids, you need more information. Instead of just *one* possibility, there are now *three* possible pairs of fighters:

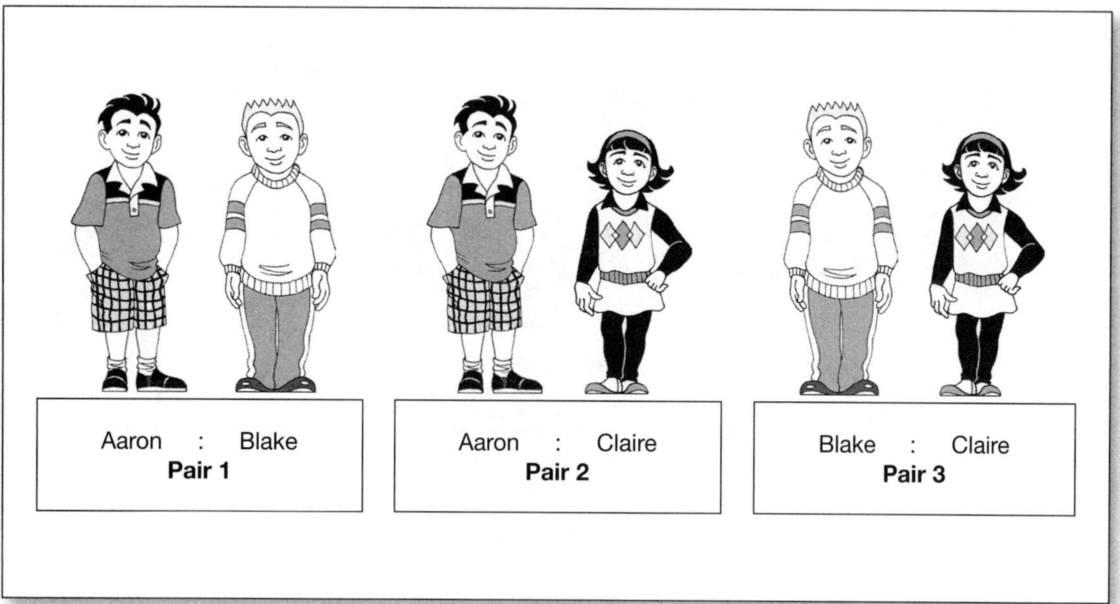

Back to our example: The ANOVA table (Table 6.3) produced a statistically significant p value (Sig. = .003), which indicates that there is a statistically significant difference detected somewhere among the three groups (*The kids are fighting!*); the post hoc table will tell us precisely *which pairs* are statistically significantly different from each other (which pair of kids is fighting). Specifically, it will reveal which group(s) outperformed which.

This brings us to the (Tukey post hoc) multiple comparisons table (Table 6.4). As with the three kids fighting, in this three-group design, there are three possible pairs of comparisons that we can assess in terms of (mean) score for the groups.

Drug A 120.57 : Drug B 122.37	Drug A 120.57 : Drug C 122.70	Drug B 122.37 : Drug C 122.70
Pair 1	**Pair 2**	**Pair 3**

We will use Table 6.1 (*Descriptives*) and Table 6.4 (*Multiple Comparisons*) to analyze the ANOVA test results. Table 6.1 lists the mean score for each of the three groups: μ(Drug A) = 120.57, μ(Drug B) = 122.37, and μ(Drug C) = 122.70. We will assess each of the three pairwise score comparisons separately.

Comparison 1—Drug A : Drug B

Table 6.4 first compares the mean score for the Drug A group with the mean score for the Drug B group, which produces a Sig.(nificance) (p) of .019. Since the p is less than the .05 α level, this tells us that for *SystolicBP,* there is a statistically significant difference between Drug A (μ = 120.57) and Drug B (μ = 122.37).

Table 6.4 ANOVA Post Hoc Multiple Comparisons Table Shows a Statistically Significant Difference Between Drug A and Drug B (p = .019).

Multiple Comparisons

SystolicBP
Tukey HSD

(I) Group	(J) Group	Mean Difference (I-J)	Std. Error	Sig.	95% Confidence Interval	
					Lower Bound	Upper Bound
Drug A	Drug B	-2.000*	.726	.019	-3.73	-.27
	Drug C	-2.333*	.726	.005	-4.06	-.60
Drug B	Drug A	2.000*	.726	.019	.27	3.73
	Drug C	-.333	.726	.891	-2.06	1.40
Drug C	Drug A	2.333*	.726	.005	.60	4.06
	Drug B	.333	.726	.891	-1.40	2.06

*. The mean difference is significant at the 0.05 level.

Comparison 2—Drug A : Drug C

The second comparison in Table 6.5 is between Drug A and Drug C, which produces a Sig.(nificance) (p) of .005. Since the p is less than the .05 α level, this tells us that for *SystolicBP,* there is a statistically significant difference between Drug A (μ = 120.57) and Drug C (μ = 122.70).

Comparison 3—Drug B : Drug C

The third comparison in Table 6.6 is between Drug B and Drug C, which produces a Sig.(nificance) (p) of .891. Since the p is greater than the .05 α level, this tells us that for *SystolicBP,* there is no statistically significant difference between Drug B (μ = 122.37) and Drug C (μ = 122.70).

This concludes the analysis of the *Multiple comparisons* (post hoc) table. You have probably noticed that we skipped analyzing half of the rows; this is because there is a double redundancy among the figures in the Sig. column. This is the kind of double redundancy that you would expect to see in a typical two-dimensional table. For example, in a multiplication table, you would see two 32s in the table because $4 \times 8 = 32$ and $8 \times 4 = 32$. Similarly, the Sig. column of the *Multiple Comparisons* table contains two p values of .005: one comparing Drug A to Drug C and the other comparing Drug C to

Table 6.5 ANOVA Post Hoc Multiple Comparisons Table Shows a Statistically Significant Difference Between Drug A and Drug C (p = .005).

Multiple Comparisons

SystolicBP
Tukey HSD

(I) Group	(J) Group	Mean Difference (I-J)	Std. Error	Sig.	95% Confidence Interval	
					Lower Bound	Upper Bound
Drug A	Drug B	-2.000*	.726	.019	-3.73	-.27
	Drug C	-2.333*	.726	.005	-4.06	-.60
Drug B	Drug A	2.000*	.726	.019	.27	3.73
	Drug C	-.333	.726	.891	-2.06	1.40
Drug C	Drug A	2.333*	.726	.005	.60	4.06
	Drug B	.333	.726	.891	-1.40	2.06

*. The mean difference is significant at the 0.05 level.

Table 6.6 ANOVA Post Hoc Multiple Comparisons Table Shows No Statistically Significant Difference Between Drug B and Drug C (p = .891).

Multiple Comparisons

SystolicBP
Tukey HSD

(I) Group	(J) Group	Mean Difference (I-J)	Std. Error	Sig.	95% Confidence Interval	
					Lower Bound	Upper Bound
Drug A	Drug B	-2.000*	.726	.019	-3.73	-.27
	Drug C	-2.333*	.726	.005	-4.06	-.60
Drug B	Drug A	2.000*	.726	.019	.27	3.73
	Drug C	-.333	.726	.891	-2.06	1.40
Drug C	Drug A	2.333*	.726	.005	.60	4.06
	Drug B	.333	.726	.891	-1.40	2.06

*. The mean difference is significant at the 0.05 level.

Drug A (Table 6.7). In addition, there are two .019 p values (Drug A : Drug B and Drug B : Drug A) and two .891 p values (Drug B : Drug C and Drug C : Drug B).

The ANOVA test can process any number of groups, provided the pretest criteria are met. As the number of groups increases, the number of (multiple) pairs of comparisons increases as well (see Table 6.8).

Table 6.7 ANOVA Post Hoc Multiple Comparisons Table Containing Double-Redundant Sig. (*p*) Values: Drug A : Drug C Produces the Same *p* Value as Drug C : Drug A ($p = .005$).

Multiple Comparisons

SystolicBP
Tukey HSD

(I) Group	(J) Group	Mean Difference (I-J)	Std. Error	Sig.	95% Confidence Interval	
					Lower Bound	Upper Bound
Drug A	Drug B	-2.000*	.726	.019	-3.73	-.27
	Drug C	-2.333*	.726	.005	-4.06	-.60
Drug B	Drug A	2.000*	.726	.019	.27	3.73
	Drug C	-.333	.726	.891	-2.06	1.40
Drug C	Drug A	2.333*	.726	.005	.60	4.06
	Drug B	.333	.726	.891	-1.40	2.06

*. The mean difference is significant at the 0.05 level.

Table 6.8 Increasing Groups Substantially Increases ANOVA Post Hoc Multiple Comparisons.

2 Groups Renders 1 Pair	3 Groups Renders 3 Pairs	4 Groups Renders 6 Pairs
$G_1:G_2$	$G_1:G_2$ $G_2:G_3$ $G_1:G_3$	$G_1:G_2$ $G_2:G_3$ $G_3:G_4$ $G_1:G_3$ $G_2:G_4$ $G_1:G_4$

NOTE: G = group.

You can easily calculate the number of (unique) pairwise comparisons the post hoc test will produce:

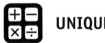

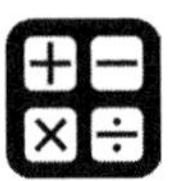

UNIQUE PAIRS FORMULA

$$G = \text{Number of groups}$$

$$\text{Number of ANOVA post hoc unique pairs} = G! \div (2 \times (G - 2)!)$$

The above formula uses the *factorial* function denoted by the exclamation mark (!). If your calculator does not have a factorial (!) button, you can calculate it manually: Simply multiply all of the integers between 1 and the specified number. For example: 3! = 1 × 2 × 3, which equals 6.

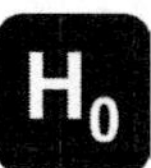

Hypothesis Resolution

To clarify the hypothesis resolution process, it is helpful to organize the findings in a table and use an asterisk to flag statistically significant difference(s) (Table 6.9).

NOTE: SPSS does not generate this table (Table 6.9) directly; you can assemble this table by gathering the means from the *Descriptives* table (Table 6.1) and the *p* values from the Sig. column in the *Multiple Comparisons* table (Table 6.4).

With this results table assembled, we can now revisit and resolve our pending hypotheses, which focus on determining the best drug for controlling moderate hypertension. To finalize this process, we will assess each hypothesis per the statistics contained in Table 6.9.

REJECT: H_0: There is no statistically significant difference in the performance of the three drugs.

ACCEPT: H_1: At least one drug (group) outperformed another.

Since we discovered a statistically significant difference among at least one pair of the drugs, we reject H_0 and accept H_1. Specifically, Drug A outperformed Drug B in lowering blood pressure ($p = .019$), and Drug A outperformed Drug C in lowering blood pressure ($p = .005$).

Incidentally, if all of the pairwise comparisons had produced *p* values that were greater than .05, then we would have accepted H_0 and rejected H_1.

Documenting Results

When documenting the results of this study, both Table 6.9 and the following verbose summary would be appropriate to include:

Table 6.9 *Results of ANOVA for SystolicBP.*

Groups	p
μ(Drug A) = 120.57 : μ(Drug B) = 122.37	.019*
μ(Drug A) = 120.57 : μ(Drug C) = 122.70	.005*
μ(Drug B) = 122.37 : μ(Drug C) = 122.70	.891

*Statistically significant difference detected between groups ($p \leq .05$).

A group of 90 patients with moderate hypertension (systolic between 130 and 140 mmHg) were recruited and randomly assigned to take Drug A, Drug B, or Drug C for 30 days.

After 1 month, patients who took Drug A had a mean systolic blood pressure of 120.57, significantly outperforming Drug B (122.37) and Drug C (122.70) using an α of .05 (see Table).

Groups	p
μ(Drug A) = 120.57 : μ(Drug B) = 122.37	.019*
μ(Drug A) = 120.57 : μ(Drug C) = 122.70	.005*
μ(Drug B) = 122.37 : μ(Drug C) = 122.70	.891

*Statistically significant difference detected between groups ($p \leq .05$).

Occasionally, a *p* value may be close to .05 (e.g., $p = .066$). In such instances, you may feel compelled to comment that the .066 *p* level is *approaching* statistical significance. While the optimism may be commendable, this is a common mistake. The term *approaching* wrongly implies that the *p* value is a dynamic variable—that it is in motion and on its way to crossing the .05 finish line, but this is not at all the case. The .066 *p* value is a static variable, meaning that it is not in motion—the .066 *p* value is no more *approaching* .05 than it is *approaching* .07. Think of the .066 *p* value as *parked;* it is not going anywhere, in the same way that a parked car is neither approaching nor departing from the car parked in front of it, no matter how close those cars are parked to each other. At best, one could state that it (the .066 *p* value) is *close* to the .05 α level and that it would be interesting to consider monitoring this variable should this experiment be repeated at some future point.

Here is a simpler way to think about this: 2 + 2 = 4, and 4 is not approaching 3 or 5; it is just 4, and it is not drifting in any direction.

OVERVIEW—KRUSKAL-WALLIS TEST

One of the pretest criteria that must be met prior to running an ANOVA states that the data from each group must be normally distributed (Figure 6.9); minor variations in the normal distribution are acceptable. Occasionally, you may encounter data that are substantially skewed (Figure 6.10), bimodal (Figure 6.11), flat (Figure 6.12), or may have some other atypical distribution. In such instances, the Kruskal-Wallis statistic is an appropriate alternative to the ANOVA test.

Figure 6.9 Normal.

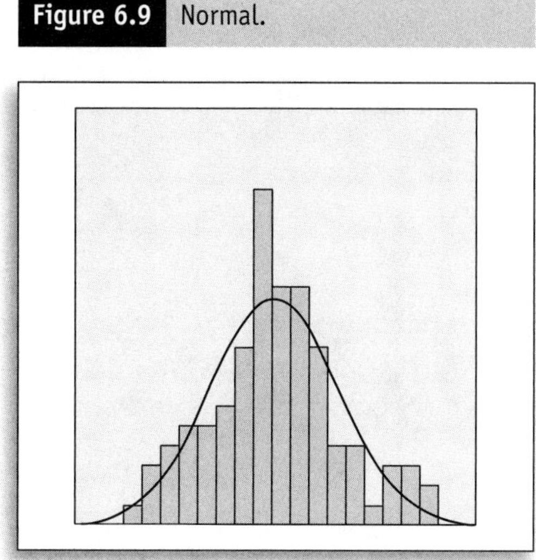

Figure 6.10 Skewed.

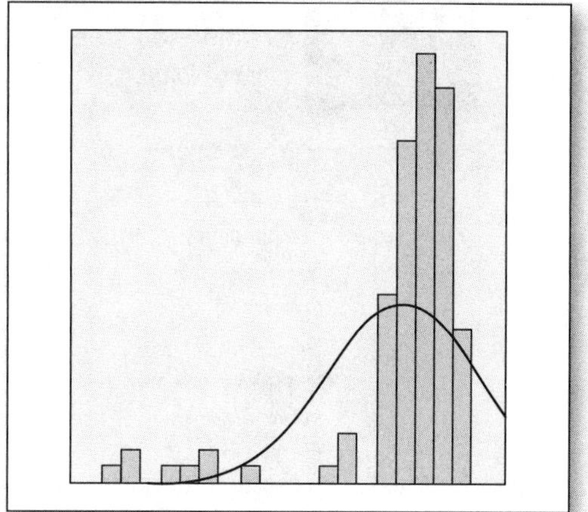

Figure 6.11 Bimodal.

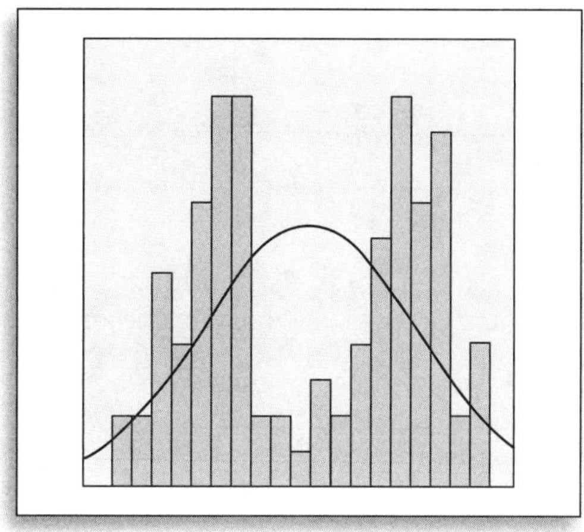

Figure 6.12 Flat.

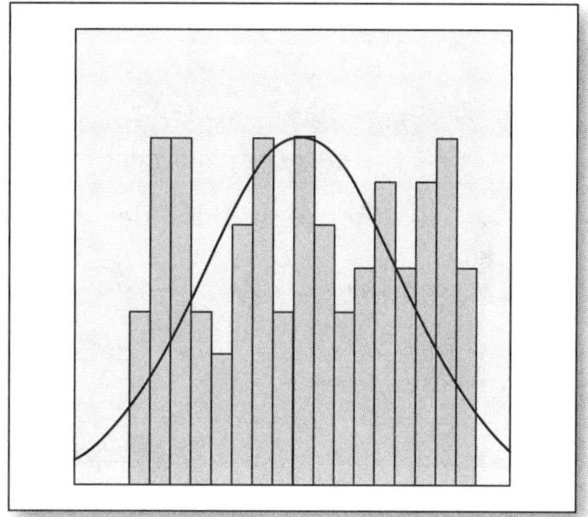

Test Run

For exemplary purposes, we will run the Kruskal-Wallis test using the same data set (**Ch 06 – Example 01 – ANOVA.sav**) even though the data are normally distributed. This will enable us to compare the results of an ANOVA test to the results produced by the Kruskal-Wallis test.

1. On the main screen, click on *Analyze, Nonparametric Tests, Legacy Dialogs, K Independent Samples* (Figure 6.13).

Figure 6.13 Ordering the Kruskal-Wallis test: Click on *Analyze, Nonparametric Tests, Legacy Dialogs, K Independent Samples.*

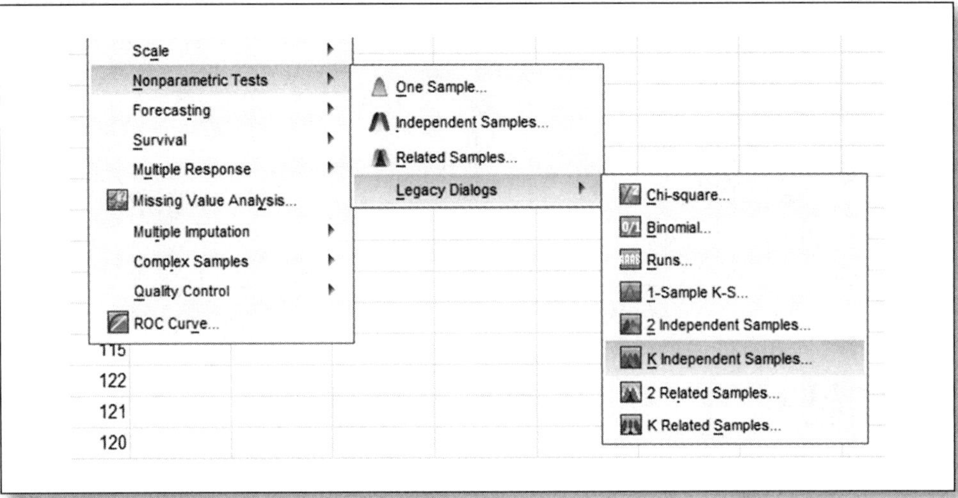

2. On the *Test for Several Independent Samples* menu, move *SystolicBP* to the *Test Variable List* window.

3. Move *Group* to the *Grouping Variable* box (Figure 6.14).

Figure 6.14 On the *Tests for Several Independent Samples* menu, move *SystolicBP* to *Test Variable List,* and move *Group* to the *Grouping Variable* box.

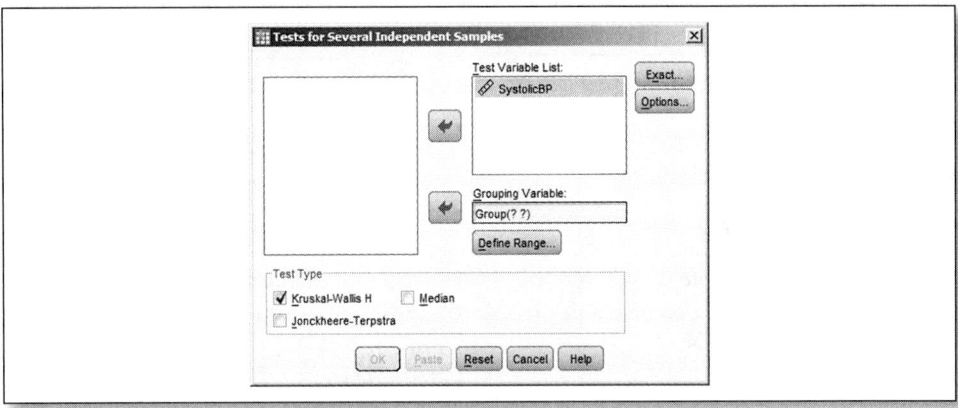

4. Click on *Group(? ?)*, then click on *Define Range.*
5. On the *Several Independent* Samples: Define Range submenu, for *Minimum,* enter *1;* for *Maximum,* enter *3* (since the groups are numbered 1 [for Drug A] through 3 [for Drug C]) (Figure 6.15).
6. Click *Continue;* this will close this submenu.

Figure 6.15 On the *Tests for Several Independent Samples* submenu, for *Minimum,* enter *1;* for *Maximum,* enter *3.*

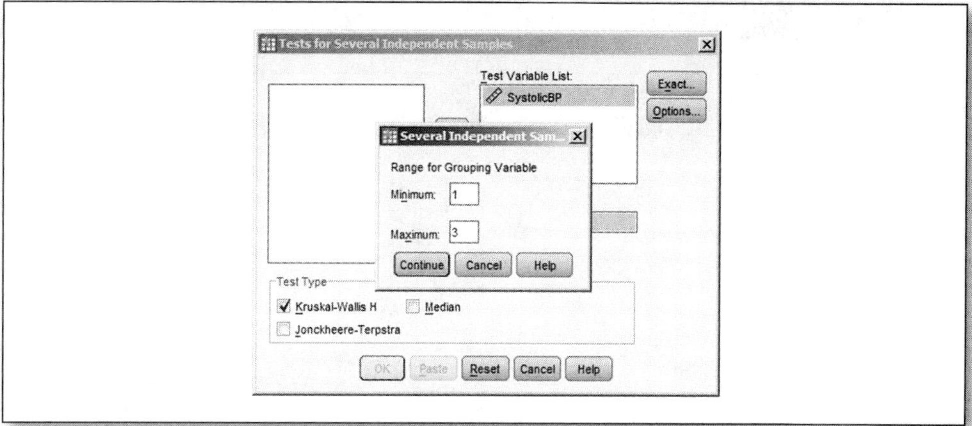

7. On the *Tests for Several Independent Samples* menu, click on *OK.*

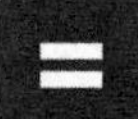

Results

The Kruskal-Wallis result is found in the *Test Statistics* table (Table 6.10); the *Asymp. Sig.* statistic rendered a *p* value of .004; since this is less than α (.05), we would conclude that there is a statistically significant difference (somewhere) among the performances of the three drugs, but we still need to conduct pairwise (post hoc type) analyses to determine which group(s) outperformed which. The ANOVA test provides a variety of post hoc options (e.g., Tukey, Sidak); although the Kruskal-Wallis test does not include a post hoc menu, we can take a few extra steps to

Table 6.10 Kruskal-Wallis *p* Value = .004.

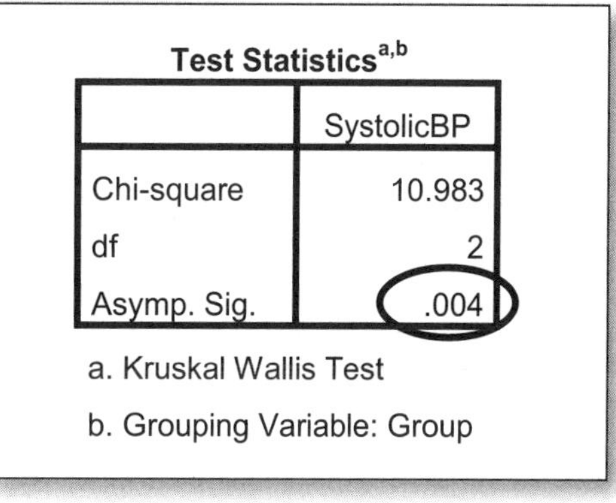

Test Statistics[a,b]

	SystolicBP
Chi-square	10.983
df	2
Asymp. Sig.	.004

a. Kruskal Wallis Test

b. Grouping Variable: Group

process pairwise comparisons among the groups using the Kruskal-Wallis test. We will accomplish this using the *Select Cases* function to select two groups at a time and run separate Kruskal-Wallis tests for each pair. First, we will select and process Drug A : Drug B, then Drug A : Drug C, and finally Drug B : Drug C.

8. Click on the *Select Cases* icon.

On the *Select Cases* menu, click on ⊙ *If condition is satisfied* (Figure 6.16).

Figure 6.16 On the Select Cases menu, click on ⊙ *If condition is satisfied,* then click on *If.*

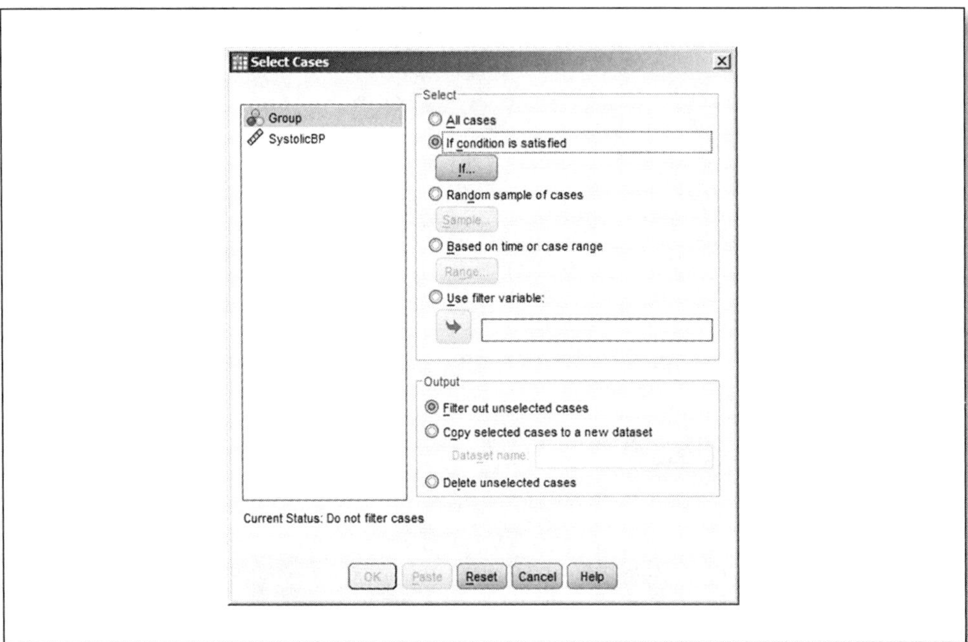

9. Click on *If.*
10. On the *Select Cases: If* menu, specify the pair of groups that you want selected (Figure 6.17):
    a. *On the first pass* through this process, enter *Group* = *1 OR Group* = *2*
    b. *On the second pass,* enter *Group* = *1 OR Group* = *3*
    c. *On the third pass,* enter *Group* = *2 OR Group* = *3*

Figure 6.17 On the *Select Cases* menu, click on ⊙ *If condition is satisfied,* then click on *If.*

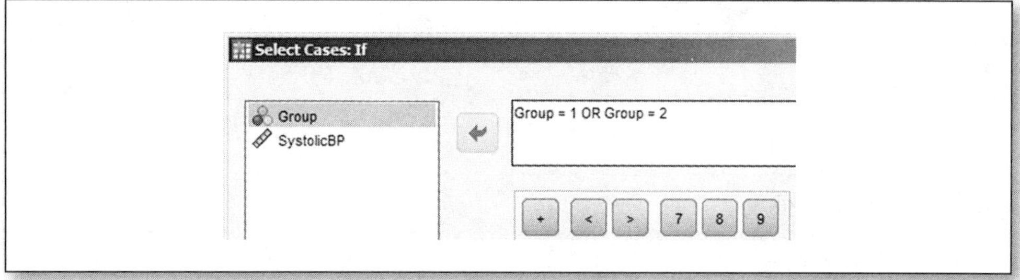

11. Click *Continue.*
12. Click *OK.*
13. Now that only two groups are selected, run the Kruskal-Wallis procedure from Step 1 and record the *p* value produced by each run; upon gathering these figures, you will be able to assemble a Kruskal-Wallis post hoc table (Table 6.11). NOTE: You can keep using the parameters specified from the previous run(s).

To finalize this discussion, consider Table 6.12, which shows the *p* values produced by the ANOVA Tukey post hoc test compared alongside the *p* values produced by the Kruskal-Wallis test.

In addition to noting the differences in the pairwise *p* values (Table 6.12), remember that the ANOVA test produced an initial *p* value of .003 (which we read before the paired post hoc tests), whereas the Kruskal-Wallis produced an initial (overall) *p* value of .004. The differences in these *p* values are due to the internal transformations that the Kruskal-Wallis test conducts on the data. If one or more substantial violations are detected when running the pretest checklist for the ANOVA, then the Kruskal-Wallis test is considered a viable alternative.

Table 6.11 Pairwise *p* Values for the Kruskal-Wallis Test (Manually Assembled).

Groups	p
Drug A : Drug B	.011*
Drug A : Drug C	.002*
Drug B : Drug C	.494

*Statistically significant difference detected between groups ($p \leq .05$).

Table 6.12 *Pairwise p Values for Kruskal-Wallis and ANOVA Post Hoc Table (Manually Assembled).*

Groups	Kruskal-Wallis p	ANOVA p
Drug A : Drug B	.011*	.019*
Drug A : Drug C	.002*	.005*
Drug B : Drug C	.494	.891

*Statistically significant difference detected between groups ($p \le .05$).

GOOD COMMON SENSE

When carrying the results of an ANOVA test into the real world, there are some practical considerations to take into account. Using this example, suppose the goal for this study was to identify a drug that would effectively reduce moderate hypertension to a systolic level of under 125 mmHg. While the findings of the ANOVA may be interesting, clearly, all three of the drugs would be considered suitable as they all met the specified criteria of reducing the systolic pressure to under 125 mmHg, and hence the p values of this test become less relevant.

Considering that the range of the three means (minimum = 120.57, maximum = 122.70) is (only) 2.13, it is plausible to dismiss this relatively minor difference in light of other real-world factors when it comes to selecting among these three drugs, such as dosage protocol (one pill a day vs. multiple dosages per day), side effects, adverse interaction(s), cost, availability, covered/not covered by insurance, and so on.

Another issue involves the capacity of the ANOVA model. Table 6.8 and the combinations formula (**Unique pairs = G! ÷ (2 × (G − 2)!)**) reveal that as more groups are included, the number of ANOVA post hoc paired comparisons increases substantially. A 5-group design would render 10 unique comparisons, 6 groups would render 15, and a 10-group design would render 45 unique comparisons along with their corresponding p values. While SPSS or any statistical software would have no problem processing these figures, there would be some real-world challenges to address: Consider the pretest criteria—in order for the results of an ANOVA test to be considered robust, there should be a minimum n of 30 per group. Hence, for a design involving 10 groups, this would require an overall n of at least 300. Furthermore, a 10-group study would render 45 unique pairwise comparisons in the ANOVA post hoc table, which, depending on the nature of the data, may be a bit unwieldy when it comes to interpretation, documentation, and overall comprehension of the results.

Key Concepts

- ANOVA
- Pretest checklist
  - Normality
  - Homogeneity of variance
  - *n*
- Post hoc tests
  - Tukey
  - Sidak
- Hypothesis resolution
- Documenting results
- Kruskal-Wallis test
- Good common sense

Practice Exercises

NOTE: These practice exercises and data sets are the same as those in **Chapter 5 – *t* Test** except instead of the two-group designs, a third group has been included to enable ANOVA processing, except for Exercises 9 and 10, which now involve four groups.

Exercise 6.1

You want to determine if meditation can reduce resting pulse rate. Participants were recruited and randomly assigned to one of three groups: Members of Group 1 (the control group) will not meditate; members of Group 2 (the first treatment group) will meditate for 30 minutes per day on Mondays, Wednesdays, and Fridays over the course of 2 weeks; and members of Group 3 (the second treatment group) will meditate for 30 minutes a day 6 days a week, Monday through Saturday. At the end, you gathered the resting pulse rates for each participant.

Data set: **Ch 06 – Exercise 01A.sav**

Codebook

Variable: Group
Definition: Group number
Type: Categorical (1 = No meditation, 2 = Meditates 3 days, 3 = Meditates 6 days)

Variable: Pulse
Definition: Pulse rate (beats per minute)
Type: Continuous

a. Write the hypotheses.
b. Run each criterion of the pretest checklist (normality, homogeneity of variance, and *n*) and discuss your findings.
c. Run the ANOVA test and document your findings (*n*s, means, and Sig. [*p* value], hypotheses resolution).

d. Write an abstract under 200 words detailing a summary of the study, the ANOVA test results, hypothesis resolution, and implications of your findings.

Repeat this exercise using data set: **Ch 06 – Exercise 01B.sav.**

Exercise 6.2

You want to determine the optimal preceptor-to-nurse ratio. Nurses will be randomly assigned to one of three groups: Group 1 will involve each preceptor working with only one nurse; in Group 2, each preceptor will work with two nurses; and in Group 3, each preceptor will work with five nurses. At the end of each shift, patients will be asked to complete the Acme Nursing Satisfaction Survey, which renders a score from 0 to 100.

Data set: **Ch 06 – Exercise 02A.sav**

Codebook

Variable:	Group
Definition:	Group number
Type:	Categorical (1 = One-to-one, 2 = Two-to-one, 3 = Five-to-one)
Variable:	ANSS
Definition:	Acme Nursing Satisfaction Survey score (0–100)
Type:	Continuous

a. Write the hypotheses.

b. Run each criterion of the pretest checklist (normality, homogeneity of variance, and *n*) and discuss your findings.

c. Run the ANOVA test and document your findings (*n*s, means, and Sig. [*p* value], hypotheses resolution).

d. Write an abstract under 200 words detailing a summary of the study, the ANOVA test results, hypothesis resolution, and implications of your findings.

Repeat this exercise using **Ch 06 – Exercise 02B.sav.**

Exercise 6.3

Clinicians at a nursing home facility want to see if giving residents a plant to tend to will help lower depression. To test this idea, the residents are randomly assigned to one of three groups: Those assigned to Group 1 will serve as the control group and will not be given a plant. Members of Group 2 will be given a small bamboo plant along with a card detailing care instructions. Members of Group 3 will be given a small cactus along with a card detailing care instructions. After 90 days, all participants will complete the Acme Depression Scale, which renders a score between 1 and 100 (1 = Low depression . . . 100 = High depression).

Data set: **Ch 06 – Exercise 03A.sav**

Codebook

Variable:	Group
Definition:	Group number
Type:	Categorical (1 = No plant, 2 = Bamboo, 3 = Cactus)
Variable:	Depress
Definition:	Acme Depression Scale (1 = Low depression . . . 100 = High depression)
Type:	Continuous

a. Write the hypotheses.

b. Run each criterion of the pretest checklist (normality, homogeneity of variance, and *n*) and discuss your findings.

c. Run the ANOVA test and document your findings (*n*s, means, and Sig. [*p* value], hypotheses resolution).

d. Write an abstract under 200 words detailing a summary of the study, the ANOVA test results, hypothesis resolution, and implications of your findings.

Repeat this exercise using **Ch 06 – Exercise 03B.sav.**

Exercise 6.4

You want to determine if chocolate enhances mood. Subjects will be recruited and randomly assigned to one of three groups: Those in Group 1 will be the control group and will eat their regular diet. Those in Group 2 will eat their usual meals and have a piece of chocolate at breakfast, lunch, and dinner over the course of a week. Those in Group 3 will eat their meals as usual and have two pieces of chocolate at breakfast, lunch, and dinner over the course of a week. At the end of the week, all participants will complete the Acme Mood Scale (1 = Extremely bad mood . . . 100 = Extremely good mood).

Data set: **Ch 06 – Exercise 04A.sav**

Codebook

Variable:	Group
Definition:	Group number
Type:	Categorical (1 = No chocolate, 2 = Chocolate [1 per meal], 3 = Chocolate [2 per meal])
Variable:	Mood
Definition:	Acme Mood Scale score (1–100)
Type:	Continuous

a. Write the hypotheses.

b. Run each criterion of the pretest checklist (normality, homogeneity of variance, and *n*) and discuss your findings.

c. Run the ANOVA test and document your findings (*ns*, means, and Sig. [*p* value], hypotheses resolution).

d. Write an abstract under 200 words detailing a summary of the study, the ANOVA test results, hypothesis resolution, and implications of your findings.

Repeat this exercise using **Ch 06 – Exercise 04B.sav.**

Exercise 6.5

During flu season, the administrators at a walk-in health clinic want to determine if providing patients with a pamphlet or a video will increase their receptivity to flu shots. Each patient will be given a ticket at the check-in desk with a 1, 2, or 3 on it; the tickets will be issued in (repeating) sequence (e.g., 1, 2, 3, 1, 2, 3, etc.). Once escorted to the exam room, patients with a number 1 ticket will serve as control participants and will not be offered any flu shot informational material. Patients with a number 2 ticket will be given a flu shot information pamphlet describing the rationale for the flu shot and flu prevention practices, emphasizing effective hand hygiene. Patients with a number 3 ticket will be shown a brief video covering the same information as contained in the pamphlet. At the end of the day, the charts were reviewed and three entries were made in the database: total number of flu shots given to patients in Group 1, total number of flu shots given to patients in Group 2, and the total number of flu shots given to patients in Group 3.

Data set: **Ch 06 – Exercise 05A.sav**

Codebook

Variable:	Group
Definition:	Group number
Type:	Categorical (1 = Nothing, 2 = Flu shot pamphlet, 3 = Flu shot video)
Variable:	Shots
Definition:	Number of flu shots given in a day for each group
Type:	Continuous

a. Write the hypotheses.

b. Run each criterion of the pretest checklist (normality, homogeneity of variance, and *n*) and discuss your findings.

c. Run the ANOVA test and document your findings (*ns*, means, and Sig. [*p* value], hypotheses resolution).

d. Write an abstract under 200 words detailing a summary of the study, the ANOVA test results, hypothesis resolution, and implications of your findings.

Repeat this exercise using **Ch 06 – Exercise 05B.sav.**

Exercise 6.6

You want to determine if introducing a video in the waiting area will help relax patients. This study will take place over 3 days: On the first day, Group 1 (the control group) will experience the waiting room as is—with the monitor off; on the second day, Group 2 will have a classic movie playing; and on the third day, Group 3 will have a scenic video playing (e.g., waterfalls, vistas, wildlife). For patients who consent to participating in this research, the nurse will anonymously copy their pulse rate to a journal along with the day number (Group).

Data set: **Ch 06 – Exercise 06A.sav**

Codebook

Variable:	Group
Definition:	Group number
Type:	Categorical (1 = Control, 2 = Classic movie, 3 = Scenic video)
Variable:	Pulse
Definition:	Pulse rate (gathered by a pulse oximeter)
Type:	Continuous

a. Write the hypotheses.

b. Run each criterion of the pretest checklist (normality, homogeneity of variance, and *n*) and discuss your findings.

c. Run the ANOVA test and document your findings (*n*s, means, and Sig. [*p* value], hypotheses resolution).

d. Write an abstract under 200 words detailing a summary of the study, the ANOVA test results, hypothesis resolution, and implications of your findings.

Repeat this exercise using **Ch 06 – Exercise 06B.sav.**

Exercise 6.7

In an effort to determine the effectiveness of light therapy to alleviate depression, you recruit a group of subjects who have been diagnosed with depression. The subjects are randomly assigned to one of three groups: Group 1 will be the control group—members of this group will receive no light therapy. Members of Group 2 will get light therapy for 1 hour on even-numbered days over the course of 1 month. Members of Group 3 will get light therapy every day for 1 hour over the course of 1 month. After 1 month, all participants will complete the Acme Mood Scale, consisting of 10 questions; this instrument renders a score between 1 and 100 (1 = Extremely bad mood . . . 100 = Extremely good mood).

Data set: **Ch 06 – Exercise 07A.sav**

Codebook

Variable:	Group
Definition:	Group number
Type:	Categorical (1 = No light therapy, 2 = Light therapy: even days, 3 = Light therapy: every day)

Variable:	Mood
Definition:	Acme Mood Scale (1 = Extremely bad mood . . . 100 = Extremely good mood)
Type:	Continuous

a. Write the hypotheses.

b. Run each criterion of the pretest checklist (normality, homogeneity of variance, and *n*) and discuss your findings.

c. Run the ANOVA test and document your findings (*n*s, means, and Sig. [*p* value], hypotheses resolution).

d. Write an abstract under 200 words detailing a summary of the study, the ANOVA test results, hypothesis resolution, and implications of your findings.

Repeat this exercise using **Ch 06 – Exercise 07B.sav.**

Exercise 6.8

It is thought that exercising early in the morning will provide better energy throughout the day. To test this idea, subjects are recruited and randomly assigned to one of three groups: Members of Group 1 will constitute the control group and not be assigned any walking. Members of Group 2 will walk from 7:00 to 7:30 a.m., Monday through Friday, over the course of 30 days. Members of Group 3 will walk from 7:00 to 8:00 a.m., Monday through Friday, over the course of 30 days. At the conclusion of the study, each participant will answer the 10 questions on the Acme End-of-the-Day Energy Scale. This instrument produces a score between 1 and 100 (1 = Extremely low energy . . . 100 = Extremely high energy).

Data set: **Ch 06 – Exercise 08A.sav**

Codebook

Variable:	Group
Definition:	Group number
Type:	Categorical (1 = No walking, 2 = Walking: 30 Minutes, 3 = Walking: 60 minutes)

Variable:	Mood
Definition:	Acme End-of-the-Day Energy Scale (1 = Extremely low energy . . . 100 = Extremely high energy)
Type:	Continuous

a. Write the hypotheses.

b. Run each criterion of the pretest checklist (normality, homogeneity of variance, and *n*) and discuss your findings.

c. Run the ANOVA test and document your findings (*n*s, means, and Sig. [*p* value], hypotheses resolution).

d. Write an abstract under 200 words detailing a summary of the study, the ANOVA test results, hypothesis resolution, and implications of your findings.

Repeat this exercise using **Ch 06 – Exercise 08B.sav.**

NOTE: Exercises 9 and 10 involve four groups each.

Exercise 6.9

In order to determine the best method for facilitating smoking cessation, patients who smoke two packs per day (40 cigarettes) are recruited and randomly assigned to one of four psychoeducational peer support groups with a qualified facilitator: Group 1 will meet once a week in an in-person setting, Group 2 will meet once a week via Internet videoconferencing, Group 3 will meet twice a week in-person, and Group 4 will meet twice a week via videoconferences. After 10 weeks, each participant will be asked how many cigarettes he or she smokes per day.

Data set: **Ch 06 – Exercise 09A.sav**

Codebook

Variable:	Group
Definition:	Group number
Type:	Categorical (1 = 1 meeting in-person, 2 = 1 meeting videoconference, 3 = 2 meetings in-person, 4 = 2 meetings videoconference)
Variable:	Smoking
Definition:	Number of cigarettes each participant smokes per day after 10 weeks
Type:	Continuous

a. Write the hypotheses.

b. Run each criterion of the pretest checklist (normality, homogeneity of variance, and *n*) and discuss your findings.

c. Run the ANOVA test and document your findings (*n*s, means, and Sig. [*p* value], hypotheses resolution).

d. Write an abstract under 200 words detailing a summary of the study, the ANOVA test results, hypothesis resolution, and implications of your findings.

Repeat this exercise using **Ch 06 – Exercise 09B.sav.**

Exercise 6.10

Due to numerous complications involving missed medication dosages, you implement a study to determine the best strategy for enhancing medication adherence. Patients who are on a daily medication regime will be recruited, receive a complimentary 1-month dosage of their regular medication(s), and randomly be assigned to one of four groups: Group 1 will serve as the control group (no treatment); Group 2 will participate in a 1-hour in-person nurse-administered medication adherence workshop; Group 3 will receive text message reminders (e.g., "It's time to take one tablet of Drug A"); Group 4 will attend the medication adherence workshop and also receive text messages. At the end of 1 month, participants will present their prescription bottle(s); the nurse will count the remaining pills and calculate the dosage adherence percentage (e.g., 0 pills remaining = 100% adherence).

Data set: **Ch 06 – Exercise 10A.sav**

Codebook

Variable:	Group
Definition:	Group number
Type:	Categorical (1 = Control, 2 = Rx workshop, 3 = Texts, 4 = Rx workshop and texts)

Variable:	RxAdhere
Definition:	Percentage of medication adherence (0–100)
Type:	Continuous

a. Write the hypotheses.

b. Run each criterion of the pretest checklist (normality, homogeneity of variance, and *n*) and discuss your findings.

c. Run the ANOVA test and document your findings (*n*s, means, and Sig. [*p* value], hypotheses resolution).

d. Write an abstract under 200 words detailing a summary of the study, the ANOVA test results, hypothesis resolution, and implications of your findings.

Repeat this exercise using **Ch 06 – Exercise 10B.sav.**

CHAPTER 7

ANCOVA

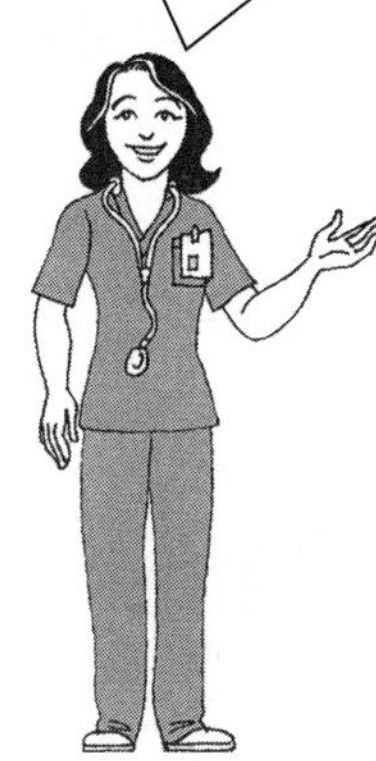
ANCOVA compares continuous variables adjusting for confounding variables.

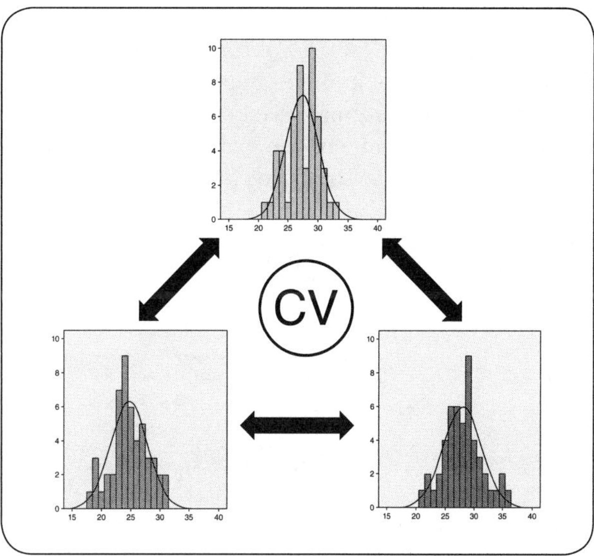
CV

Timing has a lot to do with the outcome of a rain dance.

—Cowboy proverb

LEARNING OBJECTIVES

Upon completing this chapter, you will be able to:

- Determine when it is appropriate to run an ANCOVA test
- Comprehend the characteristics of confounding variables (covariates)
- Verify that the data meet the criteria for ANCOVA processing: homogeneity of regression slopes and homogeneity of variance (Levene's test)
- Order an ANCOVA test
- Derive results from the estimates and pairwise comparisons tables
- Resolve the hypotheses
- Document the results in plain English

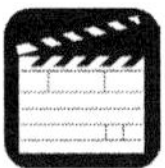

VIDEO

The tutorial video for this chapter is **Ch 07 – ANCOVA.mp4.** This video provides an overview of the ANCOVA (analysis of covariance) statistic, followed by the SPSS procedures for processing the pretest checklist, ordering the statistical run, and interpreting the results of this test using the data set: **Ch 07 – Example 01 – ANCOVA.sav.**

LAYERED LEARNING

The notion of ANCOVA is conceptually so similar to ANOVA (Chapter 6) that the same data sets will be used in the example and exercises, with one variable added to each data set. Notice that the example data set for this chapter (**Ch 07 – Example 01 – ANCOVA.sav**) is exactly the same as the example data set used for the ANOVA chapter (**(Ch 06 – Example 01 – ANOVA.sav)**), except it has a third variable (*Smoking*) included (Figure 7.1).

Figure 7.1 Excerpt from **Ch 07 – Example – ANCOVA.sav.**

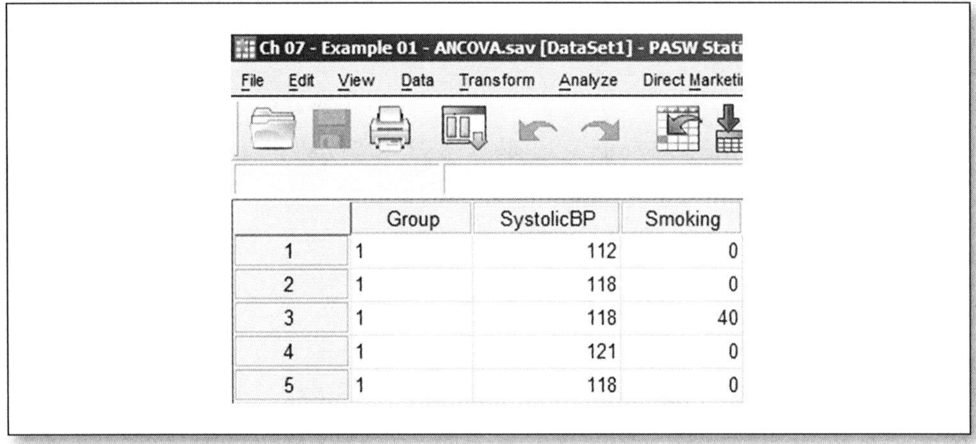

	Group	SystolicBP	Smoking
1	1	112	0
2	1	118	0
3	1	118	40
4	1	121	0
5	1	118	0

OVERVIEW—ANCOVA

The ANCOVA is similar to the ANOVA test, except ANCOVA allows us to include a covariate into the model to adjust the results for a known confounding variable.

To recap, the experimental model used in this example involves administering Drug A, Drug B, or Drug C to patients with moderate hypertension and then measuring their blood pressure. In terms of the variables, the drug (A, B, or C) is the independent variable (IV) and the systolic blood pressure is the outcome variable, technically referred to as the dependent variable (DV). In a perfect world, the experimental design could look like Figure 7.2.

Figure 7.2 Independent variable (IV) propagates change in the dependent variable (DV).

Independent Variable
Drug (A, B, C)

→

Dependent Variable
Systolic Blood Pressure

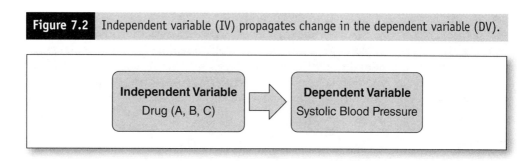

As you might expect, we do not live in a perfect world; in fact, science actively acknowledges this. It is expected that extraneous factors may influence scores as they travel from the independent variable to the dependent variable. In the language of experimental design, these factors are referred to as *confounding variables* (CV), as they can *confound* the results contained in the dependent variable. In statistical language, confounding variables are referred to as *covariates.*

In the ANOVA example, we did not identify a confounding variable, as symbolized in Figure 7.2. For the ANCOVA example, a confounding variable (*Smoking*) has been introduced: Suppose we discovered that some of the participants in the hypertension medication experiment smoke cigarettes. Cigarette smoking could be considered a confounding variable as smoking influences blood pressure. Now instead of just the independent variable (Drug A, B, or C) influencing changes in the dependent variable (systolic blood pressure), there is now an additional *confounding* factor (smoking) that can alter the data in the dependent variable (Figure 7.3).

As stated, ANCOVA is similar to an ANOVA-type model; however, ANCOVA adjusts the results according to the influence that the confounding variable (covariate) introduced. In other words, if we have data pertaining to a known confounding variable, such as the influence of smoking on blood pressure, ANCOVA can statistically adjust the results so

Figure 7.3 Independent variable (IV) and confounding variable (CV) both propagate change in the dependent variable (DV).

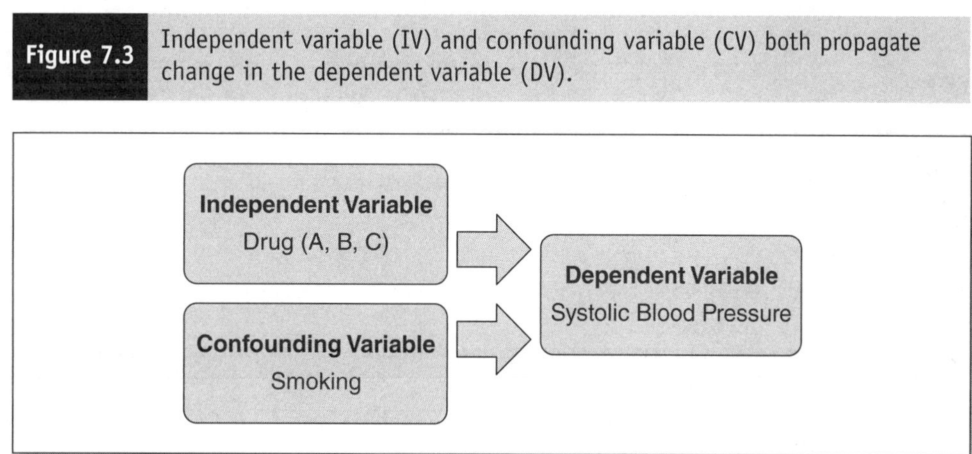

as to neutralize the effects of the identified confounding factor. This provides a cleaner image of the effect that the independent variable (Drug A, B, C) has on the dependent variable (systolic blood pressure)—as if the confounding variable (smoking) has been (statistically) removed from the picture.

The results will look as if you had ordered an ANOVA test, except the figures will be adjusted to account for the influence of the covariate (*Smoking*).

Example

The nurse manager is interested in identifying the most effective drug for managing patients with moderate hypertension (systolic between 130 mmHg and 140 mmHg). Since some of the participants smoke cigarettes, and smoking is known to affect blood pressure, we also gather the mean number of cigarettes each participant smokes per day. NOTE: In the database, where *Smoking* = *0,* this signifies a nonsmoker.

Research Question

Controlling for smoking, which is the best drug for lowering moderate hypertension: Drug A, Drug B, or Drug C?

GROUPS

The nurse manager recruits 90 volunteers who meet the criteria and consent to participate in this study. Each patient's name is written on slips of paper and placed in a hat. The nurse manager randomly draws 30 names from the hat; these patients will receive Drug A, the next 30 names drawn will get Drug B, and the remaining 30 will be given Drug C.

PROCEDURE

Each participant is brought in to the clinic for a brief visit. Their blood pressure is taken to verify that they meet the criteria (systolic between 130 mmHg and 140 mmHg), and they are given a 30-day supply of the specified medication and asked how many cigarettes they smoke on a typical day. After 30 days, each participant will return to the clinic and have his or her blood pressure taken. For purposes of this example, we will presume 100% dosage adherence.

HYPOTHESES

The null hypothesis (H_0) is phrased to anticipate that the experiment/intervention fails, indicating that *no drug outperformed any of the others*. The alternative hypothesis (H_1) states that *at least one drug did outperform another:*

H_0: There is no statistically significant difference in the performance of the three drugs.

H_1: At least one drug (group) outperformed another.

DATA SET

Use the following data set: **Ch 07 – Example – ANCOVA.sav.**

Codebook

Variable:	Group
Definition:	Group number
Type:	Categorical (1 = Drug A, 2 = Drug B, 3 = Drug C)
Variable:	SystolicBP
Definition:	Systolic blood pressure (in mmHg)
Type:	Continuous
Variable:	Smoking
Definition:	Number of cigarettes participant smokes in a typical day (0 = nonsmoker)
Type:	Continuous

PRETEST CHECKLIST

ANCOVA Pretest Checklist

☑ 1. Homogeneity of regression slopes*

☑ 2. Homogeneity of variance (Levene's test)**

*Run prior to ANCOVA test

**Results produced upon ANCOVA test run

The statistical pretest checklist for the ANCOVA involves two criteria: **(1) homogeneity of regression slopes** and **(2) homogeneity of variance (Levene's test).**

Pretest Checklist Criterion 1—Homogeneity of Regression Slopes

The homogeneity of regressions slopes test checks that the slopes of the regression lines of the variables involved are similar to each other.

1. On the main SPSS menu, click on *Analyze, General Linear Model, Univariate.*

Figure 7.4 *Analyze, General Linear Model, Univariate.*

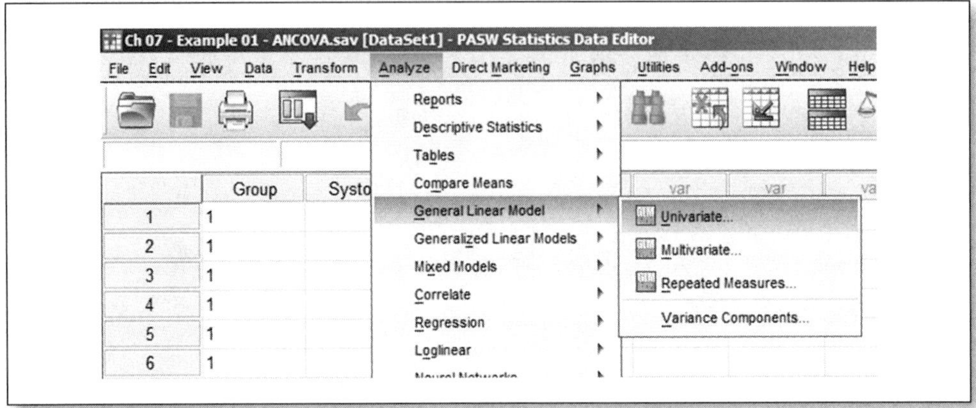

2. Move the *Group* variable into the *Fixed Factor(s)* window.
3. Move the *SystolicBP* variable into the *Dependent Variable* window.
4. Move the *Smoking* variable into the *Covariate(s)* window.
5. Click on *Model.*

Figure 7.5 *Univariate* menu.

6. Select ⊙ *Custom.*
7. Move *Group* and *Smoking* (in *Factors & Covariates* box) into *Model* box.
8. Hold down *Shift* key, and click on *Group* and *Smoking* (this will select both *Group* and *Smoking* together to signify the interaction term), and move them into the *Model* box (this should show as *Smoking*Group*).
9. Click *Continue* (this will take you back to the *Univariate* menu).
10. Click *OK.*

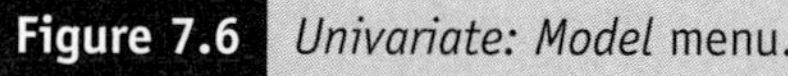

Figure 7.6 *Univariate: Model* menu.

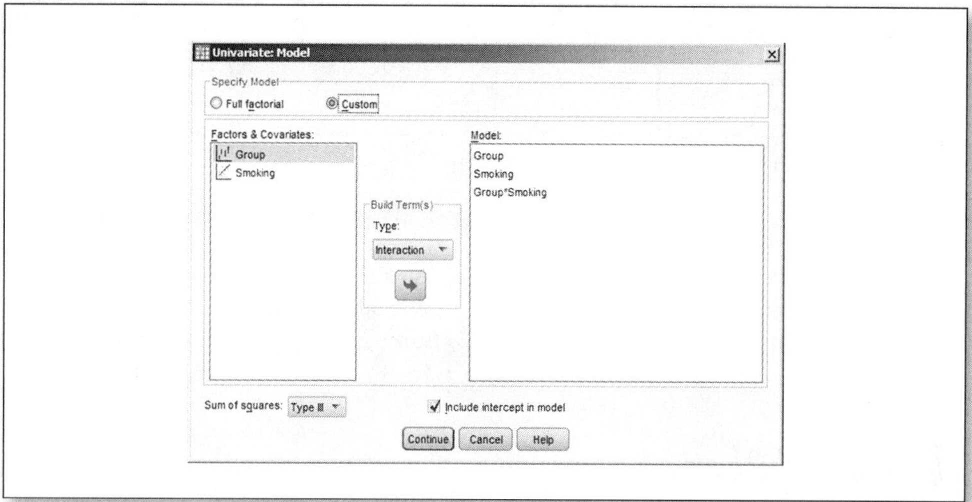

Inspect the *Test of Between-Subjects Effects* table (Table 7.1). If the *Sig.* (*p* value) for the *Group*Smoking* (interaction) term is > α (.05), then this indicates that there is no statistically significant difference in the regression slopes among the variables involved in this model. Hence, the assumption of *homogeneity of regression slopes* is satisfied. In other words, the trend of the values contained in each variable concurs (runs virtually parallel) with each other.

In this case, notice that this criterion is not satisfied; the *p* (.028) is less than .05. This violation makes sense as the covariate is somewhat atypical: The covariate in this model is *Smoking*—the number of cigarettes that each participant smokes in a typical day. Upon running descriptive statistics for *Smoking,* to better comprehend this variable, we notice that this sample consists of 91.1% (82 of 90) nonsmokers, wherein *Smoking* = 0 (Table 7.2).

As expected, this statistical anomaly is further reflected in the right (positive) skew seen on the histogram in Figure 7.7.

Table 7.1 Tests of Between-Subjects Effects.

Tests of Between-Subjects Effects

Dependent Variable:SystolicBP

Source	Type III Sum of Squares	df	Mean Square	F	Sig.
Corrected Model	168.495[a]	5	33.699	4.601	.001
Intercept	1211894.306	1	1211894.306	165447.990	.000
Group	86.804	2	43.402	5.925	.004
Smoking	7.501	1	7.501	1.024	.314
Group * Smoking	54.575	2	27.288	3.725	.028
Error	615.294	84	7.325		
Total	1336199.000	90			
Corrected Total	783.789	89			

a. R Squared = .215 (Adjusted R Squared = .168)

As with other incidents wherein the pretest criteria are not fully satisfied, we will proceed with processing the test and discuss such violations as a caveat in the Discussion section.

The remaining pretest criterion, **(2) homogeneity of variance (Levene's test),** will be processed during the **Test Run** and finalized in the **Results** section.

Table 7.2 Descriptive Statistics (Frequency Table) for *Smoking.*

Smoking

		Frequency	Percent	Valid Percent	Cumulative Percent
Valid	0	82	91.1	91.1	91.1
	20	1	1.1	1.1	92.2
	36	2	2.2	2.2	94.4
	37	1	1.1	1.1	95.6
	40	3	3.3	3.3	98.9
	60	1	1.1	1.1	100.0
	Total	90	100.0	100.0	

Figure 7.7 Histogram of *Smoking*; right (positive) skew attributable to the majority of the participants being nonsmokers (*Smoking* = 0).

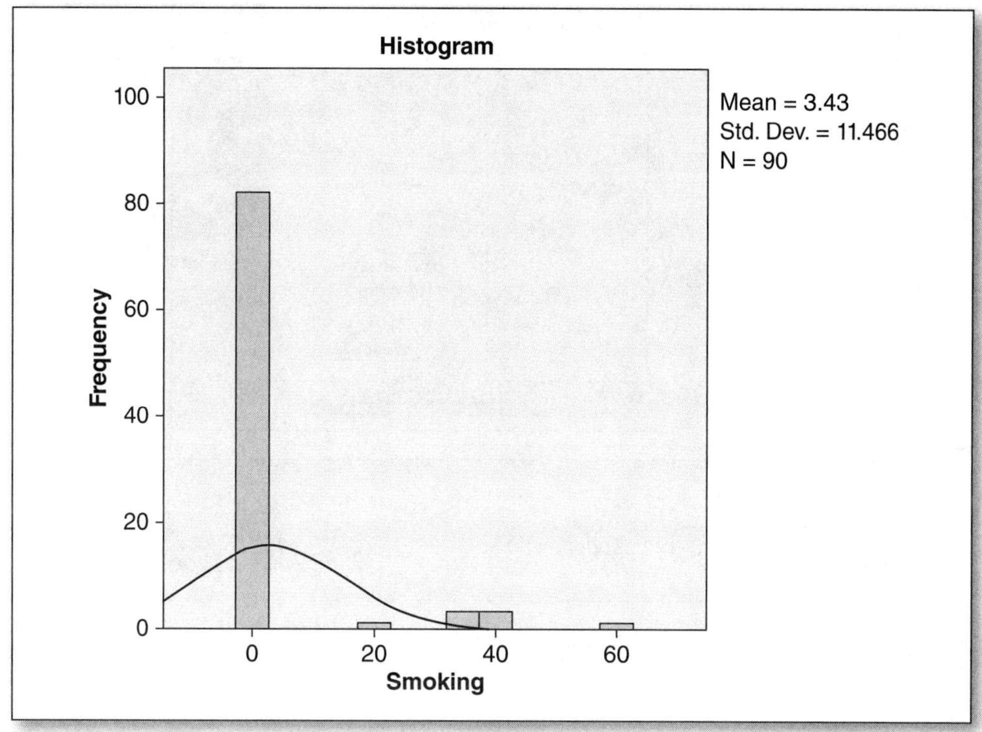

TEST RUN

1. On the main SPSS menu, click on *Analyze, General Linear Model, Univariate.*

Steps 2 to 5 may be bypassed; the variables should still reside in the proper windows from the prior procedure where we checked for the *Homogeneity of Regression Slopes*.

2. Move the *Group* variable into the *Fixed Factor(s)* window.
3. Move the *SystolicBP* variable into the *Dependent Variable* window.
4. Move the *Smoking* variable into the *Covariate(s)* window.
5. Click on *Model.*
6. Select ⊙ *Full factorial.* This will discard the model that involved the *Group*Smoking* interaction term specified earlier (Figure 7.9).

Figure 7.8 *Univariate* menu.

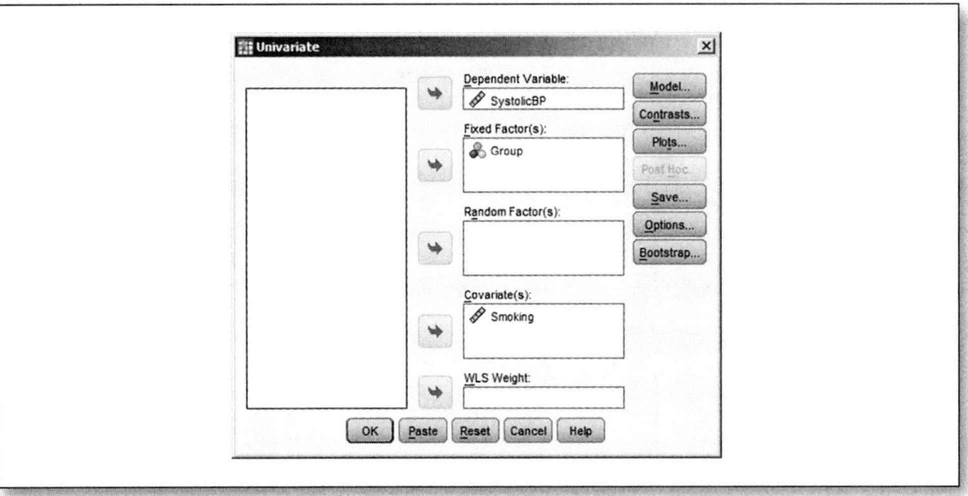

Figure 7.9 *Univariate: Model* menu.

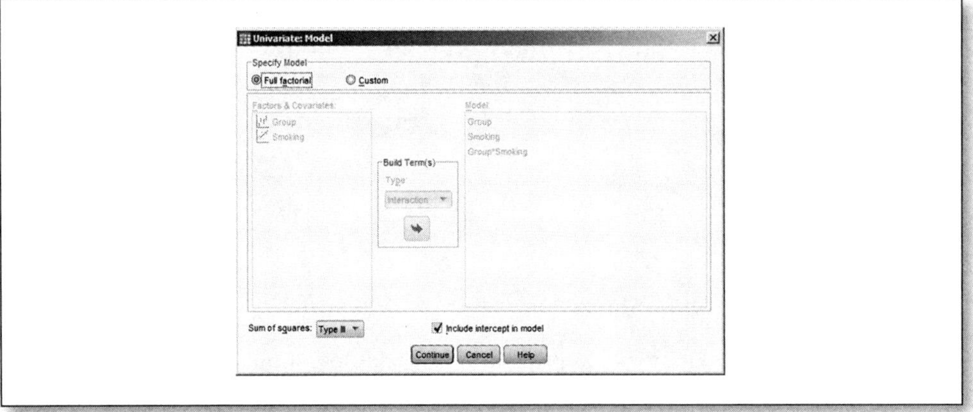

7. Click on *Continue*. This will take you back to the *Univariate* menu (Figure 7.8).

8. On the *Univariate* menu, click on *Options*.

9. In the *Factor(s) and Factor Interactions* window, move *Group* into the *Display Means for* window (Figure 7.10).

10. Check the ☑ *Compare main effects* checkbox.

11. In the *Confidence interval adjustment* pull-down menu, select *Bonferroni*.

12. In the *Display* options, check the ☑ *Homogeneity tests.*

13. Click on *Continue.*

14. Click on *OK.*

Figure 7.10 *Univariate: Options* menu.

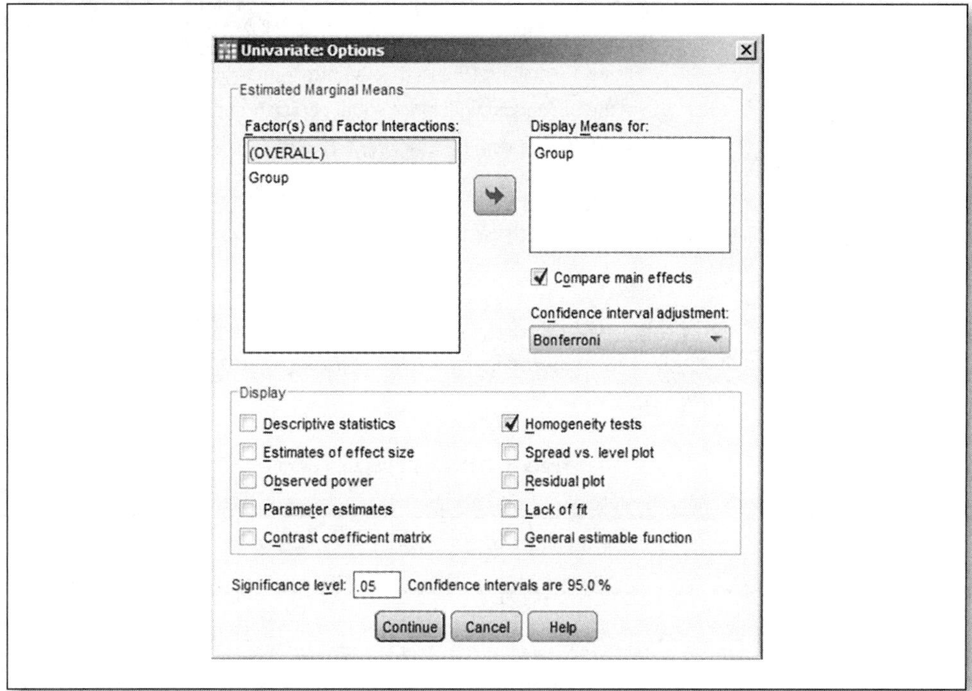

RESULTS

Pretest Checklist Criterion 2—Homogeneity of Variance (Levene's Test)

Table 7.3 shows that the Sig. (p) = .791; since this is greater than α (.05), this indicates that there is no significant difference between the variances; hence, this criterion is satisfied.

Next, we look to the *Tests of Between-Subjects Effects* table (Table 7.4); the Sig. (p) value of .004 on the *Group* row indicates that a statistically significant difference has been detected among (the adjusted means for) the groups. For specific details on which group(s) outperformed which, we look to the *Pairwise Comparisons* table (Table 7.5).

Table 7.3 Levene's Test of Equality of Error Variances Shows No Statistically Significant Difference Among the Variances ($p = .791$, $\alpha = .05$).

Levene's Test of Equality of Error Variances[a]

Dependent Variable:SystolicBP

F	df1	df2	Sig.
.235	2	87	.791

Tests the null hypothesis that the error variance of the dependent variable is equal across groups.

a. Design: Intercept + Smoking + Group

Table 7.4 *Tests of Between-Subjects Effects* Table Shows That a Significant Difference Has Been Detected Among the *Groups* ($p = .004$, $\alpha = .05$).

Tests of Between-Subjects Effects

Dependent Variable:SystolicBP

Source	Type III Sum of Squares	df	Mean Square	F	Sig.
Corrected Model	113.920[a]	3	37.973	4.875	.004
Intercept	1219483.141	1	1219483.141	156561.308	.000
Smoking	18.364	1	18.364	2.358	.128
Group	92.862	2	46.431	5.961	.004
Error	669.869	86	7.789		
Total	1336199.000	90			
Corrected Total	783.789	89			

a. R Squared = .145 (Adjusted R Squared = .116)

The *Pairwise Comparisons* table (Table 7.5) is read in the same way as the *Multiple Comparisons* table produced by the ANOVA post hoc tests. These results reveal a statistically significant difference in the adjusted means between Drug A : Drug B ($p = .034$) and between Drug A : Drug C ($p = .005$). The actual adjusted means for each (Drug) *Group* are shown in the *Estimates* table (Table 7.6).

Table 7.5 *Pairwise Comparisons* Table Shows Statistically Significant Differences Between Drug A & Drug B ($p = .034$) and Drug A & Drug C ($p = .005$).

Pairwise Comparisons

Dependent Variable:SystolicBP

(I) Dose	(J) Dose	Mean Difference (I-J)	Std. Error	Sig.[a]	95% Confidence Interval for Difference[a]	
					Lower Bound	Upper Bound
Drug A	Drug B	-1.873*	.725	.034	-3.644	-.102
	Drug C	-2.356*	.721	.005	-4.116	-.596
Drug B	Drug A	1.873*	.725	.034	.102	3.644
	Drug C	-.483	.727	1.000	-2.258	1.293
Drug C	Drug A	2.356*	.721	.005	.596	4.116
	Drug B	.483	.727	1.000	-1.293	2.258

Based on estimated marginal means

a. Adjustment for multiple comparisons: Bonferroni.

*. The mean difference is significant at the .05 level.

Table 7.6 *Estimates* Table Shows Adjusted Means for Each Group per the Influence of the *Smoking* Covariate.

Estimates

Dependent Variable:SystolicBP

Group	Mean	Std. Error	95% Confidence Interval	
			Lower Bound	Upper Bound
Drug A	120.401[a]	.510	119.387	121.415
Drug B	122.275[a]	.513	121.255	123.295
Drug C	122.757[a]	.511	121.742	123.773

a. Covariates appearing in the model are evaluated at the following values: Smoking = 3.43.

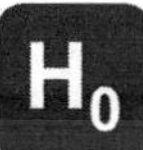

HYPOTHESIS RESOLUTION

To clarify the hypothesis resolution process, it is helpful to organize the findings in a table and use an asterisk to flag statistically significant difference(s) (Table 7.7).

NOTE: SPSS does not generate this table (Table 7.7) directly; you can assemble this table by gathering the means from the *Estimates* table (Table 7.6) and the *p* values from the Sig. column in the *Pairwise Comparisons* table (Table 7.5).

With this results table assembled, we can now revisit and resolve our pending hypotheses, which focus on determining the best drug for controlling moderate hypertension. To finalize this process, we will assess each hypothesis per the statistics contained in Table 7.7.

Table 7.7 Results of ANCOVA for SystolicBP.

Groups	p
μ(Drug A) = 120.40 : μ(Drug B) = 122.27	.034*
μ(Drug A) = 120.40 : μ(Drug C) = 122.76	.005*
μ(Drug B) = 122.27 : μ(Drug C) = 122.76	1.000

NOTE: Figures adjusted to account for cigarettes smoked per day among participants (μ = 3.4, *SD* = 11.5).

*Statistically significant difference detected between groups ($p \leq .05$).

REJECT: H_0: There is no statistically significant difference in the performance of the three drugs.

ACCEPT: H_1: At least one drug (group) outperformed another.

Since we discovered a statistically significant difference among at least one pair of the drugs, we reject H_0 and accept H_1. Specifically, Drug A outperformed Drug B in lowering blood pressure ($p = .034$), and Drug A outperformed Drug C in lowering blood pressure ($p = .005$).

Incidentally, if all of the pairwise comparisons had produced *p* values that were greater than .05, then we would have accepted H_0 and rejected H_1.

DOCUMENTING RESULTS

When documenting the results of this study, both Table 7.7 and the following verbose summary would be appropriate to include:

A group of 90 patients with moderate hypertension (systolic between 130 and 140 mmHg) were recruited and randomly assigned to take Drug A, Drug B, or Drug C for 30 days. Per concerns that smoking could influence blood pressure, we asked each participant how many cigarettes he or she smoked in a typical day and included that figure as a covariate (91.1% of the participants were nonsmokers). Note that the statistical assumption of homogeneity of regression slopes was compromised, likely due to the low prevalence of smokers that constituted the covariate.

After 1 month, patients who took Drug A had a mean systolic blood pressure of 120.40 mmHg, significantly outperforming Drug B (122.27 mmHg) and Drug C (122.76 mmHg) using an α of .05 (see Table).

Groups	p
μ(Drug A) = 120.40 : μ(Drug B) = 122.27	.034*
μ(Drug A) = 120.40 : μ(Drug C) = 122.76	.005*
μ(Drug B) = 122.27 : μ(Drug C) = 122.76	1.000

*Statistically significant difference detected between groups ($p \leq .05$). Figures adjusted to account for number of cigarettes smoked per day among participants ($\mu = 3.43$, $SD = 11.47$).

GOOD COMMON SENSE

While the ANCOVA statistic provides a system for efficiently coping with the effects of identified (measured) covariates within a multigroup design, keep in mind that the adjusted results are considered *estimated* (not perfect) values, based on the covariate data.

While it is valuable to anticipate, measure, and load a critical covariate into the ANCOVA model, it is not possible to account for and accurately measure the effects of all possible confounding variables, such as threats to internal validity, distractions, environmental impurities, and so forth.

Statistics is not about achieving perfection or proving anything; overall, it is about increasing our understanding by reducing uncertainty. ANCOVA helps to control for the effects of potential confounds, which brings us closer to achieving a clearer understanding of the IV → DV model, but it may not be possible to create a completely "clean" experiment, which would comprehensively identify and eliminate all effects that confounding variables could be having on the dependent variable.

Key Concepts

- ANCOVA
- Pretest checklist
  - Homogeneity of regression slopes
  - Homogeneity of variance (Levene's test)
- Hypothesis resolution
- Documenting results
- Good common sense

Practice Exercises

NOTE: These practice exercises and data sets are the same as those in **Chapter 6: ANOVA** except an extra (covariate) variable has been included to enable ANCOVA processing. All of the exercises involve three groups, except for Exercises 9 and 10, which involve four groups.

Exercise 7.1

You want to determine if meditation can reduce resting pulse rate. Participants were recruited and randomly assigned to one of three groups: Members of Group 1 (the control group) will not meditate; members of Group 2 (the first treatment group) will meditate for 30 minutes per day on Mondays, Wednesdays, and Fridays over the course of 2 weeks; and members of Group 3 (the second treatment group) will meditate for 30 minutes a day 6 days a week, Monday through Saturday. At the end, you gathered the resting pulse rates for each participant and daily mean antianxiety medication dosages (as the covariate).

Data set: **Ch 07 – Exercise 01A.sav**

Codebook

Variable: Group
Definition: Group number
Type: Categorical (1 = No meditation, 2 = Meditates 3 days, 3 = Meditates 6 days)

Variable: Pulse
Definition: Pulse rate (beats per minute)
Type: Continuous

Variable: Rx_anxiety
Definition: Daily dose of antianxiety medication (in milligrams)
Type: Continuous

a. Write the hypotheses.
b. Run each criterion of the pretest checklist (homogeneity of regression slopes, homogeneity of variance [Levene's test]) and discuss your findings.
c. Run the ANCOVA test and document your findings (*n*s, means, and Sig. [*p* value], hypotheses resolution).
d. Write an abstract under 200 words detailing a summary of the study, the ANCOVA test results, hypothesis resolution, and implications of your findings.

Repeat this exercise using data set: **Ch 07 – Exercise 01B.sav.**

Exercise 7.2

You want to determine the optimal preceptor-to-nurse ratio. Nurses will be randomly assigned to one of three groups: Group 1 will involve each preceptor working with only one nurse; in Group 2, each preceptor will work with two nurses; and in Group 3, each preceptor will work with five nurses. At the end of each shift, patients will be asked to complete the Acme Nursing Satisfaction Survey, which renders a score from 0 to 100, and the number of years that the preceptor nurse has been practicing (as the covariate).

Data set: **Ch 07 – Exercise 02A.sav**

Codebook

Variable:	Group
Definition:	Group number
Type:	Categorical (1 = One-to-one, 2 = Two-to-one, 3 = Five-to-one)
Variable:	ANSS
Definition:	Acme Nursing Satisfaction Survey score (0–100)
Type:	Continuous
Variable:	Preceptor_years
Definition:	Number of years the nurse has been practicing
Type:	Continuous

a. Write the hypotheses.
b. Run each criterion of the pretest checklist (homogeneity of regression slopes, homogeneity of variance [Levene's test]) and discuss your findings.
c. Run the ANCOVA test and document your findings (*ns*, means, and Sig. [*p* value], hypotheses resolution).
d. Write an abstract under 200 words detailing a summary of the study, the ANCOVA test results, hypothesis resolution, and implications of your findings.

Repeat this exercise using **Ch 07 – Exercise 02B.sav.**

Exercise 7.3

Clinicians at a nursing home facility want to see if giving residents a plant to tend to will help lower depression. To test this idea, the residents are randomly assigned to one of three groups: Those assigned to Group 1 will serve as the control group and will not be given a plant. Members of Group 2 will be given a small bamboo plant along with a card detailing care instructions. Members of Group 3 will be given a small cactus along with a card detailing care instructions. After 90 days, all participants will complete the Acme Depression Scale, which renders a score between 1 and 100 (1 = Low depression . . . 100 = High depression). Daily antidepressant medication dosages will also be recorded (as the covariate).

Data set: **Ch 07 – Exercise 03A.sav**

Codebook

Variable:	Group
Definition:	Group number
Type:	Categorical (1 = No plant, 2 = Bamboo, 3 = Cactus)

Variable: Depress
Definition: Acme Depression Scale (1 = Low depression . . . 100 = High depression)
Type: Continuous

Variable: Antidepressant_Rx
Definition: Antidepressant medication take per day (in milligrams)
Type: Continuous

a. Write the hypotheses.
b. Run each criterion of the pretest checklist (homogeneity of regression slopes, homogeneity of variance [Levene's test]) and discuss your findings.
c. Run the ANCOVA test and document your findings (*n*s, means, and Sig. [*p* value], hypotheses resolution).
d. Write an abstract under 200 words detailing a summary of the study, the ANCOVA test results, hypothesis resolution, and implications of your findings.

Repeat this exercise using **Ch 07 – Exercise 03B.sav.**

Exercise 7.4

You want to determine if chocolate enhances mood. Subjects will be recruited and randomly assigned to one of three groups: Those in Group 1 will be the control group and will eat their regular diet. Those in Group 2 will eat their usual meals and have a piece of chocolate at breakfast, lunch, and dinner over the course of a week. Those in Group 3 will eat their meals as usual and have two pieces of chocolate at breakfast, lunch, and dinner over the course of a week. At the end of the week, all participants will complete the Acme Mood Scale (1 = Extremely bad mood . . . 100 = Extremely good mood). Prior to starting this process, the AMS instrument will be administered to each participant to gather baseline mood scores (as the covariate).

Data set: **Ch 07 – Exercise 04A.sav**

Codebook

Variable: Group
Definition: Group number
Type: Categorical (1 = No chocolate, 2 = Chocolate [1 per meal], 3 = Chocolate [2 per meal])

Variable: Mood
Definition: Acme Mood Scale score (1–100)
Type: Continuous

Variable: Mood_baseline
Definition: Acme Mood Scale score at baseline (1–100)
Type: Continuous

a. Write the hypotheses.
b. Run each criterion of the pretest checklist (homogeneity of regression slopes, homogeneity of variance [Levene's test]) and discuss your findings.

c. Run the ANCOVA test and document your findings (*n*s, means, and Sig. [*p* value], hypotheses resolution).

d. Write an abstract under 200 words detailing a summary of the study, the ANCOVA test results, hypothesis resolution, and implications of your findings.

Repeat this exercise using **Ch 07 – Exercise 04B.sav.**

Exercise 7.5

During flu season, the administrators at a walk-in health clinic want to determine if providing patients with a pamphlet or a video will increase their receptivity to flu shots. Each patient will be given a ticket at the check-in desk with a 1, 2, or 3 on it; the tickets will be issued in (repeating) sequence (e.g., 1, 2, 3, 1, 2, 3, etc.). Once escorted to the exam room, patients with a number 1 ticket will serve as control participants and will not be offered any flu shot informational material. Patients with a number 2 ticket will be given a flu shot information pamphlet describing the rationale for the flu shot and flu prevention practices, emphasizing effective hand hygiene. Patients with a number 3 ticket will be shown a brief video covering the same information as contained in the pamphlet. At the end of the day, the charts were reviewed and three entries were made in the database: total number of flu shots given to patients in Group 1, total number of flu shots given to patients in Group 2, and the total number of flu shots given to patients in Group 3. Age will also be gathered (as the covariate).

Data set: **Ch 07 – Exercise 05A.sav**

Codebook

Variable:	Group
Definition:	Group number
Type:	Categorical (1 = Nothing, 2 = Flu shot pamphlet, 3 = Flu shot video)
Variable:	Shots
Definition:	Number of flu shots given in a day for each group
Type:	Continuous
Variable:	Age
Definition:	Age
Type:	Continuous

a. Write the hypotheses.

b. Run each criterion of the pretest checklist (homogeneity of regression slopes, homogeneity of variance [Levene's test]) and discuss your findings.

c. Run the ANCOVA test and document your findings (*n*s, means, and Sig. [*p* value], hypotheses resolution).

d. Write an abstract under 200 words detailing a summary of the study, the ANCOVA test results, hypothesis resolution, and implications of your findings.

Repeat this exercise using **Ch 07 – Exercise 05B.sav.**

Exercise 7.6

You want to determine if introducing a video in the waiting area will help relax patients. This study will take place over 3 days: On the first day, Group 1 (the control group) will experience the waiting room as is—with the monitor off; on the second day, Group 2 will have a classic movie playing; and on the third day, Group 3 will have a scenic video playing (e.g., waterfalls, vistas, wildlife). For patients who consent to participating in this research, the nurse will anonymously copy their pulse rate to a journal along with the day number (Group). The length of wait time (in waiting room) will also be recorded for each patient (as the covariate).

Data set: **Ch 07 – Exercise 06A.sav**

Codebook

Variable: Group
Definition: Group number
Type: Categorical (1 = Control, 2 = Classic movie, 3 = Scenic video)

Variable: Pulse
Definition: Pulse rate (gathered by a pulse oximeter)
Type: Continuous

Variable: Wait_time
Definition: Length of wait in waiting room (in minutes)
Type: Continuous

a. Write the hypotheses.
b. Run each criterion of the pretest checklist (homogeneity of regression slopes, homogeneity of variance [Levene's test]) and discuss your findings.
c. Run the ANCOVA test and document your findings (*n*s, means, and Sig. [*p* value], hypotheses resolution).
d. Write an abstract under 200 words detailing a summary of the study, the ANCOVA test results, hypothesis resolution, and implications of your findings.

Repeat this exercise using **Ch 07 – Exercise 06B.sav.**

Exercise 7.7

In an effort to determine the effectiveness of light therapy to alleviate depression, you recruit a group of subjects who have been diagnosed with depression. The subjects are randomly assigned to one of three groups: Group 1 will be the control group—members of this group will receive no light therapy. Members of Group 2 will get light therapy for 1 hour on even-numbered days over the course of 1 month. Members of Group 3 will get light therapy every day for 1 hour over the course of 1 month. After 1 month, all participants will complete the Acme Mood Scale, consisting of 10 questions; this instrument renders a score between 1 and 100 (1 = Extremely bad mood . . . 100 = Extremely good mood). Each participant's age will also be recorded (as the covariate).

Data set: **Ch 07 – Exercise 07A.sav**

Codebook

Variable: Group
Definition: Group number
Type: Categorical (1 = No light therapy, 2 = Light therapy: even days, 3 = Light therapy: every day)

Variable: Mood
Definition: Acme Mood Scale (1 = Extremely bad mood . . . 100 = Extremely good mood)
Type: Continuous

Variable: Age
Definition: Age
Type: Continuous

a. Write the hypotheses.
b. Run each criterion of the pretest checklist (homogeneity of regression slopes, homogeneity of variance [Levene's test]) and discuss your findings.
c. Run the ANCOVA test and document your findings (*n*s, means, and Sig. [*p* value], hypotheses resolution).
d. Write an abstract under 200 words detailing a summary of the study, the ANCOVA test results, hypothesis resolution, and implications of your findings.

Repeat this exercise using **Ch 07 – Exercise 07B.sav.**

Exercise 7.8

It is thought that exercising early in the morning will provide better energy throughout the day. To test this idea, subjects are recruited and randomly assigned to one of three groups: Members of Group 1 will constitute the control group and not be assigned any walking. Members of Group 2 will walk from 7:00 to 7:30 a.m., Monday through Friday, over the course of 30 days. Members of Group 3 will walk from 7:00 to 8:00 a.m., Monday through Friday, over the course of 30 days. At the conclusion of the study, each subject will answer the 10 questions on the Acme End-of-the-Day Energy Scale. This instrument produces a score between 1 and 100 (1 = Extremely low energy . . . 100 = Extremely high energy). The nurse will also record the number of sitting hours each participant has in a typical work per day (as the covariate).

Data set: **Ch 07 – Exercise 08A.sav**

Codebook

Variable: Group
Definition: Group number
Type: Categorical (1 = No walking, 2 = Walking: 30 Minutes, 3 = Walking: 60 minutes)

Variable: Mood
Definition: Acme End-of-the-Day Energy Scale (1 = Extremely low energy . . . 100 = Extremely high energy)
Type: Continuous

Variable: Sitting
Definition: Hours per day spent sitting at work
Type: Continuous

a. Write the hypotheses.
b. Run each criterion of the pretest checklist (homogeneity of regression slopes, homogeneity of variance [Levene's test]) and discuss your findings.
c. Run the ANCOVA test and document your findings (*n*s, means, and Sig. [*p* value], hypotheses resolution).
d. Write an abstract under 200 words detailing a summary of the study, the ANCOVA test results, hypothesis resolution, and implications of your findings.

Repeat this exercise using **Ch 07 – Exercise 08B.sav.**

NOTE: Exercises 9 and 10 involve four groups each.

Exercise 7.9

To determine the best method for facilitating smoking cessation, patients who smoke two packs per day (40 cigarettes) are recruited and randomly assigned to one of four psychoeducational peer support groups with a qualified facilitator: Group 1 will meet once a week in an in-person setting, Group 2 will meet once a week via Internet videoconferencing, Group 3 will meet twice a week in-person, and Group 4 will meet twice a week via videoconferences. After 10 weeks, each participant will be asked how many cigarettes he or she smokes per day and how many minutes of exercise he or she does on a typical day (as the covariate).

Data set: **Ch 07 – Exercise 09A.sav**

Codebook

Variable: Group
Definition: Group number
Type: Categorical (1 = 1 meeting in-person, 2 = 1 meeting videoconference, 3 = 2 meetings in-person, 4 = 2 meetings videoconference)

Variable: Smoking
Definition: Number of cigarettes each participant smokes per day after 10 weeks
Type: Continuous

Variable: Exercise
Definition: Number of minutes of exercise per day
Type: Continuous

a. Write the hypotheses.

b. Run each criterion of the pretest checklist (homogeneity of regression slopes, homogeneity of variance [Levene's test]) and discuss your findings.

c. Run the ANCOVA test and document your findings (*ns*, means, and Sig. [*p* value], hypotheses resolution).

d. Write an abstract under 200 words detailing a summary of the study, the ANCOVA test results, hypothesis resolution, and implications of your findings.

Repeat this exercise using **Ch 07 – Exercise 09B.sav.**

Exercise 7.10

Due to numerous complications involving missed medication dosages, you implement a study to determine the best strategy for enhancing medication adherence. Patients who are on a daily medication regime will be recruited, receive a complimentary 1-month dosage of their regular medication(s), and randomly assigned to one of four groups: Group 1 will serve as the control group (no treatment); Group 2 will participate in a 1-hour in-person nurse-administered medication adherence workshop; Group 3 will receive text message reminders (e.g., *It's time to take one tablet of Drug A*); Group 4 will attend the medication adherence workshop and also receive text messages. At the end of 1 month, participants will present their prescription bottle(s); the nurse will count the remaining pills and calculate the dosage adherence percentage (e.g., 0 pills remaining = 100% adherence). The total number of pills that each participant is prescribed to take per day will also be recorded (as the covariate).

Data set: **Ch 07 – Exercise 10A.sav**

Codebook

Variable: Group
Definition: Group number
Type: Categorical (1 = Control, 2 = Rx workshop, 3 = Texts, 4 = Rx workshop and texts)

Variable: RxAdhere
Definition: Percentage of medication adherence (0–100)
Type: Continuous

Variable: Pills_prescribed
Definition: Total number of pills prescribed per day
Type: Continuous

a. Write the hypotheses.

b. Run each criterion of the pretest checklist (homogeneity of regression slopes, homogeneity of variance [Levene's test]) and discuss your findings.

c. Run the ANCOVA test and document your findings (*ns*, means, and Sig. [*p* value], hypotheses resolution).

d. Write an abstract under 200 words detailing a summary of the study, the ANCOVA test results, hypothesis resolution, and implications of your findings.

Repeat this exercise using **Ch 07 – Exercise 10B.sav.**

CHAPTER 8

MANOVA

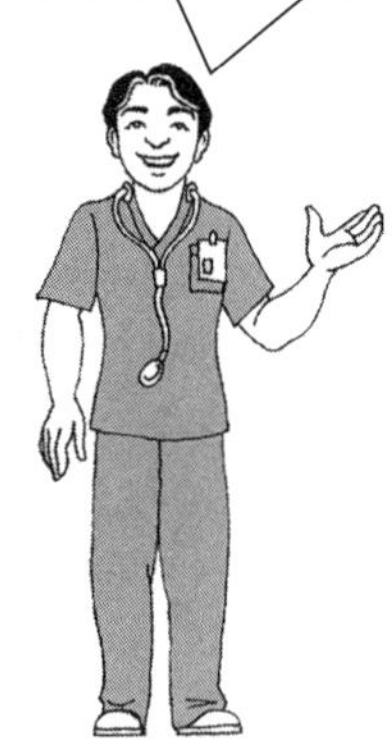
MANOVA compares the groups when there's more than one continuous outcome.

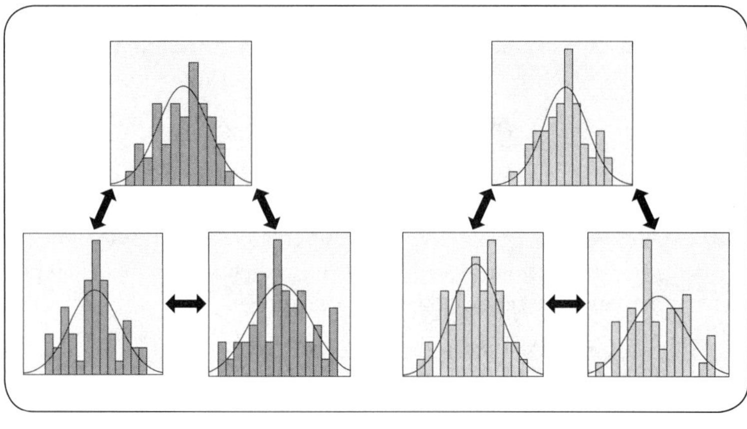

Forget about style; worry about results.

—Bobby Orr

LEARNING OBJECTIVES

Upon completing this chapter, you will be able to:

- Determine when it is appropriate to run a MANOVA test
- Verify that the data meet the criteria for MANOVA processing: sample size, normality, moderate correlation, homogeneity of variance-covariance (Box's *M* test), and homogeneity of variance (Levene's test)
- Order a MANOVA test
- Derive results from the estimates and pairwise comparisons tables
- Resolve the hypotheses
- Document the results in plain English

VIDEO

The tutorial video for this chapter is **Ch 08 – MANOVA.mp4.** This video provides an overview of the MANOVA (multiple analysis of variance) statistic, followed by the SPSS procedures for processing the pretest checklist, ordering the statistical run, and interpreting the results of this test using the data set: **Ch 08 – Example 01 – MANOVA.sav.**

LAYERED LEARNING

The notion of MANOVA builds on the concept of ANOVA (Chapter 6); hence, the same data sets will be used in the example and exercises, with one variable added to each data set. Notice that the example data set for this chapter (**Ch 08 – Example 01 – MANOVA.sav**) is exactly the same as the example data set used for the ANOVA chapter (**Ch 06 – Example 01 – ANOVA.sav**), except it has a third variable (*Pulse*) included (Figure 8.1).

Figure 8.1 Excerpt from **Ch 08 – Example – MANOVA.sav.**

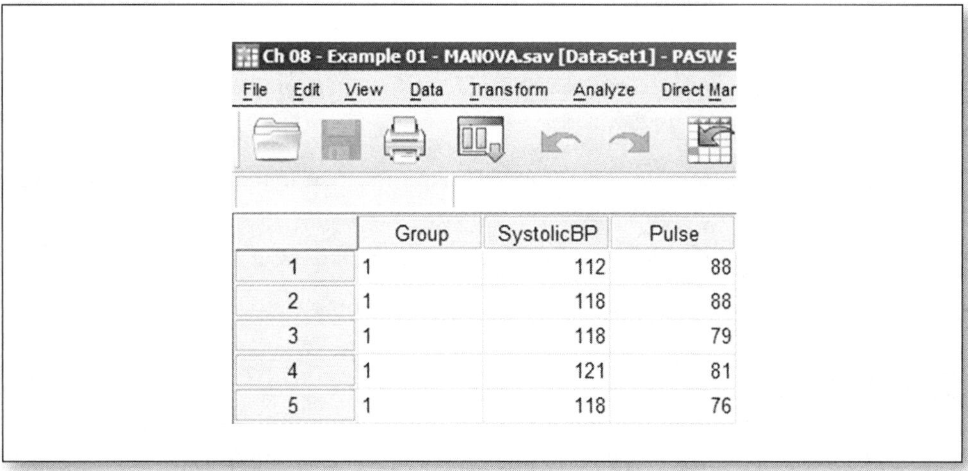

	Group	SystolicBP	Pulse
1	1	112	88
2	1	118	88
3	1	118	79
4	1	121	81
5	1	118	76

OVERVIEW—MANOVA

The MANOVA is similar to the ANOVA test, except MANOVA allows us to assess more than one outcome (dependent) variable.

To recap, the experimental model used in the ANOVA example involved administering *Drug A, Drug B,* or *Drug C* to patients with moderate hypertension and then measuring *one* outcome—their blood pressure (*SystolicBP*)—to compare the effectiveness of each drug. Suppose, in addition to assessing the drugs' effect on blood pressure, we also wanted to compare these drugs to determine if they may have an effect on a *second* outcome variable, such as pulse rate (*Pulse*). Basically, this MANOVA would be akin to running two separate ANOVAs:

- $ANOVA_1$: *(Drug A, Drug B, Drug C)* : (*SystolicBP*)
- $ANOVA_2$: (*Drug A, Drug B, Drug C*) : (*Pulse*)

The disadvantage of running two separate ANOVAs (one for *SystolicBP* and another for *Pulse*) is that doing so would substantially increase the likelihood of committing a Type I error (as detailed at the ★ icon on page **94**).

The MANOVA will basically perform these two ANOVA tests as a single procedure. The results will look as if you had ordered two separate ANOVA tests: (1) comparing the three drugs in terms of their effects on *SystolicBP* and (2) comparing the three drugs in terms of their effect on *Pulse*. For a preview of the MANOVA results, see pages **177** and **178**.

Example

The nurse manager is interested in identifying the most effective drug for managing patients with moderate hypertension (systolic between 130 mmHg and 140 mmHg). Considering that some drugs can have an effect on the patient's pulse rate, data on the pulse rate will be gathered as well.

Research Questions

Since this example involves two outcome (dependent) variables, it is appropriate to have two research questions:

Q_1: Which is the best drug for lowering moderate hypertension: Drug A, Drug B, or Drug C?

(NOTE: Q_1 is the same research question as was used in the ANOVA example.)

Q_2: How do these drugs compare in terms of their effect on pulse?

GROUPS

The nurse manager recruits 90 volunteers who meet the criteria and consent to participate in this study. Each patient's name is written on slips of paper and placed in a hat. The nurse manager randomly draws 30 names from the hat; these patients will receive Drug A, the next 30 names drawn will get Drug B, and the remaining 30 will be given Drug C.

PROCEDURE

Each participant is brought in to the clinic for a brief visit. Their blood pressure is taken to verify that they meet the criteria (systolic between 130 mmHg and 140 mmHg), and they are given a 30-day supply of the specified medication. After 30 days, each participant will return to the clinic and have his or her blood pressure and pulse taken. For purposes of this example, we will presume 100% dosage adherence.

HYPOTHESES

Since this study involves two outcome (dependent) variables (*SystolicBP* and *Pulse*), two sets of hypotheses are constructed: H_0 and H_1 pertain to blood pressure; H_0 and H_2 pertain to pulse.

H_0: Drugs A, B, and C have equal effects on blood pressure and pulse rate.

H_1: At least one drug (group) outperformed another in controlling blood pressure.

H_2: At least one drug (group) had a unique effect on pulse rate.

DATA SET

Use the following data set: **Ch 08 – Example 01 – MANOVA.sav.**

Codebook

Variable: Group
Definition: Group number
Type: Categorical (1 = Drug A, 2 = Drug B, 3 = Drug C)

Variable: SystolicBP
Definition: Systolic blood pressure (in mmHg)
Type: Continuous

Variable: Pulse
Definition: Pulse rate measured by a pulse oximeter (in beats per minute)
Type: Continuous

PRETEST CHECKLIST

MANOVA Pretest Checklist

☑ 1. *n* quota*

☑ 2. Normality*

☑ 3. Moderate correlation*

☑ 4. Homogeneity of variance-covariance (Box's *M* test)**

☑ 5. Homogeneity of variance (Levene's test)**

*Run prior to MANOVA test

**Results produced upon MANOVA test run

Considering the (behind-the-scenes) internal complexity of the MANOVA statistic, five pretest criteria need to be assessed to better ensure the robustness of the findings: **(1) *n* quota, (2) normality, (3) moderate correlation, (4) homogeneity of variance-covariance (Box's *M* test),** and **(5) homogeneity of variance (Levene's test)**.

Pretest Checklist Criterion 1—*n* Quota

As with the *t* test and ANOVA, the MANOVA becomes more stable with a larger sample. An *n* of at least 30 per group is advised.

1. On the SPSS main menu, click on *Analyze, Descriptive Statistics, Frequencies* (Figure 8.2).

Figure 8.2 *Analyze, Descriptive Statistics, Frequencies.*

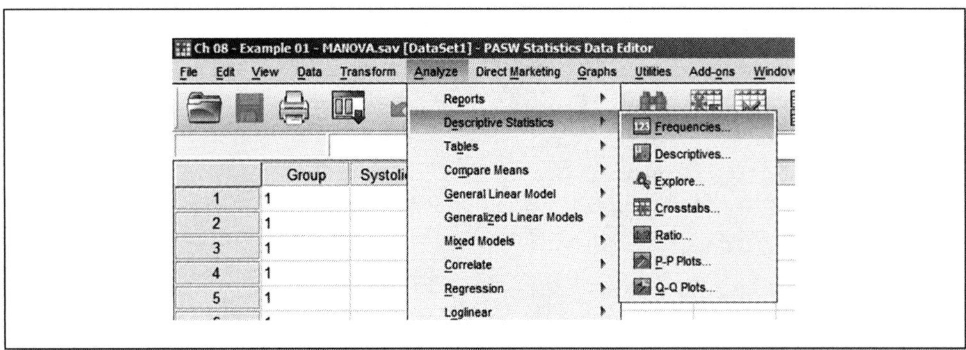

2. Move the *Group* variable into the *Variable(s)* window.
3. Click on *OK* (Figure 8.3).

Figure 8.3 *Frequencies* menu.

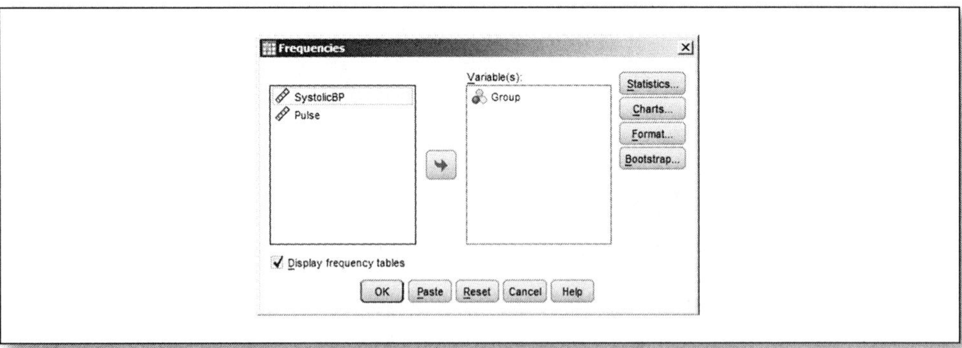

Table 8.1 *Frequencies* Table for *Group*; *n* (Frequency) ≥ 30 for Each Group.

Group

		Frequency	Percent	Valid Percent	Cumulative Percent
Valid	Drug A	30	33.3	33.3	33.3
	Drug B	30	33.3	33.3	66.7
	Drug C	30	33.3	33.3	100.0
	Total	90	100.0	100.0	

The *Frequency* table indicates 30 participants per group (Table 8.1); hence, this criterion is satisfied.

Pretest Checklist Criterion 2—Normality

When assessing the normality criteria for ANOVA, it involved examining three separate normal curves: *SystolicBP* for *Drug A, SystolicBP* for *Drug B,* and *SystolicBP* for *Drug C.* Considering that an additional outcome variable (*Pulse*) is included in the MANOVA model, we need to examine three additional histograms to check for normality: *Pulse* for *Drug A, Pulse* for *Drug B,* and *Pulse* for *Drug C:*

1. Use the *Select Cases* icon to select the records pertaining to *Drug A;* the selection criteria would be *Group = 1.*

   For more details on this procedure, refer to Chapter 4 ("SPSS—Descriptive Statistics: Continuous Variable (Age) Select by Categorical Variable (Gender)—Females Only"); see the star (★) icon on page **66**—instead of *Gender = 1,* specify *Group = 1.*

2. Run a histogram (with normal curve) on the variables *SystolicBP* and *Pulse;* SPSS can process charts for several variables in a single order (see Figure 8.4).

   For more details on this procedure, refer to Chapter 4 ("SPSS—Descriptive Statistics: Continuous Variables (Age)"); see the star (★) icon on page **58**—on the *Frequencies* menu, instead of moving *Age* into the *Variable(s)* window, move *SystolicBP* and *Pulse* (Figure 8.4).

Figure 8.4 On the *Frequencies* menu, load *SystolicBP* and *Pulse* into the *Variable(s)* window to produce (separate histograms with normal curve) *Charts* for these two variables.

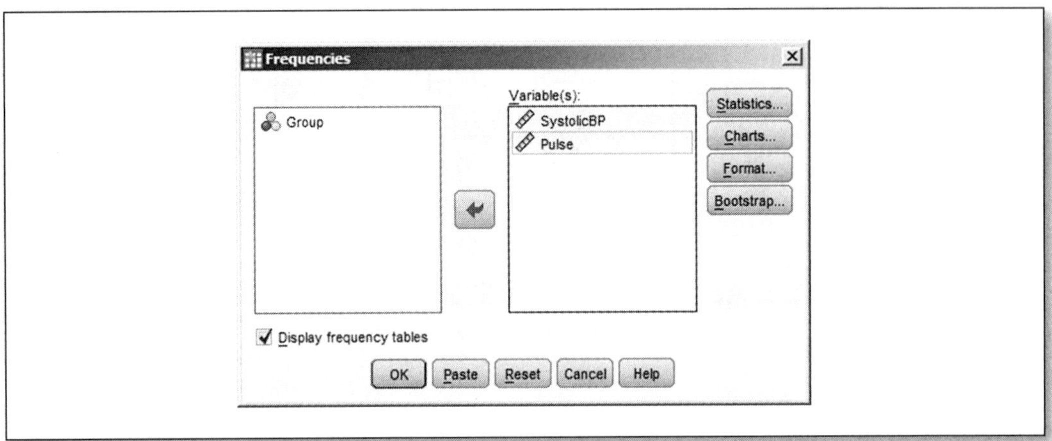

3. Repeat the process for the *Drug B* group (*Group* = 2).
4. Repeat the process a final time for the *Drug C* group (*Group* = 3).

This will produce six histograms with normal curves (Figures 8.5–8.10). The symmetry of the bell-shaped curve on each of these histograms satisfies the criterion of normality among these variables.

Figure 8.5 Histogram of *SystolicBP* for *Drug A*.

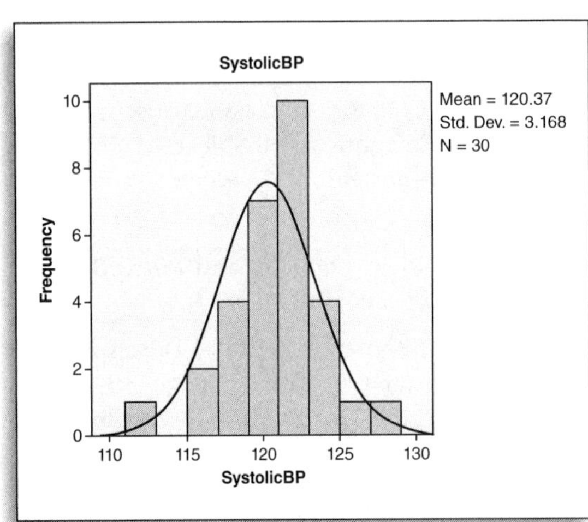

Figure 8.6 Histogram of *Pulse* for *Drug A*.

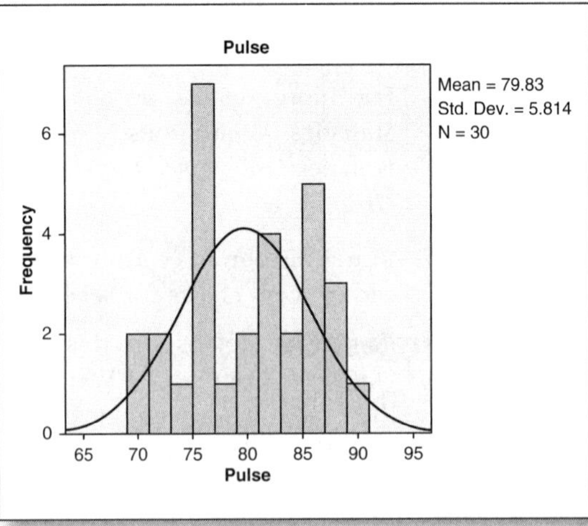

Figure 8.7 Histogram of *SystolicBP* for *Drug B.*

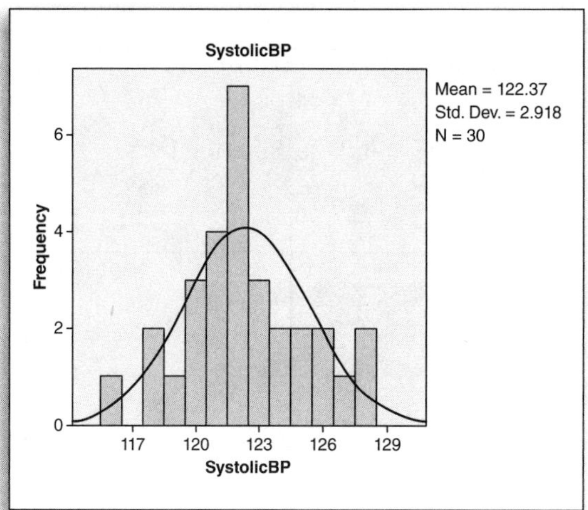

Figure 8.8 Histogram of *Pulse* for *Drug B.*

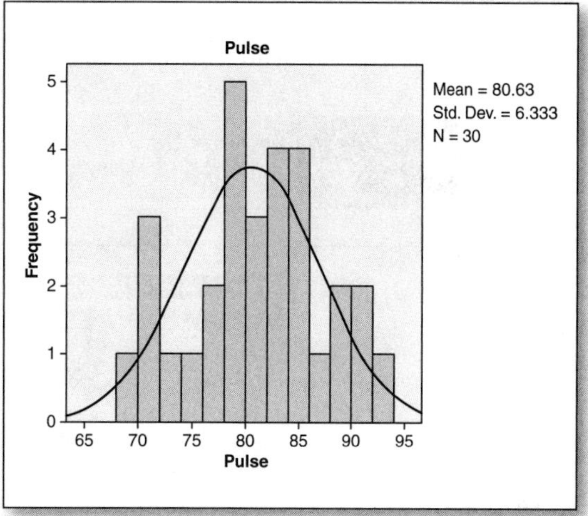

Figure 8.9 Histogram of *SystolicBP* for *Drug C.*

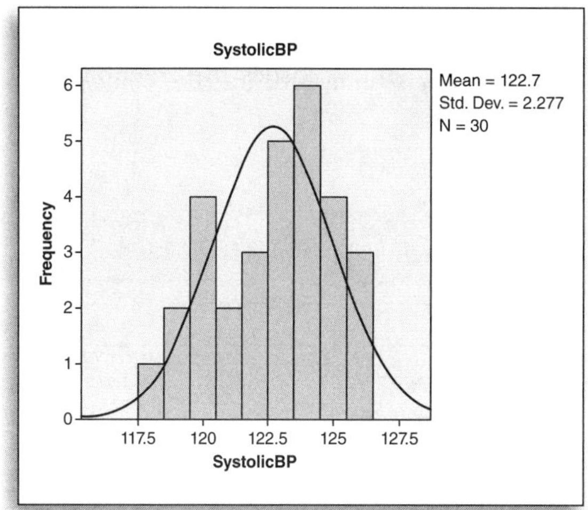

Figure 8.10 Histogram of *Pulse* for *Drug C.*

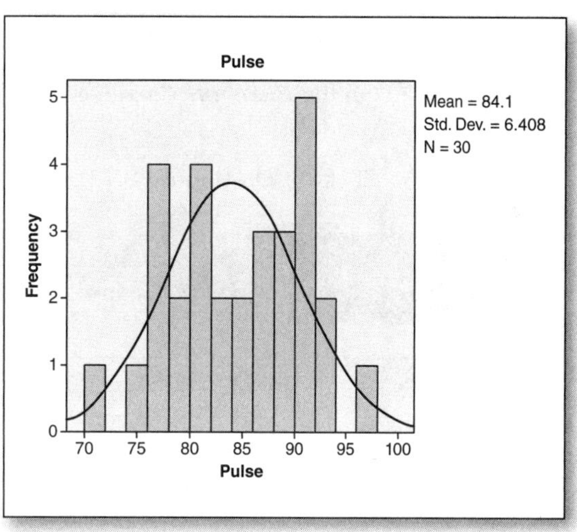

Pretest Checklist Criterion 3—Moderate Correlation

The variables (*SystolicBP* and *Pulse*) must be moderately correlated. This concept is covered thoroughly in Chapter 11: Correlation and Regression, but for now, consider correlation, which ranges from –1 to +1 indicates the extent to which two variables are associated with each other. A correlation score that is further from 0 (near –1 or +1) indicates a stronger association between the variables, whereas a correlation score nearer to 0 indicates a weaker association.

To run a correlational analysis between *SystolicBP* and *Pulse:*

1. On the main screen, click on *Analyze*, *Correlate*, *Bivariate* (Figure 8.11).

Figure 8.11 To order the correlation between *SystolicBP* and *Pulse,* click on *Analyze, Correlate, Bivariate.*

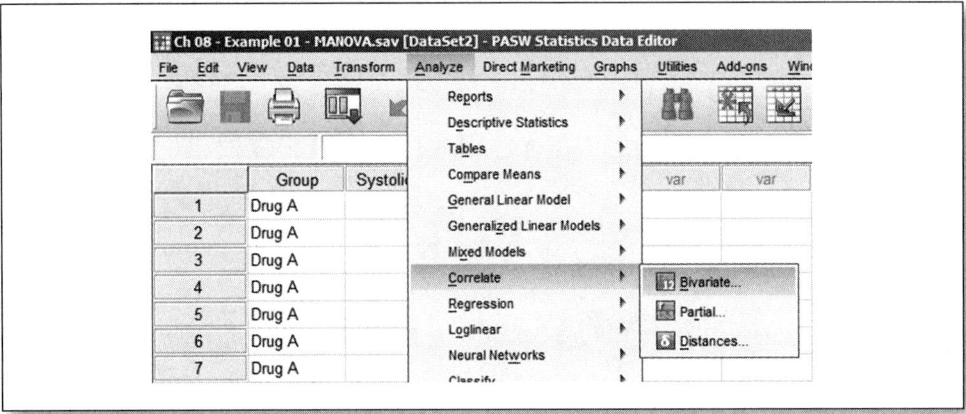

2. On the *Bivariate Correlations* menu, move *SystolicBP* and *Pulse* into the *Variables* window.

3. Click on *OK* (Figure 8.12).

Figure 8.12 On the *Bivariate Correlation* menu, load *SystolicBP* and *Pulse* into the *Variables* window.

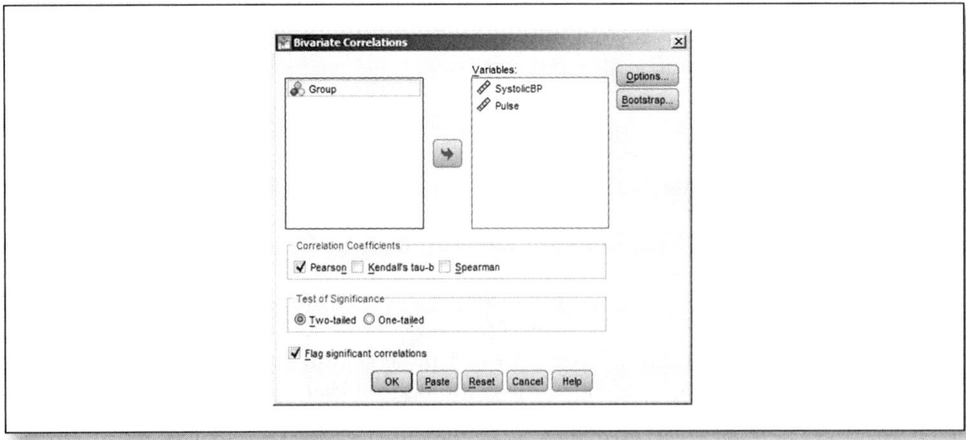

Table 8.2 *Correlations* Table Shows a .339 (Pearson) Correlation for the Two Outcome Variables, *SystolicBP* : *Pulse*.

Correlations

		SystolicBP	Pulse
SystolicBP	Pearson Correlation	1	.339**
	Sig. (2-tailed)		.001
	N	90	90
Pulse	Pearson Correlation	.339**	1
	Sig. (2-tailed)	.001	
	N	90	90

** Correlation is significant at the 0.01 level (2-tailed).

This criterion specifies that there must be a *moderate* correlation between the variables, meaning that the correlation needs to be between −.9 and −.3 or between .3 and .9 (Figure 8.13). Correlations that are between −.3 and .3 are considered too weak, whereas correlations that are less than −.9 or greater than .9 are considered too strongly correlated, which is referred to as *multicollinearity* (pronounced *multi-coe-lyn-ee-air-it-tee*). When variables are very highly correlated with each other (e.g., glove size : hand size), including both in the statistical model basically constitutes double-loading the formula. The rule of thumb for handling multicollinearity is that since the two variables contain such similar values, just select one of them to process, and leave the other out of the model. Typically, the decision as to which one to keep and which to leave out involves considering the characteristics of the variables in question (e.g., reliability, ease of access to the data, time/economic costs of gathering the variables).

Figure 8.13 Moderate correlation is −9 . . . −.3, and +.3 . . . +.9.

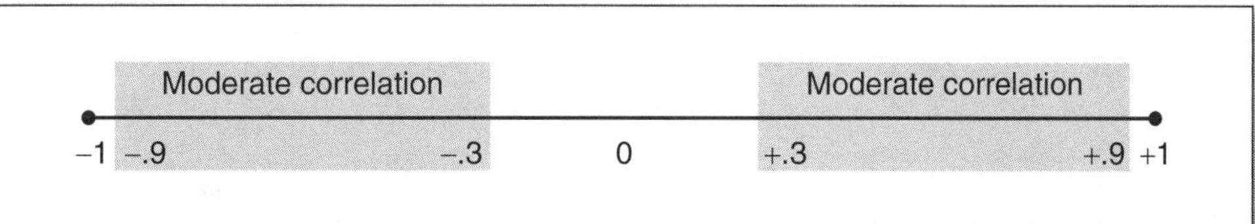

The remaining two pretest criteria, **(4) homogeneity of variance-covariance (Box's *M* test)** and **(5) homogeneity of variance (Levene's test)**, will be processed during the **Test Run** and finalized in the **Results** section.

TEST RUN

1. On the SPSS main menu, click on *Analyze, General Linear Model, Multivariate* (Figure 8.14).

Figure 8.14 To order a MANOVA test, click on *Analyze, General Linear Model, Multivariate.*

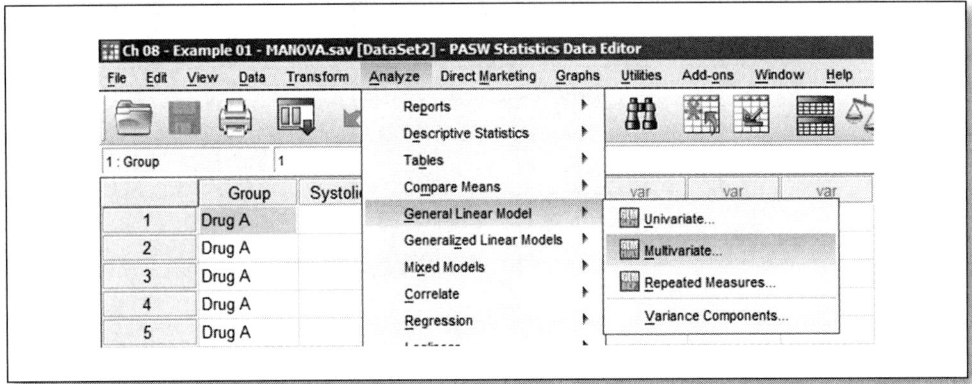

2. On the *Multivariate* menu (Figure 8.15), move *SystolicBP* and *Pulse* to the *Dependent Variables* window.
3. Move *Group* to the *Fixed Factor(s)* window.

Figure 8.15 Move *SystolicBP* and *Pulse* to the *Dependent Variables* window and *Group* to the *Fixed Factor(s)* window.

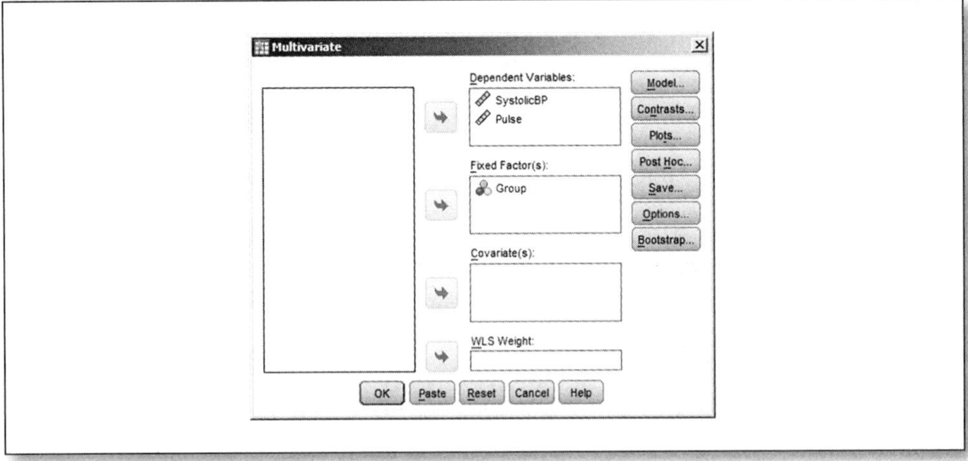

4. Click on *Post Hoc*.

5. On the *Multivariate: Post Hoc* menu (Figure 8.16), move *Group* from the *Factor(s)* window to the *Post Hoc Tests for* window.

6. On the *Equal Variances Assumed* options, check ☑ *Bonferroni*.

Figure 8.16 Move *Group* to the *Post Hoc Tests for* window, and check ☑ *Bonferroni*.

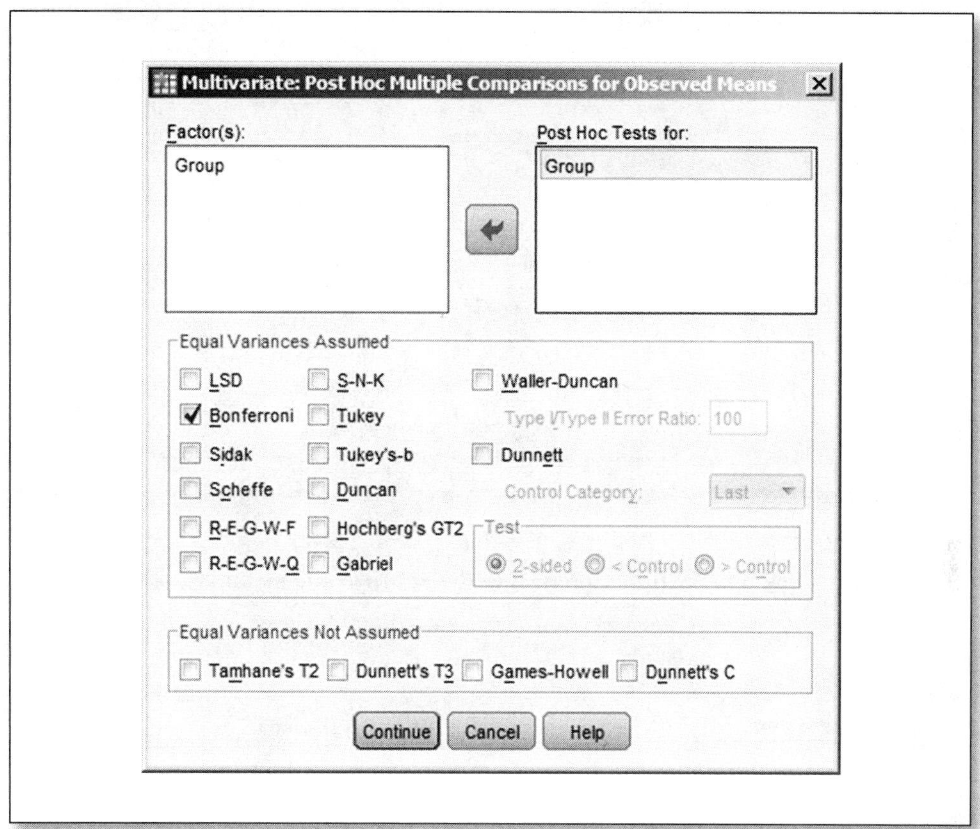

7. Click on *Continue* to return to the *Multivariate* menu.

8. On the *Multivariate* menu, click on *Options*.

9. On the *Multivariate: Options* menu (Figure 8.17), move *Group* into the *Display Means for* window.

10. Check ☑ *Homogeneity tests*.

Figure 8.17 On the *Multivariates: Options* menu, move *Group* into the *Display Means for* window, and check ☑ *Homogeneity tests.*

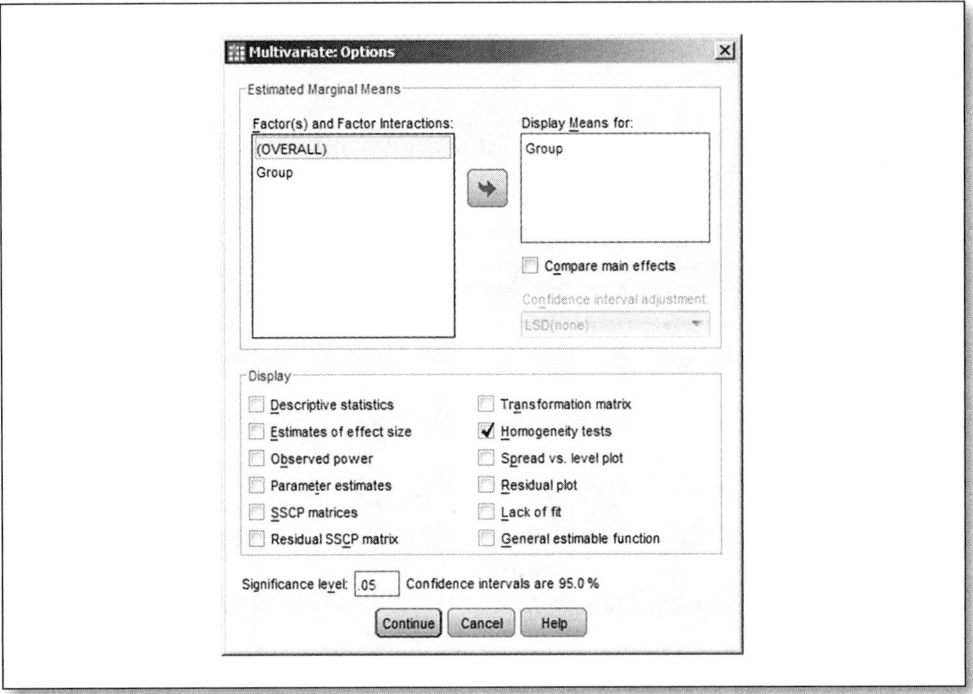

11. Click on *Continue* to return to the *Multivariate* menu.
12. On the *Multivariate* menu, click on *OK.*

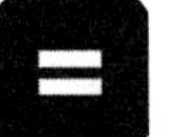

RESULTS

Pretest Checklist Criterion 4—Homogeneity of Variance-Covariance (Box's *M* Test)

To assess the homogeneity of variance-covariance, we look to *Box's Test of Equality of Covariance Matrices* (Table 8.3), which rendered a Sig. (p) = .703; since this is greater than the α (.001) associated with this test, this indicates that there is no significant difference between the variance-covariances in this model, and hence, this pretest criterion is satisfied.

Table 8.3 Box's *M* Test (*Box's Test of Equality of Covariance Matrices* Table) Shows No Statistically Significant Difference Among the Variances ($p = .703$, $\alpha = .001$).

Box's Test of Equality of Covariance Matrices[a]

Box's M	3.937
F	.634
df1	6
df2	188642.769
Sig.	.703

Tests the null hypothesis that the observed covariance matrices of the dependent variables are equal across groups.

a. Design: Intercept + Group

Pretest Checklist Criterion 5—Homogeneity of Variance (Levene's Test)

Next, the homogeneity of variance test checks to see that there is no statistically significant difference in the variances among the three groups (*Drug A, Drug B,* and *Drug C*) for each of the two outcome variables: *SystolicBP* and *Pulse*.

Levene's Test of Equality of Error Variances (Table 8.4) shows a Sig. (*p*) of .656 for *SystolicBP* and .765 for *Pulse*. Since these *p* values are greater than α (.05), this indicates that there is no statistically significant difference among the groups (*Drug A, Drug B, Drug C*) for the two outcome variables (*SystolicBP* and *Pulse*), and hence, this criterion is satisfied.

Proceeding with the results of the MANOVA test, the first table to inspect is the *Multivariate Tests* (Table 8.5); notice the four statistics pertaining to the *Group* variable: *Pillai's Trace* (symbol is "V"), *Wilks' Lambda* (symbol is "Λ"—the Greek letter, lambda), *Hotelling's Trace* (symbol is "T"), and *Roy's Largest Root* (symbol is "Θ"—the Greek letter, theta). Usually, these four will produce fairly similar *p* values; of these four, Pillai's Trace is considered to be preferred in that it is the most conservative and the most robust in terms of possible violations to the pretest checklist criteria (assumptions).

Table 8.4 *Levene's Test of Equality of Error Variances* shows a Sig. (p) of .656 for *SystolicBP* and .765 for *Pulse.*

Levene's Test of Equality of Error Variances[a]

	F	df1	df2	Sig.
SystolicBP	.423	2	87	.656
Pulse	.268	2	87	.765

Tests the null hypothesis that the error variance of the dependent variable is equal across groups.

a. Design: Intercept + Group

NOTE: Since these p values are greater than α (.05), this indicates that there is no statistically significant difference in the variances among the groups (*Drug A, Drug B, Drug C*) for the two outcome variables (*SystolicBP* and *Pulse*).

Table 8.5 *Multivariate Tests: Pillai's Trace* rendered a Sig. (p) = .003 (α = .05), Indicating That at Least One Statistically Significant Difference Has Been Detected Among the Pairs of Variables.

Multivariate Tests[c]

Effect		Value	F	Hypothesis df	Error df	Sig.
Intercept	Pillai's Trace	.999	83436.130[a]	2.000	86.000	.000
	Wilks' Lambda	.001	83436.130[a]	2.000	86.000	.000
	Hotelling's Trace	1940.375	83436.130[a]	2.000	86.000	.000
	Roy's Largest Root	1940.375	83436.130[a]	2.000	86.000	.000
Group	Pillai's Trace	.178	4.256	4.000	174.000	.003
	Wilks' Lambda	.828	4.266[a]	4.000	172.000	.003
	Hotelling's Trace	.201	4.274	4.000	170.000	.003
	Roy's Largest Root	.155	6.752[b]	2.000	87.000	.002

a. Exact statistic

b. The statistic is an upper bound on F that yields a lower bound on the significance level.

c. Design: Intercept + Group

Pillai's Trace indicates Sig. (p) = .003, which is less than the .05 α level, indicating that a statistically significant difference has been detected among the pairs of groups (*Drug A, Drug B, Drug C*) for the outcome (dependent) variables *SystolicBP* and *Pulse.*

To finalize this analysis, we look to the *Multiple Comparisons* table (Table 8.6) to determine which group(s) performed statistically significantly different from which and the *Estimates* table for the means (Table 8.7). Notice that the *Multiple Comparisons* table (Table 8.6) resembles two ANOVA Multiple Comparisons tables, wherein the top half of the table shows the three pairwise comparisons (*Drug A, Drug B, Drug C*) for *SystolicBP,* and the bottom half shows a separate set of comparisons for *Pulse.*

Despite all of these data being presented on a single table, this does not compound the complexity of the documentation process. The results will be documented as if we had conducted two separate ANOVA tests: one for *SystolicBP* (wherein pairs that are significantly different are identified with ovals) and another for *Pulse* (where rectangles are used).

Table 8.6 *Multiple Comparisons* Table Shows Pairwise Group Comparisons (*Drug A, Drug B, Drug C*) for Each of the Two Outcome Variables (*SystolicBP* at the Top and *Pulse* at the Bottom).

Multiple Comparisons

Bonferroni

Dependent Variable	(I) Group	(J) Group	Mean Difference (I-J)	Std. Error	Sig.	95% Confidence Interval	
						Lower Bound	Upper Bound
SystolicBP	Drug A	Drug B	-2.00*	.726	.022	-3.77	-.23
		Drug C	-2.33*	.726	.006	-4.11	-.56
	Drug B	Drug A	2.00*	.726	.022	.23	3.77
		Drug C	-.33	.726	1.000	-2.11	1.44
	Drug C	Drug A	2.33*	.726	.006	.56	4.11
		Drug B	.33	.726	1.000	-1.44	2.11
Pulse	Drug A	Drug B	-.53	1.608	1.000	-4.46	3.39
		Drug C	-4.17*	1.608	.034	-8.09	-.24
	Drug B	Drug A	.53	1.608	1.000	-3.39	4.46
		Drug C	-3.63	1.608	.079	-7.56	.29
	Drug C	Drug A	4.17*	1.608	.034	.24	8.09
		Drug B	3.63	1.608	.079	-.29	7.56

Based on observed means.

The error term is Mean Square(Error) = 38.805.

*. The mean difference is significant at the .05 level.

Table 8.7 Group *Estimates* Table Shows the Means From Each *Group* (*Drug A, Drug B, Drug C*) for Each of the Outcome Variables (*SystolicBP* at the Top and *Pulse* at the Bottom).

Estimates

Dependent Variable	Group	Mean	Std. Error	95% Confidence Interval Lower Bound	95% Confidence Interval Upper Bound
SystolicBP	Drug A	120.367	.514	119.346	121.387
	Drug B	122.367	.514	121.346	123.387
	Drug C	122.700	.514	121.679	123.721
Pulse	Drug A	79.933	1.137	77.673	82.194
	Drug B	80.467	1.137	78.206	82.727
	Drug C	84.100	1.137	81.839	86.361

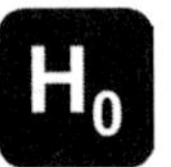

HYPOTHESIS RESOLUTION

To clarify the hypothesis resolution process, it is helpful to organize the findings in a table and use an asterisk to flag statistically significant difference(s) (Table 8.8).

Table 8.8 Results of MANOVA for *SystolicBP* and *Pulse.*

	MANOVA Summary Table	p
Systolic BP	μ(Drug A) = 120.37 : μ(Drug B) = 122.37	.022*
Systolic BP	μ(Drug A) = 120.37 : μ(Drug C) = 122.70	.006*
Systolic BP	μ(Drug B) = 122.37 : μ(Drug C) = 122.70	1.000
Pulse	μ(Drug A) = 79.93 : μ(Drug B) = 80.47	1.000
Pulse	μ(Drug A) = 79.93 : μ(Drug C) = 84.10	.034*
Pulse	μ(Drug B) = 80.47 : μ(Drug C) = 84.10	.079

NOTE: SPSS does not generate this table (Table 8.8) directly; you can assemble this table by gathering the means from the *Estimates* table (Table 8.7) and the *p* values from the Sig. column in the *Multiple Comparisons* table (Table 8.6).

*Statistically significant ($p \leq .05$).

With this results table assembled, consider the hypothesis resolution as if you had run two separate ANOVA tests.

REJECT: H_0: Drugs A, B, and C have equal effects on blood pressure and pulse rate.

ACCEPT: H_1: At least one drug (group) outperformed another in controlling blood pressure.

ACCEPT: H_2: At least one drug (group) had a unique effect on pulse rate.

Since a statistically significant difference was discovered among at least one pair of the drugs, we reject H_0 and accept H_1. Specifically, Drug A outperformed Drug B in lowering blood pressure ($p = .022$), and Drug A outperformed Drug C in lowering blood pressure ($p = .006$).

Additionally, it was found that the pulse rate of those who took Drug A was significantly different ($p = .034$) compared to those who took Drug C; hence, we reject H_0 (which is already rejected) and accept H_2.

DOCUMENTING RESULTS

When documenting the results of this study, both Table 8.8 and the following verbose summary would be appropriate to include:

A group of 90 patients with moderate hypertension (systolic between 130 and 140 mmHg) were recruited and randomly assigned to take Drug A, Drug B, or Drug C for 30 days.

After 1 month, patients who took Drug A had a mean systolic blood pressure of 120.37 mmHg, significantly outperforming Drug B (122.37 mmHg) ($p = .022$) and Drug C (122.70 mmHg) ($p = .006$) using an α of .05 (see Table). There was not a significant difference between Drugs B and C.

Additionally, it was found that the mean resting pulse rate of those who took Drug A (79.93 bpm) was significantly lower than those who took Drug C (84.10 bpm) ($p = .034$, $\alpha = .05$). There were no other significant differences in pulse rates between the drug groups.

Note: In the above documentation, notice that the second paragraph addresses the *SystolicBP* results, and the third paragraph (separately) discusses the *Pulse* rate results.

	Summary Table	**p**
Systolic BP	μ(Drug A) = 120.37 : μ(Drug B) = 122.37	.022*
Systolic BP	μ(Drug A) = 120.37 : μ(Drug C) = 122.70	.006*
Systolic BP	μ(Drug B) = 122.37 : μ(Drug C) = 122.70	1.000

(Continued)

(Continued)

Pulse	μ(Drug A) = 79.93 : μ(Drug B) = 80.47	1.000
Pulse	μ(Drug A) = 79.93 : μ(Drug C) = 84.10	.034*
Pulse	μ(Drug B) = 80.47 : μ(Drug C) = 84.10	.079

*Statistically significant ($p \leq .05$).

GOOD COMMON SENSE

One of the pretest criteria for running a quality MANOVA involves checking that the outcome (dependent) variables (*SystolicBP* and *Pulse*) are moderately correlated; they also need to be *conceptually* correlated. In the example that we processed, it is reasonable to consider the possible effect that an antihypertensive drug may have on the pulse rate; hence, the decision to include *Pulse* in this MANOVA conceptually makes sense. Conversely, gathering data on *SystolicBP* and *foot size* would constitute an implausible MANOVA model: It is unreasonable to presume that administering an antihypertensive drug would have any effect on the length of the patient's foot. Despite the obvious implausibility of this model, it may be that *SystolicBP* and *foot size* pass the moderate correlation test, but any such correlation should be reasonably dismissed as spurious (coincidental, but not pertinent).

Another point worth considering is that at the onset of this study, the participants were screened; all of the participants had a baseline systolic blood pressure between 130 and 140 mmHg; however, this design did not specify gathering a baseline pulse rate (although it could have). As such, the documentation of the results involving the pulse rate needs to be handled appropriately: The MANOVA revealed that those who took Drug A had the lowest mean pulse rate (79.93 bpm) compared to those who took Drug B (80.47 bpm) and those who took Drug C (84.10 bpm); however, since baseline pulse data were not gathered, it is not possible to determine precisely what effect the drug(s) had on the pulse rate. There are a variety of possibilities:

(1) Drug A lowered pulse; Drugs B and C lowered pulse but not as much as Drug A.

(2) Drug A lowered pulse; Drugs B and C had no effect on pulse.

(3) Drug A lowered pulse; Drugs B and C increased pulse.

(4) Drug A had no effect on pulse; Drugs B and C increased pulse.

(5) Drug A increased pulse; Drugs B and C increased pulse more than Drug A.

Given the experimental design and the data that are available, the above (pulse rate) possibilities are unresolvable; take appropriate care when phrasing such results. Alternatively, consider the advantage of gathering pretest data on outcome (dependent) variables, when feasible, to help reduce potentially ambiguous results.

Key Concepts

- MANOVA
- Pretest checklist
  - Sample size
  - Normality
  - Moderate correlation
  - Homogeneity of variance-covariance (Box's *M* test)
  - Homogeneity of variance (Levene's test)
- Hypothesis resolution
- Documenting results
- Good common sense

Practice Exercises

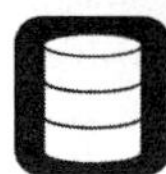

NOTE: These practice exercises and data sets are the same as those in **Chapter 6: ANOVA** except an extra outcome (dependent) variable has been included to enable MANOVA processing. All of the exercises involve three groups, except for Exercises 9 and 10, which involve four groups.

Exercise 8.1

You want to determine if meditation can reduce resting pulse rate. Participants were recruited and randomly assigned to one of three groups: Members of Group 1 (the control group) will not meditate; members of Group 2 (the first treatment group) will meditate for 30 minutes per day on Mondays, Wednesdays, and Fridays over the course of 2 weeks; and members of Group 3 (the second treatment group) will meditate for 30 minutes a day 6 days a week, Monday through Saturday. At the end, you gathered the resting pulse rates for each participant and administer the Acme Life Stress Index—a self-administered instrument (0 = No stress . . . 70 = High stress).

Data set: **Ch 08 – Exercise 01A.sav**

Codebook

Variable: Group
Definition: Group number
Type: Categorical (1 = No meditation, 2 = Meditates 3 days, 3 = Meditates 6 days)

Variable: Pulse
Definition: Pulse rate (beats per minute)
Type: Continuous

Variable: Stress
Definition: Acme Life Stress Index (0 = No stress . . . 70 = High stress)
Type: Continuous

a. Write the hypotheses.

b. Run each criterion of the pretest checklist (*n* quota, normality, moderate correlation, homogeneity of variance-covariance [Box's *M* test], and homogeneity of variance [Levene's test]) and discuss your findings.

c. Run the MANOVA test and document your findings (*n*s, means, and Sig. [*p* value], hypotheses resolution).

d. Write an abstract under 200 words detailing a summary of the study, the MANOVA test results, hypothesis resolution, and implications of your findings.

Repeat this exercise using data set: **Ch 08 – Exercise 01B.sav.**

Exercise 8.2

You want to determine the optimal preceptor-to-nurse ratio. Nurses will be randomly assigned to one of three groups: Group 1 will involve each preceptor working with only one nurse; in Group 2, each preceptor will work with two nurses; and in Group 3, each preceptor will work with five nurses. At the end of each shift, patients will be asked to complete the Acme Nursing Satisfaction Survey, which renders a score from 0 to 100, and the number of charting errors or omissions made during that shift per independent chart audit.

Data set: **Ch 08 – Exercise 02A.sav**

Codebook

Variable: Group
Definition: Group number
Type: Categorical (1 = One-to-one, 2 = Two-to-one, 3 = Five-to-one)

Variable: ANSS
Definition: Acme Nursing Satisfaction Survey score (0–100)
Type: Continuous

Variable: Chart_errors
Definition: Number of charting errors or omissions
Type: Continuous

a. Write the hypotheses.

b. Run each criterion of the pretest checklist (*n* quota, normality, moderate correlation, homogeneity of variance-covariance [Box's *M* test], and homogeneity of variance [Levene's test]) and discuss your findings.

c. Run the MANOVA test and document your findings (*n*s, means, and Sig. [*p* value], hypotheses resolution).

d. Write an abstract under 200 words detailing a summary of the study, the MANOVA test results, hypothesis resolution, and implications of your findings.

Repeat this exercise using **Ch 08 – Exercise 02B.sav.**

Exercise 8.3

Clinicians at a nursing home facility want to see if giving residents a plant to tend to will help lower depression. To test this idea, the residents are randomly assigned to one of three groups: Those assigned to Group 1 will serve as the control group and will not be given a plant. Members of Group 2 will be given a small bamboo plant along with a card detailing care instructions. Members of Group 3 will be given a small cactus along with a card detailing care instructions. After 90 days, all participants will complete the Acme Depression Scale, which renders a score between 1 and 100 (1 = Low depression . . . 100 = High depression). The staff will also keep track of the socialization of each participant (number of hours per day each resident is outside his or her room).

Data set: **Ch 08 – Exercise 03A.sav**

Codebook

Variable:	Group
Definition:	Group number
Type:	Categorical (1 = No plant, 2 = Bamboo, 3 = Cactus)
Variable:	Depress
Definition:	Acme Depression Scale (1 = Low depression . . . 100 = High depression)
Type:	Continuous
Variable:	Social_hours
Definition:	The mean number of hours per day the resident is out of his or her room (rounded to half-hour)
Type:	Continuous

a. Write the hypotheses.

b. Run each criterion of the pretest checklist (*n* quota, normality, moderate correlation, homogeneity of variance-covariance [Box's *M* test], and homogeneity of variance [Levene's test]) and discuss your findings.

c. Run the MANOVA test and document your findings (*n*s, means, and Sig. [*p* value], hypotheses resolution).

d. Write an abstract under 200 words detailing a summary of the study, the MANOVA test results, hypothesis resolution, and implications of your findings.

Repeat this exercise using **Ch 08 – Exercise 03B.sav.**

Exercise 8.4

You want to determine if chocolate enhances mood. Subjects will be recruited and randomly assigned to one of three groups: Those in Group 1 will be the control group and will eat their regular diet. Those in Group 2 will eat their usual meals and have a piece of chocolate at breakfast, lunch, and dinner over the course of a week. Those in Group 3 will eat their meals as usual and have two pieces of chocolate at breakfast, lunch, and dinner over the course of a week. At the end of the week, all participants will complete the Acme Mood Scale (1 = Extremely bad mood . . . 100 = Extremely good mood). Participants will maintain a written sleep journal, detailing the sleeping hours—the mean sleep hours per night will be entered into the database for each participant.

Data set: **Ch 08 – Exercise 04A.sav**

Codebook

Variable:	Group
Definition:	Group number
Type:	Categorical (1 = No chocolate, 2 = Chocolate [1 per meal], 3 = Chocolate [2 per meal])
Variable:	Mood
Definition:	Acme Mood Scale score (1–100)
Type:	Continuous
Variable:	Sleep
Definition:	Mean hours of sleep per night (rounded to half-hour)
Type:	Continuous

a. Write the hypotheses.

b. Run each criterion of the pretest checklist (n quota, normality, moderate correlation, homogeneity of variance-covariance [Box's M test], and homogeneity of variance [Levene's test]) and discuss your findings.

c. Run the MANOVA test and document your findings (ns, means, and Sig. [p value], hypotheses resolution).

d. Write an abstract under 200 words detailing a summary of the study, the MANOVA test results, hypothesis resolution, and implications of your findings.

Repeat this exercise using **Ch 08 – Exercise 04B.sav.**

Exercise 8.5

During flu season, the administrators at a walk-in health clinic want to determine if providing patients with a pamphlet or a video will increase their receptivity to flu shots. Each patient will be given a ticket at the check-in desk with a 1, 2, or 3 on it; the tickets will be issued in (repeating) sequence (e.g., 1, 2, 3, 1, 2, 3, etc.). Once escorted to the exam room, patients with a number 1 ticket will serve as control participants and will not be offered any flu shot informational material. Patients with a number 2 ticket will be given a flu shot information pamphlet describing the rationale for the flu shot and flu prevention practices, emphasizing effective hand hygiene. Patients with a number 3 ticket will be shown a brief video covering the same information as contained in the pamphlet. At the end of the day, the charts were reviewed and three entries were made in the database: total number of flu shots given to patients in Group 1, total number of flu shots given to patients in Group 2, and the total number of flu shots given to patients in Group 3. Ninety days after each patient appointment, the nurse researcher will send each patient the Acme Flu Symptom Survey (0 = No flu symptoms . . . 7 = Strong flu symptoms), which asks about flu symptoms over the 90 days, and compute the mean for each of the three groups for each day.

Data set: **Ch 08 – Exercise 05A.sav**

Codebook

Variable:	Group
Definition:	Group number
Type:	Categorical (1 = Nothing, 2 = Flu shot pamphlet, 3 = Flu shot video)
Variable:	Shots
Definition:	Number of flu shots given in a day for each group
Type:	Continuous
Variable:	Flu_symptoms
Definition:	Mean of Acme Flu Symptom Survey (0 = No flu symptoms . . . 7 = Strong flu symptoms) for each group, 90 days after appointment
Type:	Continuous

a. Write the hypotheses.
b. Run each criterion of the pretest checklist (*n* quota, normality, moderate correlation, homogeneity of variance-covariance [Box's *M* test], and homogeneity of variance [Levene's test]) and discuss your findings.
c. Run the MANOVA test and document your findings (*n*s, means, and Sig. [*p* value], hypotheses resolution).
d. Write an abstract under 200 words detailing a summary of the study, the MANOVA test results, hypothesis resolution, and implications of your findings.

Repeat this exercise using **Ch 08 – Exercise 05B.sav.**

Exercise 8.6

You want to determine if introducing a video in the waiting area will help relax patients. This study will take place over 3 days: On the first day, Group 1 (the control group) will experience the waiting room as is—with the monitor off; on the second day, Group 2 will have a classic movie playing; and on the third day, Group 3 will have a scenic video playing (e.g., waterfalls, vistas, wildlife). For patients who consent to participating in this research, the nurse will anonymously copy their pulse rate and O_2 level (as gathered by a pulse oximeter) to a journal along with the day number (Group).

Data set: **Ch 08 – Exercise 06A.sav**

Codebook

Variable:	Group
Definition:	Group number
Type:	Categorical (1 = Control, 2 = Classic movie, 3 = Scenic video)

Variable: Pulse
Definition: Pulse rate (gathered by a pulse oximeter)
Type: Continuous

Variable: O2
Definition: O_2 level (gathered by pulse oximeter)
Type: Continuous

a. Write the hypotheses.

b. Run each criterion of the pretest checklist (*n* quota, normality, moderate correlation, homogeneity of variance-covariance [Box's *M* test], and homogeneity of variance [Levene's test]) and discuss your findings.

c. Run the MANOVA test and document your findings (*n*s, means, and Sig. [*p* value], hypotheses resolution).

d. Write an abstract under 200 words detailing a summary of the study, the MANOVA test results, hypothesis resolution, and implications of your findings.

Repeat this exercise using **Ch 08 – Exercise 06B.sav.**

Exercise 8.7

In an effort to determine the effectiveness of light therapy to alleviate depression, you recruit a group of subjects who have been diagnosed with depression. The subjects are randomly assigned to one of three groups: Group 1 will be the control group—members of this group will receive no light therapy. Members of Group 2 will get light therapy for 1 hour on even-numbered days over the course of 1 month. Members of Group 3 will get light therapy every day for 1 hour over the course of 1 month. After 1 month, all participants will complete the Acme Mood Scale, consisting of 10 questions; this instrument renders a score between 1 and 100 (1 = Extremely bad mood . . . 100 = Extremely good mood). Additionally, each participant will respond to the Acme Self Care Survey—a self-administered survey (5 = Strong self-neglect . . . 30 = Strong self-care).

Data set: **Ch 08 – Exercise 07A.sav**

Codebook

Variable: Group
Definition: Group number
Type: Categorical (1 = No light therapy, 2 = Light therapy: even days, 3 = Light therapy: every day)

Variable: Mood
Definition: Acme Mood Scale (1 = Extremely bad mood . . . 100 = Extremely good mood)
Type: Continuous

Variable: Self_care
Definition: Acme Self Care Survey (5 = Strong self-neglect . . . 30 = Strong self-care)
Type: Continuous

a. Write the hypotheses.

b. Run each criterion of the pretest checklist (*n* quota, normality, moderate correlation, homogeneity of variance-covariance [Box's *M* test], and homogeneity of variance [Levene's test]) and discuss your findings.

c. Run the MANOVA test and document your findings (*n*s, means, and Sig. [*p* value], hypotheses resolution).

d. Write an abstract under 200 words detailing a summary of the study, the MANOVA test results, hypothesis resolution, and implications of your findings.

Repeat this exercise using **Ch 08 – Exercise 07B.sav.**

Exercise 8.8

It is thought that exercising early in the morning will provide better energy throughout the day. To test this idea, subjects are recruited and randomly assigned to one of three groups: Members of Group 1 will constitute the control group and not be assigned any walking. Members of Group 2 will walk from 7:00 to 7:30 a.m., Monday through Friday, over the course of 30 days. Members of Group 3 will walk from 7:00 to 8:00 a.m., Monday through Friday, over the course of 30 days. At the conclusion of the study, each subject will answer the 10 questions on the Acme End-of-the-Day Energy Scale. This instrument produces a score between 1 and 100 (1 = Extremely low energy . . . 100 = Extremely high energy). The nurse will also record the number of sick days each participant has had over the past 30 days.

Data set: **Ch 08 – Exercise 08A.sav**

Codebook

Variable: Group
Definition: Group number
Type: Categorical (1 = No walking, 2 = Walking: 30 Minutes, 3 = Walking: 60 minutes)

Variable: Mood
Definition: Acme End-of-the-Day Energy Scale (1 = Extremely low energy . . . 100 = Extremely high energy)
Type: Continuous

Variable: Sick_days
Definition: Number of sick days over the past 30 days
Type: Continuous

a. Write the hypotheses.

b. Run each criterion of the pretest checklist (*n* quota, normality, moderate correlation, homogeneity of variance-covariance [Box's *M* test], and homogeneity of variance [Levene's test]) and discuss your findings.

c. Run the MANOVA test and document your findings (*n*s, means, and Sig. [*p* value], hypotheses resolution).

d. Write an abstract under 200 words detailing a summary of the study, the MANOVA test results, hypothesis resolution, and implications of your findings.

Repeat this exercise using **Ch 08 – Exercise 08B.sav.**

NOTE: Exercises 9 and 10 involve four groups each.

Exercise 8.9

To determine the best method for facilitating smoking cessation, patients who smoke two packs per day (40 cigarettes) are recruited and randomly assigned to one of four psycho-educational peer support groups with a qualified facilitator: Group 1 will meet once a week in an in-person setting, Group 2 will meet once a week via Internet videoconferencing, Group 3 will meet twice a week in-person, and Group 4 will meet twice a week via videoconferences. After 10 weeks, each participant will be asked how many cigarettes he or she smokes per day and how much weight he or she has lost or gained.

Data set: **Ch 08 – Exercise 09A.sav**

Codebook

Variable: Group
Definition: Group number
Type: Categorical (1 = 1 meeting in-person, 2 = 1 meeting videoconference, 3 = 2 meetings in-person, 4 = 2 meetings videoconference)

Variable: Smoking
Definition: Number of cigarettes each participant smokes per day after 10 weeks
Type: Continuous

Variable: Weight_change
Definition: Difference in weight (in pounds) from start to end

(NOTE: Negative value indicates weight loss; positive value indicates weight gain)

Type: Continuous

a. Write the hypotheses.

b. Run each criterion of the pretest checklist (*n* quota, normality, moderate correlation, homogeneity of variance-covariance [Box's *M* test], and homogeneity of variance [Levene's test]) and discuss your findings.

c. Run the MANOVA test and document your findings (*n*s, means, and Sig. [*p* value], hypotheses resolution).

d. Write an abstract under 200 words detailing a summary of the study, the MANOVA test results, hypothesis resolution, and implications of your findings.

Repeat this exercise using **Ch 08 – Exercise 09B.sav.**

Exercise 8.10

Due to numerous complications involving missed medication dosages, you implement a study to determine the best strategy for enhancing medication adherence. Patients who are on a daily medication regime will be recruited, receive a complimentary 1-month dosage of their regular medication(s), and randomly assigned to one of four groups: Group 1 will serve as the control group (no treatment); Group 2 will participate in a 1-hour in-person nurse-administered medication adherence workshop; Group 3 will receive text message reminders (e.g., "It's time to take one tablet of Drug A"); Group 4 will attend the medication adherence workshop and also receive text messages. At the end of 1 month, participants will present their prescription bottle(s); the nurse will count the remaining pills and calculate the dosage adherence percentage (e.g., 0 pills remaining = 100% adherence). At the conclusion of the month, each participant will answer the Acme Health Outlook Survey—a self-administered instrument to measure how pessimistic/optimistic one feels about his or her health (1 = Strong negative outlook . . . 20 = Strong positive outlook).

Data set: **Ch 08 – Exercise 10A.sav**

Codebook

Variable:	Group
Definition:	Group number
Type:	Categorical (1 = Control, 2 = Rx workshop, 3 = Texts, 4 = Rx workshop and texts)
Variable:	RxAdhere
Definition:	Percentage of medication adherence (0–100)
Type:	Continuous
Variable:	Health_outlook
Definition:	Score on Acme Health Outlook Survey (1 = Strong negative outlook . . . 20 = Strong positive outlook)
Type:	Continuous

a. Write the hypotheses.

b. Run each criterion of the pretest checklist (*n* quota, normality, moderate correlation, homogeneity of variance-covariance [Box's *M* test], and homogeneity of variance [Levene's test]) and discuss your findings.

c. Run the MANOVA test and document your findings (*n*s, means, and Sig. [*p* value], hypotheses resolution).

d. Write an abstract under 200 words detailing a summary of the study, the MANOVA test results, hypothesis resolution, and implications of your findings.

Repeat this exercise using **Ch 08 – Exercise 10B.sav.**

PART IV

Measuring Differences Over Time

These chapters provide statistics for detecting change(s) in a continuous variable over time using a single group.

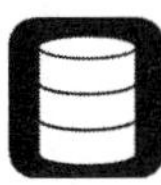

LAYERED LEARNING

Chapter 9: Paired *t* Test and Wilcoxon Test: The **paired *t* test** is generally used to gather data on a variable before and after an intervention to determine if the performance on the posttest is significantly better than the pretest. In the event that the data are not fully suitable to run a **paired *t* test,** the **Wilcoxon test** provides an alternative.

Chapter 10: ANOVA Repeated Measures is similar to the **paired *t* test,** but it is capable of assessing a variable over *more than two time points.*

CHAPTER 9

Paired *t* Test and Wilcoxon Test

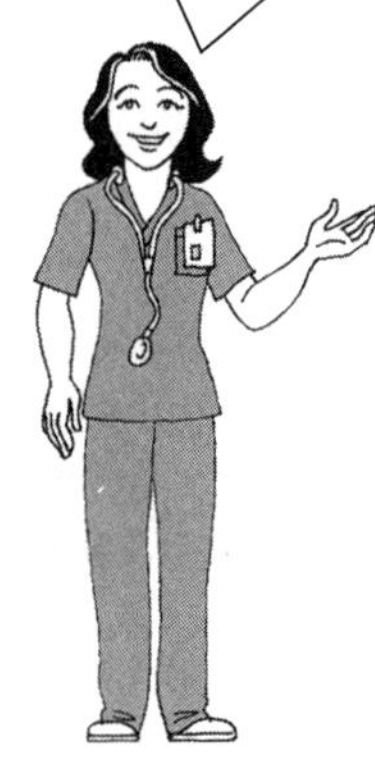

To compare pretest to posttest for continuous variables, run a **Paired t Test**.

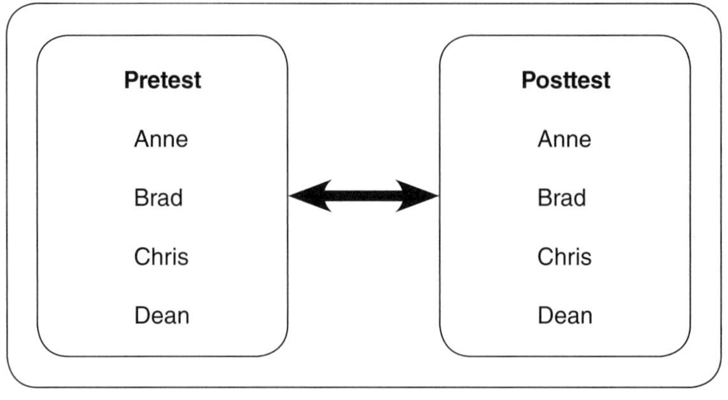

Things never happen the same way twice.

—C. S. Lewis

LEARNING OBJECTIVES

Upon completing this chapter, you will be able to:

- Determine when it is appropriate to run a paired *t* test
- Verify that the data meet the criteria for paired *t* test processing: normality of differences
- Order a paired *t* test
- Interpret test results
- Resolve the hypotheses
- Know when and how to run and interpret the Wilcoxon test
- Document the results in plain English
- Calculate and document the Δ% formula

TUTORIAL VIDEO

The tutorial videos for this chapter are **Ch 09 – Paired t Test.mp4** and **Ch 09 – Wilcoxon Test.mp4.** These videos provide an overview of these tests, followed by the SPSS procedures for processing the pretest checklist, ordering the statistical run, and interpreting the results using the data set: **Ch 09 – Example 01 – Paired t Test.sav.**

OVERVIEW—PAIRED *t* TEST

The *t* test and ANOVA test were appropriate for conducting research using a classic experimental model, which involves random assignment of participants to a control group and at least one other (treatment) group. There will be times when such rigorous designs are not feasible due to limited resources (e.g., low *n,* limited staff, lack of facilities, budget constraints, etc.). The paired *t* test provides an alternate approach that can be used to test the effectiveness of an implementation using a single group that does not require a sizable *n.*

Pretest/Posttest Design

The design associated with the paired *t* test is typically referred to as a *pretest/posttest design,* also known as a *simple time-series design,* or *O X O design* (O = observation, X = treatment) (Figure 9.1).

Figure 9.1 Pretest/posttest design.

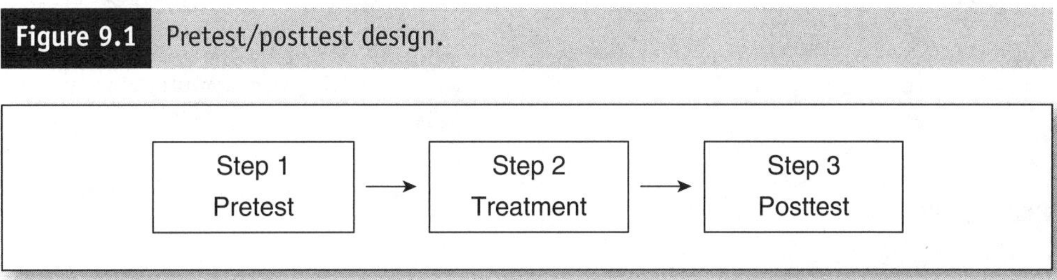

This design consists of one group and three steps:

Step 1: Pretest

Begin by gathering a quantitative metric, and attach each participant's name or ID to the score. The score needs to be a continuous variable. This could be an existing score or a test that you administer. This will be the *pretest* score, sometimes referred to as the *baseline* score, indicating the level that each participant was at prior to exposing him or her to the treatment. For the *t* test processing, it is important that the participant's name or ID is included with his or her responses (the pretest score for each participant will need to be paired with his or her posttest score). Essentially, each subject acts as his or her own control group.

Step 2: Treatment

Execute the treatment (e.g., intervention, change in condition, training, etc.).

Step 3: Posttest

Administer the same test that was used in Step 1 (pretest) to the same people and record the participant's name or ID with the score.

The paired *t* test analysis produces three critical pieces of information: (1) the mean pretest score, (2) the mean posttest score, and (3) the *p* value. If the *p* value is less than or equal to the specified α level (.05), then this indicates that there is a statistically significant difference between the pretest score and the posttest score, suggesting that the treatment made an impact.

Example

The nurse who is leading the smoking cessation group wants to determine the effectiveness of the intervention.

Research Question

The question is as follows: Will providing a 1-hour smoking cessation seminar help to reduce smoking among the participants?

Groups

As stated earlier, part of the utility of the paired *t* test is that it can function with just one group. The (one) group will consist of 40 participants who want to stop smoking.

Procedure

Step 1: Pretest

The week before the smoking cessation seminar, each participant is issued a special cigarette lighter equipped to digitally record the date and time each time it is lit—each light counts as one cigarette smoked. After 7 days, each participant will bring his or her lighter to the smoking cessation seminar. The data from each lighter will be downloaded into a database where a daily (baseline) smoking mean will be computed and entered as the *pretest* (mean daily smoking) score for each participant. The data on each lighter will be cleared and then returned to the participants.

Step 2: Treatment

The nurse administers the 1-hour smoking cessation seminar.

Step 3: Posttest

After 1 week, the participants return with their lighters; data from the second week are downloaded, and the mean daily smoking rate for each participant is computed and entered into the database as the *posttest* score.

Hypotheses

H_0: The smoking cessation seminar is not effective in reducing smoking.

H_1: The smoking cessation seminar is effective in reducing smoking.

Data Set

Use the following data set: **Ch 09 – Example 01 – Paired t Test.sav.**

Codebook

Variable:	Initials
Definition:	Initials of each participant (first, middle, last)
Type:	Alphanumeric
Variable:	Pretest
Definition:	Baseline average number of cigarettes smoked daily (over 7 days)
Type:	Continuous
Variable:	Posttest
Definition:	Average number of cigarettes smoked daily (over 7 days) after smoking cessation treatment
Type:	Continuous

Pretest Checklist

Paired *t* Test Pretest Checklist

☑ 1. Normality of differences*

*Run prior to paired *t* test

Pretest Checklist Criterion 1—Normality of Differences

To run a paired *t* test, only one pretest criterion must be satisfied: The difference between the *Pretest* scores and the *Posttest* scores must be normally distributed. This process involves two steps:

(1) We will have SPSS compute a new variable (*Diff*), which will contain the difference between each *Pretest* score and the corresponding *Posttest* score for each record (*Diff* = *Posttest* – *Pretest*).

(2) We will run a histogram with a normal curve for *Diff* and inspect the curve for normality.

1. On the main screen, click on Transform, Compute Variable (Figure 9.2).

Figure 9.2 Select *Transform, Compute Variable*

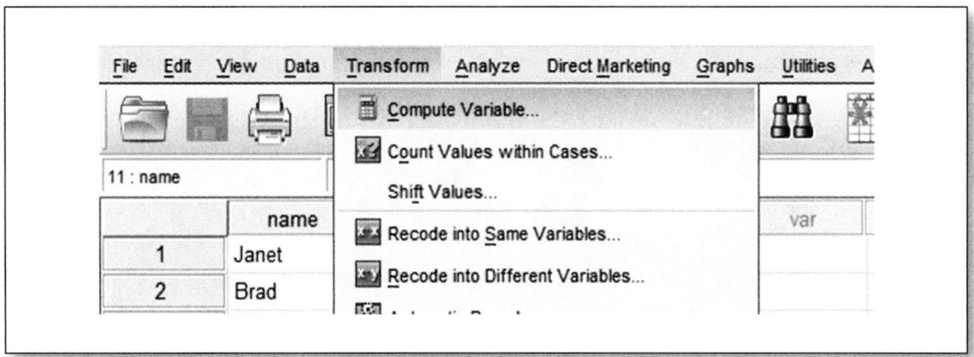

2. On the Compute Variable menu (Figure 9.3). Enter Diff in the Target Variable box. Enter Posttest – Pretest in the Numeric Expression box. You can type in the variables Posttest and Pretest, double-click on them, or use the arrow key to copy them from the left box to the right box.

NOTE: For this procedure, you can enter *Posttest – Pretest or Pretest – Posttest*; either is fine.

3. Click the OK button to process this menu.

Notice that this operation created a new variable, *Diff* (Figure 9.4), which equals the *Posttest* – *Pretest* for each row. We can now order the histogram with a normal curve for the *Diff* variable. This is the same procedure used as part of the pretest checklist for the *t* test and ANOVA. For more details on this procedure, refer to Chapter 4 ("SPSS—Descriptive Statistics: Continuous Variables (Age)"); see the star (★) icon on page **58**.

Alternatively, the following steps will produce a histogram with a normal curve for *Diff:*

1. From the main screen, select *Analyze, Descriptive Statistics, Frequencies*; this will take you to the *Frequencies* menu.

2. On the *Frequencies* menu, move *Diff* from the left window to the right (*Variables*) window.

3. Click on the *Charts* button; this will take you to the *Charts* menu.

Figure 9.3 *Compute Variable* menu.

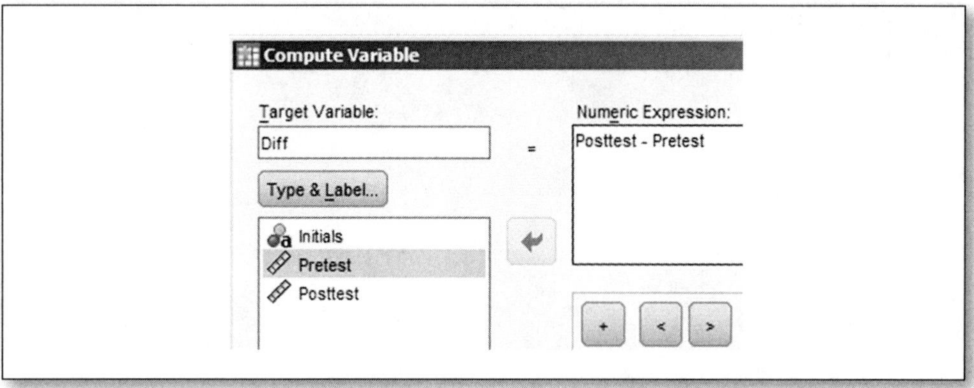

Figure 9.4 *Data View* reveals new variable: *Diff* (derived from Posttest – Pretest).

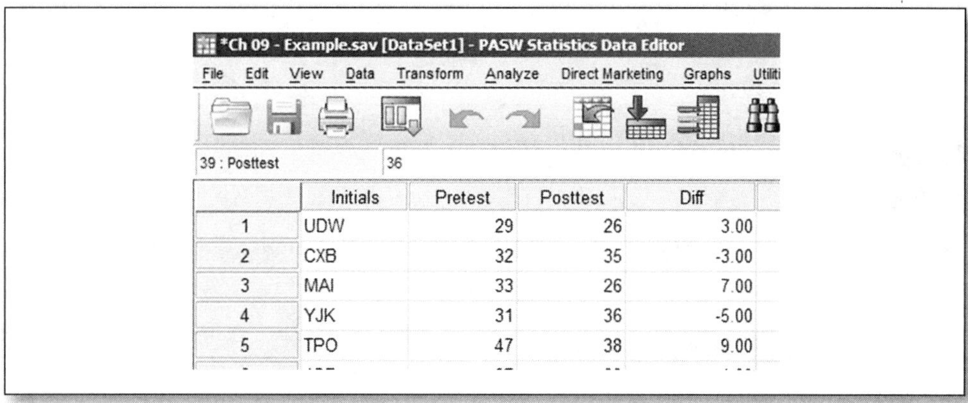

4. Click on the *Histograms* button, and check the *Show normal curve on histogram* checkbox.
5. Click on the *Continue* button; this will return you to the *Frequencies* menu.
6. Click on the *OK* button, and the system will produce a histogram with a normal curve for the *Diff* variable (Figure 9.5).

The normal curve for *Diff* (Figure 9.5) presents as a reasonably symmetrical bell shape—hence, we would say that the difference between the *Pretest* and *Posttest* scores meets the criteria of normality.

Figure 9.5 Histogram with normal curve for *Diff*

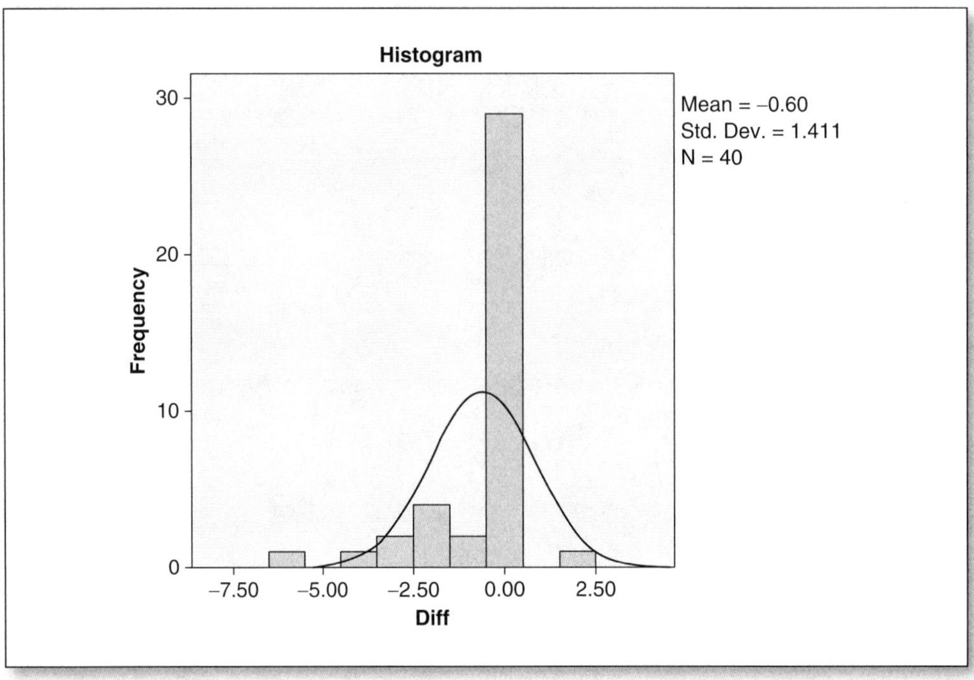

Test Run

1. Click on Analyze, Compare Means, Paired-Samples T Test (Figure 9.6).

Figure 9.6 Order paired *t* test.

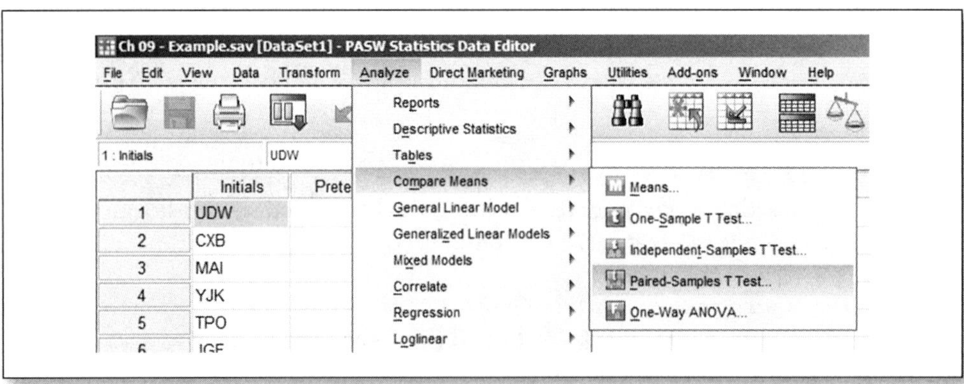

This will take you to the *Paired-Samples T Test* menu (Figure 9.7).

Figure 9.7 Paired-samples *t* test menu.

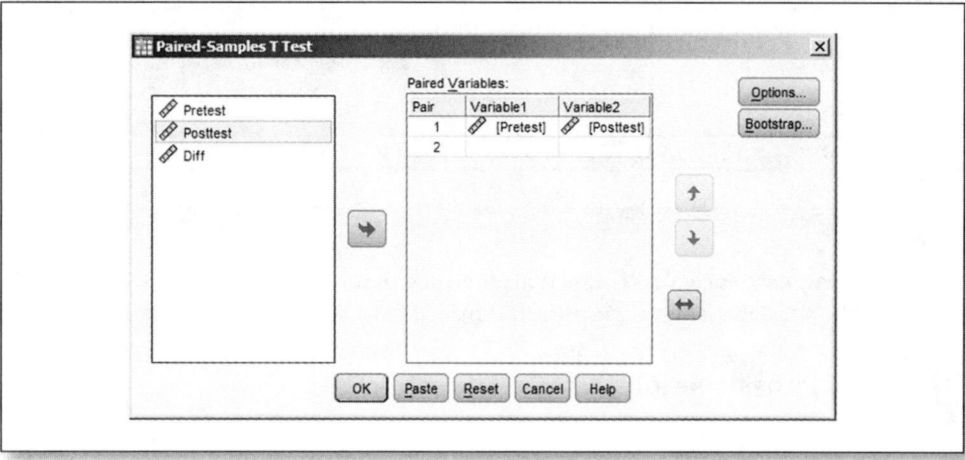

2. On the Paired-Samples T Test menu (Figure 9.7), copy the *Pretest* variable from the left window to the right window (under *Variable1*); next, copy the *Posttest* variable from the left window to the right window (under *Variable2*).

3. Click on *OK*.

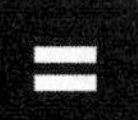

Results

The results of the paired *t* test are read from two tables: The *paired-samples statistics test* (Table 9.1) reports the means for each group: μ(Pretest) = 29.40 and μ(Posttest) = 28.80. The table also shows the corresponding *ns* and standard deviations.

Table 9.1 Paired-Samples (Summary) Statistics for *Pretest* and *Posttest*.

Paired-Samples Statistics

		Mean	N	Std. Deviation	Std. Error Mean
Pair 1	Pretest	29.40	40	6.109	.966
	Posttest	28.80	40	6.277	.992

The *Paired-Samples Test* (Table 9.2) focuses on the difference between the mean of the *Pretest* (μ = 29.40) and the mean of the *Posttest* (μ = 28.80) scores, which is .600 (29.40 − 28.80 = .600). The last column (Sig.) shows that the *p* value is .010 for this

Table 9.2 Paired-Samples Test Results.

Paired-Samples Test

	Paired Differences					t	df	Sig. (2-tailed)
				95% Confidence Interval of the Difference				
	Mean	Std. Deviation	Std. Error Mean	Lower	Upper			
Pair 1 Pretest - Posttest	.600	1.411	.223	.149	1.051	2.690	39	.010

comparison; since .010 is less than the specified α level of .05, we would conclude that there is a statistically significant difference between the *Pretest* and *Posttest* scores.

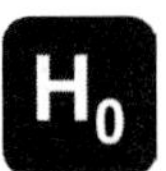

Hypothesis Resolution

H_0: The smoking cessation seminar is not effective in reducing smoking.

H_1: The smoking cessation seminar is effective in reducing smoking.

Since the *p* value (.010) is less than the specified α level (.05), this suggests that the .6 decrease in the mean number of cigarettes smoked per day (from 29.40 to 28.80) is statistically significant. In terms of the hypotheses, we would reject H_0 and not reject H_1.

Document Results

The paired *t* test is a fairly straightforward process; as such, the documentation is typically concise:

Each of the 40 participants in our smoking cessation program was issued a cigarette lighter equipped with technology to digitally record the date and time of each light. We compared daily average smoking figures for the week before and week after our program. After the first week of the intervention, participants smoked an average of .6 fewer cigarettes (down from 29.4 to 28.8), which is a statistically significant decrease in daily smoking (p = .01, α = .05).

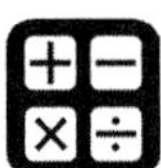

Δ% Formula

The change from *Pretest* to *Posttest* can also be expressed clearly as a percentage using the Δ% formula (Δ is the Greek letter delta, which symbolizes *change*). SPSS does not provide the Δ%, but you can easily process this formula on any calculator, simply by plugging two variables into the equation: **Δ% = (New − Old) ÷ Old × 100,** where the *Old* value is *Pretest* mean (29.4), and the *New* value is *Posttest* mean (28.8) (Table 9.3).

NOTE: In this example, the Δ% formula produced a *negative* value (Δ% = −2.04), which translates to a 2.04% *decrease* from *Pretest* to *Posttest*. Conversely, a *positive* Δ% (e.g., Δ% = 2.04), would indicate a 2.04% *increase* from *Pretest* to *Posttest*.

In terms of documentation, you could include the Δ% = −2.04 as is or express it verbosely: *We observed a 2.04% decrease in smoking, from a baseline mean of 29.4 cigarettes per day (measured over the week prior to our program), down to 28.8 after the first week of our program.*

Table 9.3 Δ% Formula Computes Change Percentage.

Δ% Formula
Δ% = (New − Old) ÷ Old × 100
Δ% = (28.8 − 29.4) ÷ 29.4 × 100
Δ% = (−.6) ÷ 29.4 × 100
Δ% = −.0204 × 100
Δ% = −2.04

OVERVIEW—WILCOXON TEST

Remember that the pretest criteria that must be assessed prior to running a paired *t* test require that the difference between each pair of scores must be computed (which produced the *Diff* variable) and that those differences (contained in the *Diff* variable) must be normally distributed (Figure 9.8); minor variations in the normal distribution are acceptable. Occasionally, you may encounter data that are substantially skewed (Figure 9.9), bimodal (Figure 9.10), flat (Figure 9.11), or may have some other atypical distribution. In such instances, the Wilcoxon statistic is an appropriate alternative to the paired *t* test.

Figure 9.8 Normal.

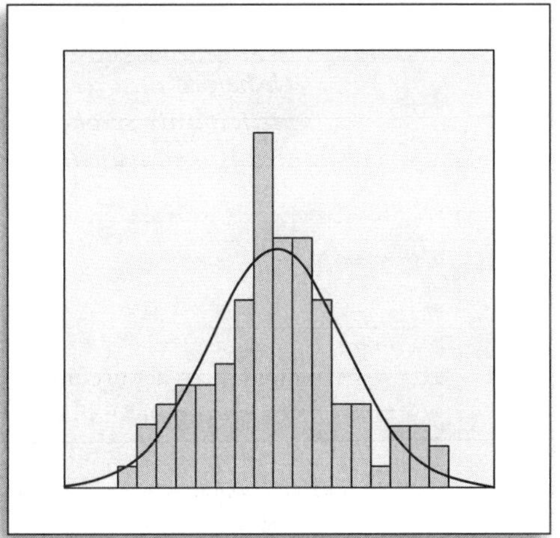

Figure 9.9 Skewed.

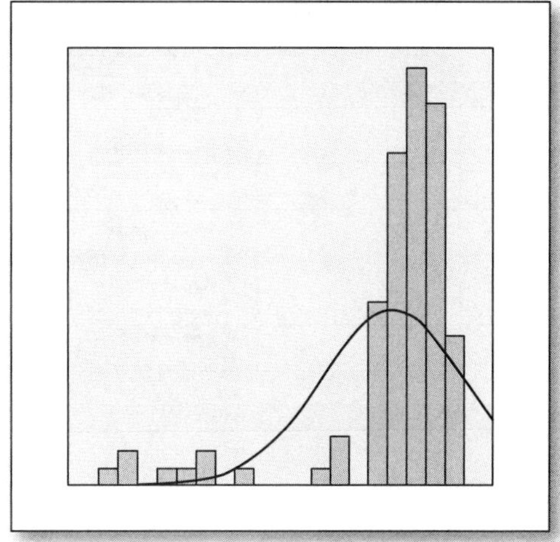

Figure 9.10 Bimodal.

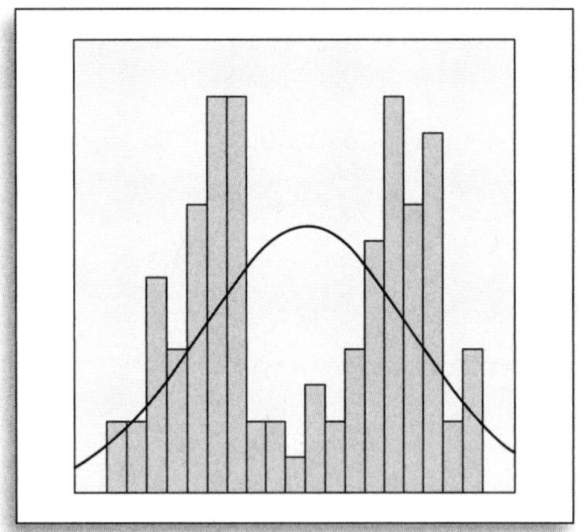

Figure 9.11 Flat.

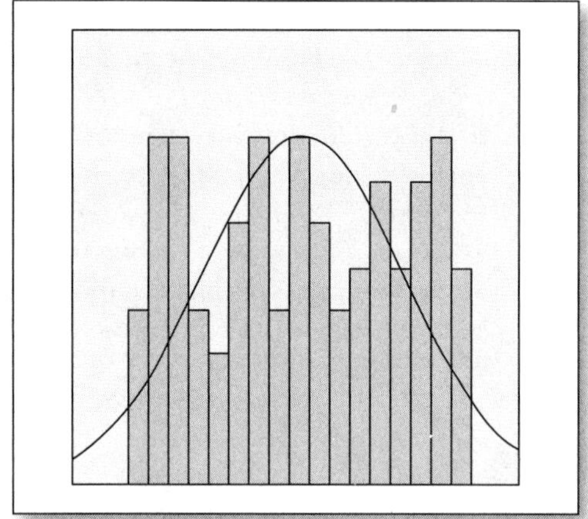

Test Run

For exemplary purposes, we will run the Wilcoxon test using the same data set (**Ch 09 – Example 01 – Paired t Test.sav**) even though the data are normally distributed. This will enable us to compare the results of a paired *t* test to the results produced by the Wilcoxon test.

1. On the main screen, click on *Analyze, Nonparametric Tests, Legacy Dialogs, 2 Related Samples* (Figure 9.12).

Figure 9.12 Ordering the Wilcoxon: click on *Analyze, Nonparametric Tests, Legacy Dialogs, 2 Related Samples.*

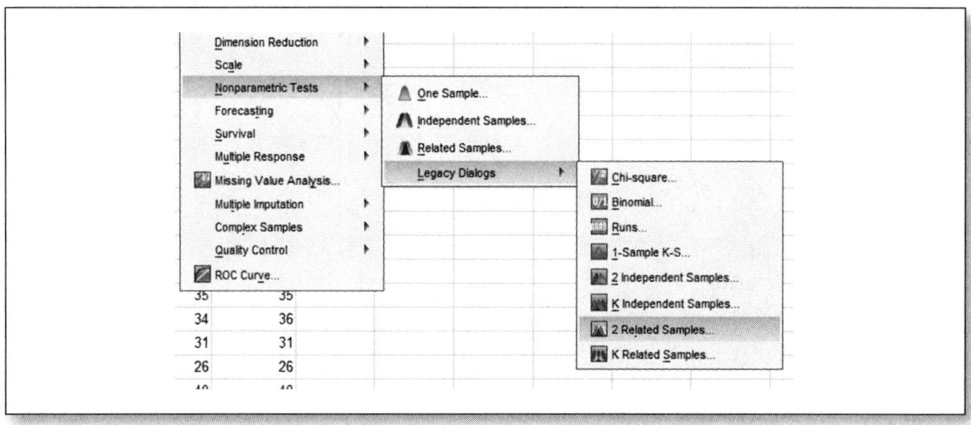

2. On the *Two-Related-Samples Tests* menu (Figure 9.13), move *Pretest* to *Variable1*.
3. Move *Posttest* to *Variable2*.
4. Click on *OK*.

Figure 9.13 On the *Two-Related-Samples Tests* menu, move *Pretest* to *Variable1* and *Posttest* to *Variable 2*.

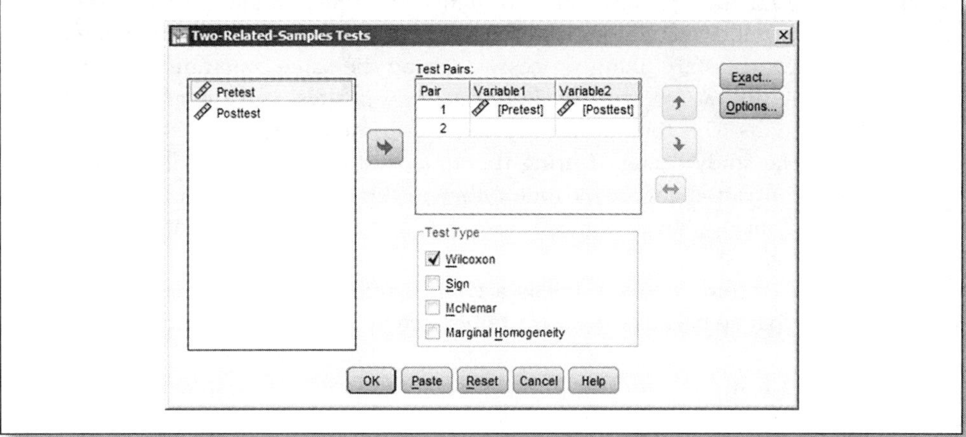

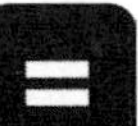

Results

The Wilcoxon test result is found on the *Test Statistics* table (Table 9.4); the *Asymp. Sig. (2-tailed)* statistic rendered a *p* value of .012; since this is less than α (.05), we would conclude that there is a statistically significant difference between the scores of the pretest and the posttest.

Referring back, remember that the paired *t* test produced a *p* value of .010. The differences in these *p* values are due to the internal transformations that the Wilcoxon test conducts on the data. If a substantial violation in the normality criteria is detected when running the pretest checklist for the paired *t* test, then the Wilcoxon test is considered a viable alternative.

Table 9.4 Wilcoxon *p* Value = .012.

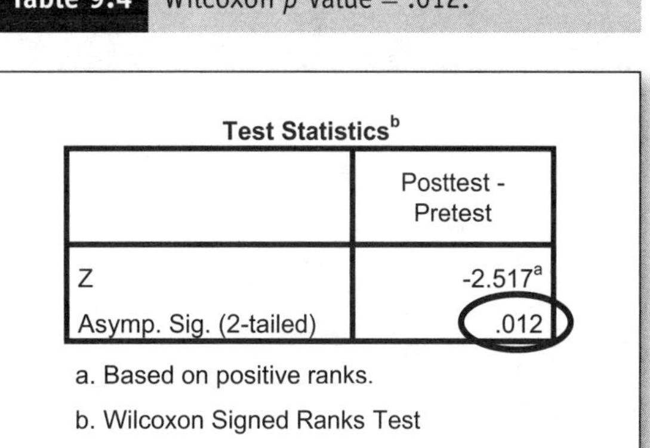

Test Statistics[b]

	Posttest - Pretest
Z	-2.517[a]
Asymp. Sig. (2-tailed)	.012

a. Based on positive ranks.

b. Wilcoxon Signed Ranks Test

GOOD COMMON SENSE

For simplicity, the example used in this chapter focused exclusively on weekly smoking, but you may opt to gather additional pre/post data (e.g., job satisfaction survey scores, stress, (over) eating, drinking, other substance usage, etc.) and conduct separate paired *t* tests on those metrics as well. Such findings may shed light on other relevant variables; since this intervention involves reducing/eliminating smoking, it may be wise to include additional pretest/posttest metrics that gather data on other possibly relevant topics such as irritability, sleep hours, social/coworker relations, and so on.

When opting for the pretest/posttest design and corresponding paired *t* test, the potential for historical confounds must be considered. In a classic experimental design, the control group and treatment group(s) are being processed during the same timeframe, but when using the paired *t* test, the pretest (control/baseline) data and posttest (treatment) data are collected at different time points. This time difference may involve minutes, hours, weeks, or even months, depending on the study design. During this time, history does not stand still; things outside your investigation can change over time either in the individual or in the environment (e.g., personal issues, sociopolitical events, season, etc.), which could potentially affect the pretest or posttest scores.

Additionally, in some cases, there is a chance that participants may show improvement in the posttest, partly because they are familiar with it—they remember it from the pretest phase.

The paired *t* test has other applications beyond pretest/posttest designs. The paired *t* test may be used when two continuous variables are gathered, each from the same person, provided that both variables are used to measure the same outcome, which are scaled the same. For example, suppose you wanted to determine the accuracy of a new ear thermometer compared to an oral thermometer, which is known to produce stable readings. You could take both measures (*Ear* and *Oral* temperature) from each patient in a group, and instead of naming the variables *Pretest* and *Posttest,* they would be named (and processed) as *Ear* and *Oral*.

Key Concepts

- Paired *t* test
- Paired *t* test designs (synonyms):
  - Pretest/treatment/posttest
  - Pretest/posttest design
  - Simple time-series design
  - O-X-O design
- Histogram with a normal curve
- Paired *t* test with multiple metrics
- Δ%
- Historical confound
- Wilcoxon test
- Good common sense

Practice Exercises

Exercise 9.1

Nursing students are given a list of 60 pills that they need to visually identify. Students are issued a deck of 60 flashcards with the picture of the pill on one side and the name of the pill on the other side. Before studying, students are instructed to record their *Pretest* score—the number of pills they correctly identify from the picture (0–60) on their first pass through the deck. After 30 minutes of studying the cards that they got wrong, the student is instructed to shuffle all of the cards and record his or her *Posttest* pill identification score (0–60).

Data set: **Ch 09 – Exercise 01A.sav**

Codebook

Variable:	ID
Definition:	Student ID (first and last initials)
Type:	Alphanumeric
Variable:	Pretest
Definition:	Number of pills correctly identified on the first attempt
Type:	Continuous
Variable:	Enrolled
Definition:	Number of pills correctly identified on the second attempt
Type:	Continuous

a. Write the hypotheses.

b. Run the criteria of the pretest checklist (normality for *Posttest* – *Pretest*) and discuss your findings.

c. Run the paired *t* test and document your findings (means and Sig. [*p* value], hypothesis resolution).

d. Write an abstract under 200 words detailing a summary of the study, the paired *t* test results, hypothesis resolution, and implications of your findings.

Repeat this exercise using data set: **Ch 09 – Exercise 01B.sav.**

Exercise 9.2

Prior to a Heart Health presentation, you administer a survey asking participants to indicate how many times they used the stairs (as opposed to the elevator) in the past week. A week after the lecture, you resurvey the attendees.

Data set: **Ch 09 – Exercise 02A.sav**

Codebook

Variable: ID
Definition: Participant ID code
Type: Alphanumeric

Variable: Pretest
Definition: Number of times steps were used in the week before the seminar
Type: Continuous

Variable: Posttest
Definition: Number of times the steps were used in the week after the seminar
Type: Continuous

a. Write the hypotheses.
b. Run the criteria of the pretest checklist (normality for *Posttest – Pretest*) and discuss your findings.
c. Run the paired *t* test and document your findings (means and Sig. [*p* value], hypothesis resolution).
d. Write an abstract under 200 words detailing a summary of the study, the paired *t* test results, hypothesis resolution, and implications of your findings.

Repeat this exercise using data set: **Ch 09 – Exercise 02B.sav.**

Exercise 9.3

In an effort to reduce the medication dosage(s) needed to manage patients diagnosed with generalized anxiety disorder (GAD), meditation therapy was introduced as an ancillary method of relaxation. The session involved a briefing on meditation, followed by a 30-minute guided meditation exercise. The nurse who was leading this training recorded the pulse rates of each participant before and after the training.

Data set: **Ch 09 – Exercise 03A.sav**

Codebook

Variable: ID
Definition: Participant ID
Type: Alphanumeric

Variable: Pretest
Definition: Pulse rate before the training
Type: Continuous

Variable: Posttest
Definition: Pulse rate after the training
Type: Continuous

a. Write the hypotheses.

b. Run the criteria of the pretest checklist (normality for *Posttest – Pretest*) and discuss your findings.

c. Run the paired *t* test and document your findings (means and Sig. [*p* value], hypothesis resolution).

d. Write an abstract under 200 words detailing a summary of the study, the paired *t* test results, hypothesis resolution, and implications of your findings.

Repeat this exercise using data set: **Ch 09 – Exercise 03B.sav.**

Exercise 9.4

The staff at a mental health clinic wants to determine if their current form of short-term therapy substantially reduces depression. Prior to treatment, each patient will be asked to complete the Acme Depression Inventory (ADI), which renders a score from 0 to 75 (0 = low depression . . . 75 = high depression). Patients will also be asked to complete the same instrument at the conclusion of their final appointment.

Data set: **Ch 09 – Exercise 04A.sav**

Codebook:

Variable: ID
Definition: Participant ID
Type: Alphanumeric

Variable: Pretest
Definition: ADI score before treatment
Type: Continuous

Variable: Posttest
Definition: ADI score after treatment
Type: Continuous

a. Write the hypotheses.

b. Run the criteria of the pretest checklist (normality for *Posttest – Pretest*) and discuss your findings.

c. Run the paired *t* test and document your findings (means and Sig. [*p* value], hypothesis resolution).

d. Write an abstract under 200 words detailing a summary of the study, the paired *t* test results, hypothesis resolution, and implications of your findings.

Repeat this exercise using data set: **Ch 09 – Exercise 04B.sav.**

Exercise 9.5

In a clinical nursing course, each student is paired with a nurse who is an expert on setting up IVs. The student will make his or her (baseline) first attempt with no instruction; the preceptor will score the quality of the work on a 0–10 scale (0 = none of the steps in the procedure done correctly . . . 10 = all steps in the procedure done perfectly); this score will be recorded as IV_1. After the first attempt, the preceptor will give constructive feedback along with corresponding tutorials. Each student will do a second IV setup and receive another score, which will be recorded as IV_2, and receive feedback from the preceptor.

Data set: **Ch 09 – Exercise 05A.sav**

Codebook

Variable:	ID
Definition:	Participant ID
Type:	Alphanumeric
Variable:	IV_1
Definition:	Proficiency score on first IV setup
Type:	Continuous
Variable:	IV_2
Definition:	Proficiency score on second IV setup (after receiving feedback)
Type:	Continuous

NOTE: The variable names *IV_1* and *IV_2* pertain to *Pretest* and *Posttest* data, respectively; do not let the different variable names throw you.

a. Write the hypotheses.

b. Run the criteria of the pretest checklist (normality for *IV_2 – IV_1*) and discuss your findings.

c. Run the paired *t* test and document your findings (means and Sig. [*p* value], hypothesis resolution).

d. Write an abstract under 200 words detailing a summary of the study, the paired *t* test results, hypothesis resolution, and implications of your findings.

Repeat this exercise using data set: **Ch 09 – Exercise 05B.sav.**

Exercise 9.6

The administrators of a nursing school want to assess students' grades (in percent) over two academic terms.

Data set: **Ch 09 – Exercise 06A.sav**

Codebook

Variable: ID
Definition: Student ID
Type: Alphanumeric

Variable: Term_1
Definition: Mean academic score from first term
Type: Continuous

Variable: Term_2
Definition: Mean academic score from second term
Type: Continuous

NOTE: The variable names *Term_1* and *Term_2* pertain to *Pretest* and *Posttest,* respectively; do not let the different variable names throw you.

a. Write the hypotheses.
b. Run the criteria of the pretest checklist (normality for *Term_2 – Term_1*) and discuss your findings.
c. Run the paired *t* test and document your findings (means and Sig. [*p* value], hypothesis resolution).
d. Write an abstract under 200 words detailing a summary of the study, the paired *t* test results, hypothesis resolution, and implications of your findings.

Repeat this exercise using data set: **Ch 09 – Exercise 06B.sav.**

Exercise 9.7

Acme Brand allergy medicine claims that its product reduces allergy-related sneezing. To test this claim, you recruit a group of allergy patients who are not currently taking any medications for their allergies and ask them to count the number of times they sneeze per day. The next day, each participant takes the Acme allergy medicine in the morning as directed and keeps a (separate) sneeze tally for that day too.

Data set: **Ch 09 – Exercise 07A.sav**

Codebook

Variable: ID
Definition: Participant ID
Type: Alphanumeric

Variable: Pretest
Definition: Number of sneezes per day
Type: Continuous

Variable: Posttest
Definition: Number of sneezes per day
Type: Continuous

a. Write the hypotheses.
b. Run the criteria of the pretest checklist (normality for *Posttest – Pretest*) and discuss your findings.
c. Run the paired *t* test and document your findings (means and Sig. [*p* value], hypothesis resolution).
d. Write an abstract under 200 words detailing a summary of the study, the paired *t* test results, hypothesis resolution, and implications of your findings.

Repeat this exercise using data set: **Ch 09 – Exercise 07B.sav.**

Exercise 9.8

An herbalist interested in natural remedies wants to assess the effectiveness of an herbal tea in reducing fever. The investigator recruits a group of patients who have fever and records the temperature for each person. Next, each participant is given one cup of the tea. An hour later, the investigator takes each participant's temperature again.

Data set: **Ch 09 – Exercise 08A.sav**

Codebook

Variable: ID
Definition: Participant ID
Type: Alphanumeric

Variable: Pretest
Definition: Body temperature before tea
Type: Continuous

Variable: Posttest
Definition: Body temperature after tea
Type: Continuous

a. Write the hypotheses.
b. Run the criteria of the pretest checklist (normality for *Posttest – Pretest*) and discuss your findings.
c. Run the paired *t* test and document your findings (means and Sig. [*p* value], hypothesis resolution).
d. Write an abstract under 200 words detailing a summary of the study, the paired *t* test results, hypothesis resolution, and implications of your findings.

Repeat this exercise using data set: **Ch 09 – Exercise 08B.sav.**

Exercise 9.9

In an effort to discover ways to boost morale, the nurse manager wants to assess the effects that fresh gourmet coffee has on attitude. The nurses on each ward agree to partake in this study. At the beginning of their shift, each nurse is asked to complete the Acme Attitude Survey (AAS), a 10-question instrument that renders a score ranging from 0 to 10 (0 = very bad attitude . . . 10 = very good attitude). Next, the nurses are given free unlimited access to the coffee machine at each nursing station as they proceed with their nursing duties. Four hours later, the nurse manager administers the AAS to the nurses a second time.

Data set: **Ch 09 – Exercise 09A.sav**

Codebook

Variable: ID
Definition: Participant ID
Type: Alphanumeric

Variable: Pretest
Definition: Baseline attitude (AAS score)
Type: Continuous

Variable: Posttest
Definition: Attitude (AAS score) 4 hours into shift (with coffee)
Type: Continuous

a. Write the hypotheses.
b. Run the criteria of the pretest checklist (normality for *Posttest – Pretest*) and discuss your findings.
c. Run the paired *t* test and document your findings (means and Sig. [*p* value], hypothesis resolution).
d. Write an abstract under 200 words detailing a summary of the study, the paired *t* test results, hypothesis resolution, and implications of your findings.

Repeat this exercise using data set: **Ch 09 – Exercise 09B.sav.**

Exercise 9.10

In addition to providing dialysis to inpatients, Acme Hospital has an outpatient hemodialysis center. Outpatients are scheduled for treatment three times per week (Monday, Wednesday, and Friday or Tuesday, Thursday, and Saturday). The nurse manager of the center has identified patients with a history of missed appointments and has implemented an Adherence Coaching program, wherein a nurse on staff works with vulnerable patients to provide education, emotional support, and roundtrip transportation assistance (transit tokens, taxi vouchers, shuttle service), along with phone calls to track progress, clear roadblocks, and provide positive emotional support. Weekly appointment keeping is tracked (0–3 appointments kept).

Data set: **Ch 09 – Exercise 10A.sav**

Codebook

Variable:	ID
Definition:	Participant ID
Type:	Alphanumeric
Variable:	Baseline
Definition:	Weekly appointments kept before Adherence Coaching
Type:	Continuous
Variable:	With_Coaching
Definition:	Weekly appointments kept with Adherence Coaching
Type:	Continuous

NOTE: The variable names *Baseline* and *With_Coaching* pertain to *Pretest* and *Posttest,* respectively; do not let the different variable names throw you.

a. Write the hypotheses.
b. Run the criteria of the pretest checklist (normality for *With_Coaching – Baseline*) and discuss your findings.
c. Run the paired *t* test and document your findings (means and Sig. [*p* value], hypothesis resolution).
d. Write an abstract under 200 words detailing a summary of the study, the paired *t* test results, hypothesis resolution, and implications of your findings.

Repeat this exercise using data set: **Ch 09 – Exercise 10B.sav.**

CHAPTER 10

ANOVA Repeated Measures

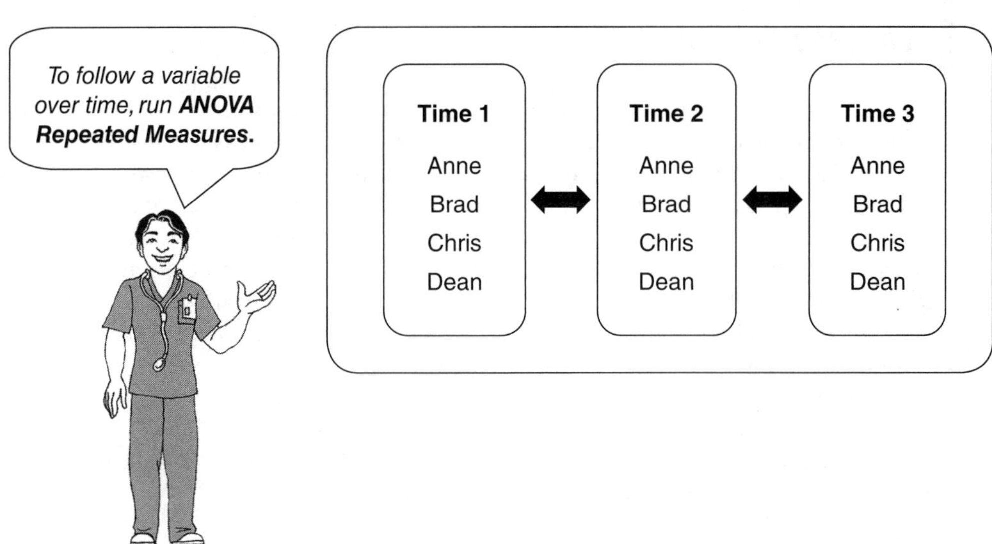

The only reason for time is so that everything doesn't happen at once.

—Albert Einstein

LEARNING OBJECTIVES

Upon completing this chapter, you will be able to:

- Determine when it is appropriate to run an ANOVA repeated-measures test
- Verify that the data meet the criteria for ANOVA repeated-measures test processing: Mauchly's test of sphericity
- Order an ANOVA repeated-measures test
- Interpret test results
- Resolve the hypotheses
- Document the results in plain English
- Comprehend the versatility of repeated-measures designs

TUTORIAL VIDEO

The tutorial video for this chapter is **Ch 10 – ANOVA Repeated Measures.mp4.** This video provides an overview of the ANOVA repeated-measures statistic, followed by the SPSS procedures for processing the pretest checklist, ordering the statistical run, and interpreting the results of this test using the data set: **Ch 10 – Example 01 – ANOVA Repeated Measures.sav.**

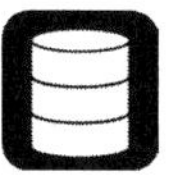

LAYERED LEARNING

If you mastered the paired *t* test, then you can consider yourself more than halfway there when it comes to comprehending the ANOVA repeated-measures test. Whereas the paired *t* test involves measuring the same thing at *two* time points (*pretest* vs. *posttest*), the ANOVA repeated-measures test does exactly the same thing, except it accommodates more than *two* time points—for example, (1) a score gathered at 7:00 a.m. to establish a baseline, followed immediately by the treatment; (2) a score gathered at 9:00 a.m. to detect the initial effectiveness of the treatment; and (3) a score gathered at 11:00 a.m. to check for sustainability—this will tell us if the effects of the treatment endure over time, beyond the (first) 9:00 a.m. posttest. The ANOVA repeated measures is a versatile upgrade to the paired *t* test, as it lends itself to more elaborate longitudinal designs involving any number of measures gathered over any duration. This will be discussed more thoroughly at the conclusion of the chapter, but first we will begin with a more detailed overview of the ANOVA repeated-measures test.

OVERVIEW—ANOVA REPEATED MEASURES

Before embarking on the ANOVA repeated-measures test, we will briefly revisit the paired *t* test. The paired *t* test is typically thought of as the statistic used to measure change from *pretest* to *posttest,* which can render some valuable information regarding the effect of the treatment, situated (in time) between the *pretest* and *posttest*. Another way to think about the labels *pretest* and *posttest* is to conceive them in terms of time: The variable labeled *pretest* could plausibly be renamed as $Time_1$, and the variable *posttest* could be renamed as $Time_2$. With this in mind, we can move into the ANOVA repeated-measures test.

Essentially, the findings of the paired *t* test end at the *posttest* ($Time_2$), but what if we wanted to know *what happens next?* In the example used in Chapter 9, the paired *t* test revealed that those who participated in the smoking cessation seminar smoked (statistically) significantly fewer cigarettes in the week after the session, but that is *all* we know. Considering that smoking is a chronic condition, it would be useful if we had a way to track the progress of these participants over time—beyond the posttest; ANOVA repeated measures enables us to do just that.

Just as the ANOVA test compares the mean from each group to every other group ($Group_1$: $Group_2$, $Group_1$: $Group_3$, $Group_2$: $Group_3$) and produces corresponding *p* values, the ANOVA repeated-measures test compares the mean from each time point to every other time point ($Time_1$: $Time_2$, $Time_1$: $Time_3$, $Time_2$: $Time_3$) and produces corresponding *p* values for each pair of times.

To build on the similarity between the *paired t test* and the *ANOVA repeated-measures test,* this chapter will use the same example that was used in Chapter 9 with some slight enhancements:

- The (SPSS) variables are renamed from *Pretest* and *Posttest* to *Week1* and *Week2,* respectively; all the data contained within those variables are the same.
- A new variable, *Week3,* is now included.

We will use the O X O O (O = observation, X = treatment) (quasi) experimental design for this example, which will consist of the weekly smoking means taken at $Week_1$, $Week_2$, and $Week_3$ (Figure 10.1).

This design will enable us to determine

- the baseline daily smoking rate ($Week_1$);
- the initial effectiveness of the smoking cessation treatment (comparing $Week_1$ to $Week_2$);
- if the effect of the treatment is sustained over time (comparing $Week_2$ to $Week_3$); and
- if, over time, the decrease in smoking was maintained or if smokers reverted back to their baseline smoking rate (comparing $Week_1$ to $Week_3$).

Figure 10.1 Repeated-measures design (0 X 0 0) to assess short-term sustainability. 0 = observation; X = treatment.

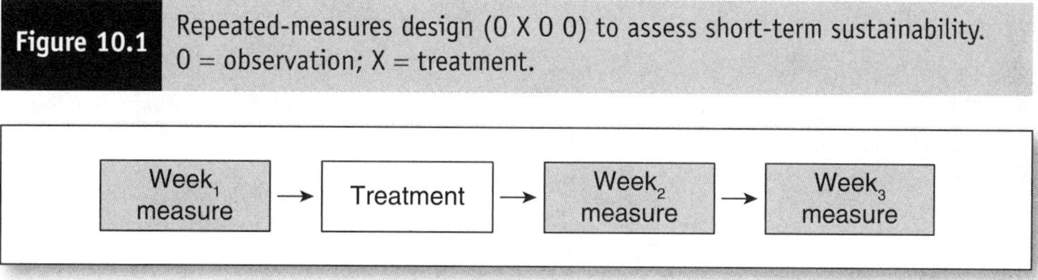

Example

The nurse who is leading the smoking cessation group wants to determine the effectiveness of the intervention over time.

Research Question

The question is: Will providing a 1-hour smoking cessation seminar help to reduce smoking among the participants?

Groups

The (one) group will consist of 40 participants who want to stop smoking.

Procedure

Step 1—*Week*$_1$: The week before the smoking cessation seminar, each participant is issued a special cigarette lighter equipped to digitally record the date and time each time it is lit. After 7 days, each participant will bring his or her lighter to the smoking cessation seminar. The data from each lighter will be downloaded into a database where a daily (baseline) smoking mean will be computed and entered as the *Week*$_1$ (mean daily smoking) score for each participant. The data on each lighter will be cleared and then returned to the participants.

Step 2—Treatment: The nurse administers the 1-hour smoking cessation seminar.

Step 3—*Week*$_2$: After 1 week, the participants return with their lighters; data from the second week are downloaded, and the mean daily smoking rate for each participant is computed and entered into the database as the *Week*$_2$ score.

Step 4—*Week*$_3$: One week later, the participants return with their lighters; data from the third week are downloaded, and the mean daily smoking rate for each participant is computed and entered into the database as the *Week*$_3$ score.

Hypotheses

H_0: The smoking cessation seminar is not effective in reducing smoking.

H_1: The smoking cessation seminar is effective in reducing smoking.

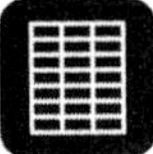

Data Set

Use the following data set: **Ch 10 – Example 01 – ANOVA Repeated Measures .sav.**

Codebook

Variable: Initials
Definition: Initials of each participant (first, middle, last)
Type: Alphanumeric

Variable: Week1
Definition: Baseline average number of cigarettes smoked daily (over days 1–7)
Type: Continuous

Variable: Week2
Definition: Average number of cigarettes smoked daily (over days 8–14)
Type: Continuous

Variable: Week3
Definition: Average number of cigarettes smoked daily (over days 15–21)
Type: Continuous

NOTE: *Week1* = *Pretest* (from Chapter 9: Paired *t* Test), *Week2* = *Posttest* (from Chapter 9: Paired *t* Test), and *Week3* is new.

Pretest Checklist

ANOVA Repeated-Measures Pretest Checklist

☑ 1. Mauchly's test of sphericity*

*Results produced upon ANOVA repeated-measures test run

Pretest Checklist Criterion 1—Mauchly's Test of Sphericity

To run an ANOVA repeated-measures test, we need to check that the variances from each of the time points are similar. We check for this using Mauchly's test of sphericity. If this test produces a *p* value that is greater than .05, then this tells us that there is no statistically significant difference among the variances from the data gathered at the (three) time points, indicating that this criterion is satisfied.

This test will be processed during the **Test Run** and finalized in the **Results** section.

NOTE: Occasionally, this test renders a *p* value that is less than .05; in such cases, proceed with the ANOVA repeated-measures test, and include a statement pertaining to this (imperfect) finding when documenting the results.

Test Run

1. To run the ANOVA repeated measures, from the *Data View* screen, click on *Analyze, General Linear Model, Repeated Measures* (Figure 10.2).

Figure 10.2 Order ANOVA repeated-measures test.

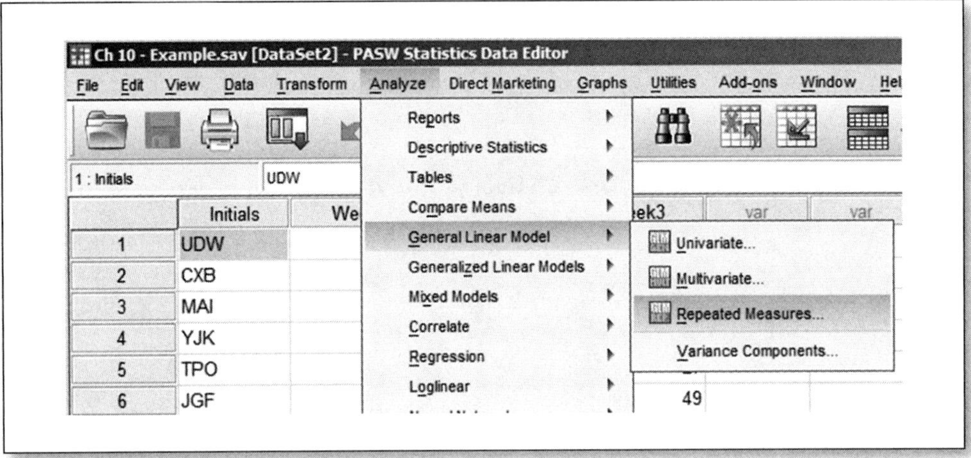

2. This will take you to the *Repeated Measure Define Factor(s)* menu (Figure 10.3).

Figure 10.3 *Repeated Measures Define Factor(s)* menu.

Repeated Measures Define Factor(s)

Within-Subject Factor Name: Time

Number of Levels: 3

Add

Change

Remove

Measure Name:

Add

Change

Remove

Define Reset Cancel Help

3. In the *Within-Subject Factor Name* box, erase *factor1* and type in *Time*. In the *Number of Levels* box, enter *3,* indicating that we will be comparing measurements taken from *three* time points. Click on *Add,* then click on *Define*. This will take you to the *Repeated Measures* menu (Figure 10.4).

Figure 10.4 *Repeated Measures* menu.

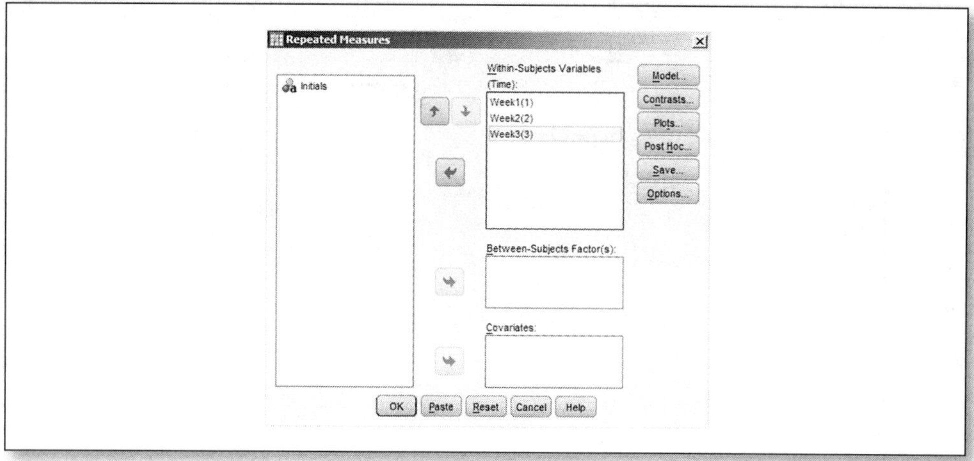

4. On the *Repeated Measures* menu, move the variables *Week1, Week2,* and *Week3* from the left box to the *Within-Subjects Variables (Time)* box; be sure to keep them in order, then click on *Options* (Figure 10.4). This will take you to the *Repeated Measures: Options* menu (Figure 10.5).

Figure 10.5 *Repeated Measures: Options* menu.

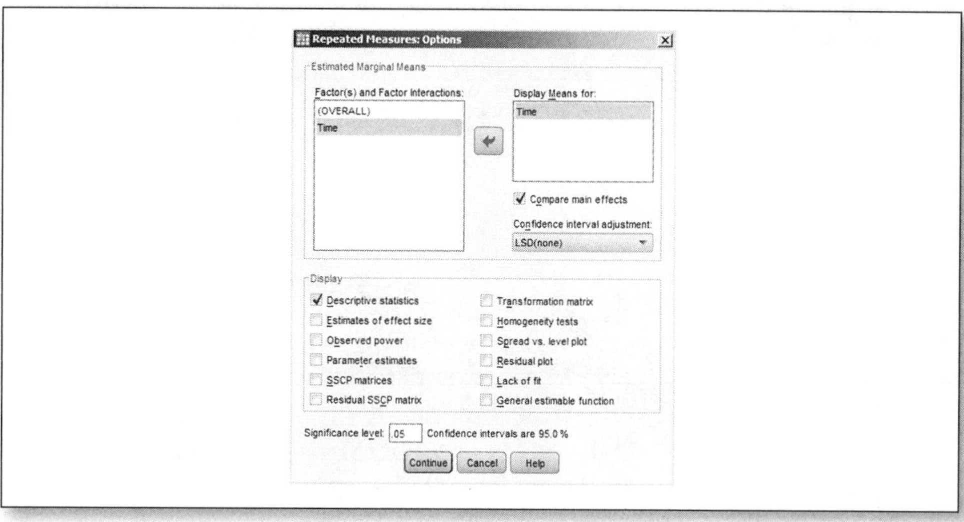

5. Move *Time* from the *Factor(s) and Factor Interactions* box to the *Display Means for* box. Check the ☑ *Compare main effects* option and the ☑ *Descriptive statistics* option, then click *Continue*. This will take you back to the *Repeated Measures* menu (Figure 10.6).

Figure 10.6 *Repeated Measures* menu.

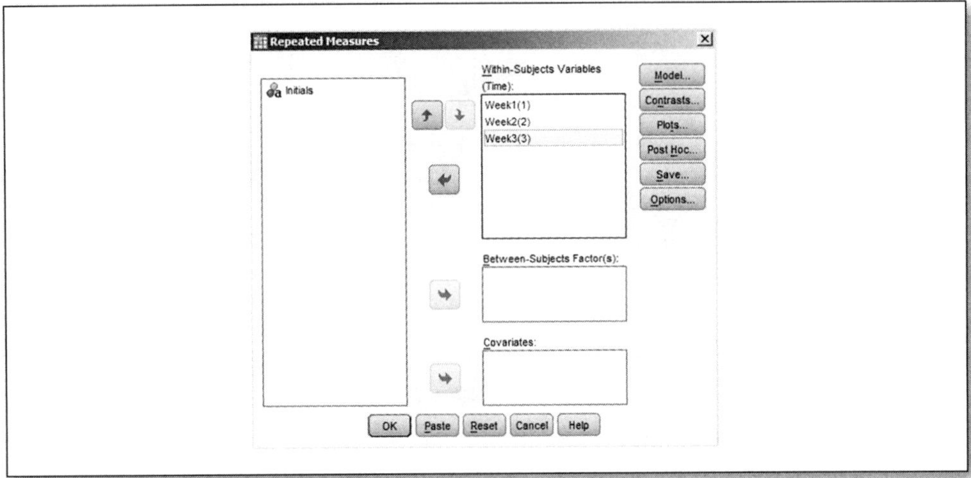

6. On the *Repeated Measures* menu, click on *Plots*. This will take you to the *Repeated Measures: Profile Plots* menu (Figure 10.7).

7. Next, we will order a line graph that will show how the data changed over the three time points (Week$_1$ to Week$_2$ to Week$_3$). On the *Repeated Measures:*

Figure 10.7 *Repeated Measures: Profile Plots* menu.

Repeated Measures: Profile Plots
Factors:
Time
Horizontal Axis:
Separate Lines:
Separate Plots:
Plots:
Add
Change
Remove
Time
Continue
Cancel
Help

Profile Plots menu, move *Time* from the *Factors* box to the *Horizontal Axis* box, then click on *Add*. Finally, click on *Continue*. This will take you back to the *Repeated Measures* menu (Figure 10.8).

8. On the *Repeated Measures* menu, click on *OK*, and the data will be processed.

Figure 10.8 *Repeated Measures* menu.

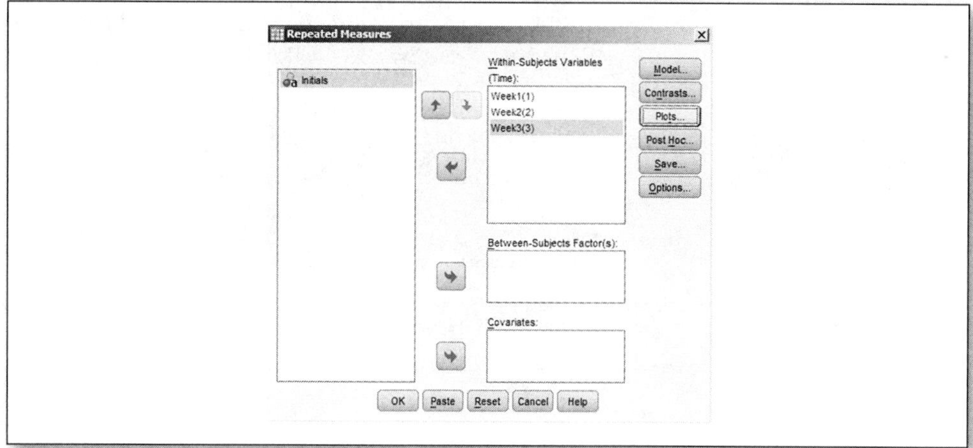

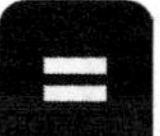

Results

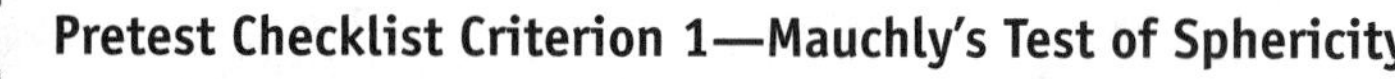

Pretest Checklist Criterion 1—Mauchly's Test of Sphericity

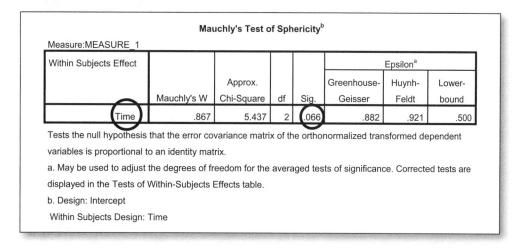

We can now finalize the pretest checklist; look at the *Mauchly's Test of Sphericity* table (Table 10.1), specifically, focus on the Sig. (p) value, which is .066. Since this is

Table 10.1 *Mauchly's Test of Sphericity* Table [Sig. (p) > α (.05)] Indicates a Pass.

Mauchly's Test of Sphericity[b]

Measure:MEASURE_1

Within Subjects Effect					Epsilon[a]		
	Mauchly's W	Approx. Chi-Square	df	Sig.	Greenhouse-Geisser	Huynh-Feldt	Lower-bound
Time	.867	5.437	2	.066	.882	.921	.500

Tests the null hypothesis that the error covariance matrix of the orthonormalized transformed dependent variables is proportional to an identity matrix.

a. May be used to adjust the degrees of freedom for the averaged tests of significance. Corrected tests are displayed in the Tests of Within-Subjects Effects table.

b. Design: Intercept

Within Subjects Design: Time

greater than the α level of .05, this tells us that there is no statistically significant difference between the variances of the data gathered at the three time points; hence, this pretest criterion is satisfied.

Next, inspect the *Tests of Within-Subjects Effects* table (Table 10.2), focusing on the *Time, Sphericity Assumed Sig.* (*p*) value, .015. Since this is less than the α level (.05), this indicates that the mean of one of the *Weeks* is significantly different from the mean of one of the other *Weeks*.

The mean for each *Week* is shown in the *Descriptive Statistics* table (Table 10.3). The *Pairwise Comparisons* table (Tables 10.4, 10.5, and 10.6) indicates which *Week* outperformed which (other) *Week*(s) as indicated by the *p* values.

Table 10.2 Tests of Within-Subjects Effects Table.

Tests of Within-Subjects Effects

Measure:MEASURE_1

Source		Type III Sum of Squares	df	Mean Square	F	Sig.
Time	Sphericity Assumed	13.867	2	6.933	4.428	.015
	Greenhouse-Geisser	13.867	1.765	7.858	4.428	.019
	Huynh-Feldt	13.867	1.842	7.528	4.428	.018
	Lower-bound	13.867	1.000	13.867	4.428	.042
Error(Time)	Sphericity Assumed	122.133	78	1.566		
	Greenhouse-Geisser	122.133	68.825	1.775		
	Huynh-Feldt	122.133	71.840	1.700		
	Lower-bound	122.133	39.000	3.132		

NOTE: For *Time, Sphericity Assumed* Sig. (*p*) < α (.05), indicating that there is a statistically significant difference (somewhere) among the pairs of *Weeks*.

Table 10.3 Descriptive Statistics Table Provides the Mean for Each Week.

Descriptive Statistics

	Mean	Std. Deviation	N
Week1	29.40	6.109	40
Week2	28.80	6.277	40
Week3	28.60	6.531	40

Table 10.4 Pairwise Comparisons—*Week*$_1$: *Week*$_2$.

Pairwise Comparisons

Measure:MEASURE_1

(I) Time	(J) Time	Mean Difference (I-J)	Std. Error	Sig.[a]	95% Confidence Interval for Difference[a] Lower Bound	Upper Bound
1	2	.600*	.223	.010	.149	1.051
	3	.800*	.306	.013	.180	1.420
2	1	-.600*	.223	.010	-1.051	-.149
	3	.200	.302	.512	-.411	.811
3	1	-.800*	.306	.013	-1.420	-.180
	2	-.200	.302	.512	-.811	.411

Based on estimated marginal means

*. The mean difference is significant at the .05 level.

a. Adjustment for multiple comparisons: Least Significant Difference (equivalent to no adjustments).

Table 10.5 Pairwise Comparisons—*Week*$_2$: *Week*$_3$.

Pairwise Comparisons

Measure:MEASURE_1

(I) Time	(J) Time	Mean Difference (I-J)	Std. Error	Sig.[a]	95% Confidence Interval for Difference[a] Lower Bound	Upper Bound
1	2	.600*	.223	.010	.149	1.051
	3	.800*	.306	.013	.180	1.420
2	1	-.600*	.223	.010	-1.051	-.149
	3	.200	.302	.512	-.411	.811
3	1	-.800*	.306	.013	-1.420	-.180
	2	-.200	.302	.512	-.811	.411

Based on estimated marginal means

*. The mean difference is significant at the .05 level.

a. Adjustment for multiple comparisons: Least Significant Difference (equivalent to no adjustments).

Table 10.6 Pairwise Comparisons—*Week*$_1$: *Week*$_3$.

Pairwise Comparisons

Measure:MEASURE_1

(I) Time	(J) Time	Mean Difference (I-J)	Std. Error	Sig.[a]	95% Confidence Interval for Difference[a] Lower Bound	Upper Bound
1	2	.600*	.223	.010	.149	1.051
	3	.800*	.306	.013	.180	1.420
2	1	-.600*	.223	.010	-1.051	-.149
	3	.200	.302	.512	-.411	.811
3	1	-.800*	.306	.013	-1.420	-.180
	2	-.200	.302	.512	-.811	.411

Based on estimated marginal means

*. The mean difference is significant at the .05 level.

a. Adjustment for multiple comparisons: Least Significant Difference (equivalent to no adjustments).

The best way to comprehend the story of how the cigarette smoking changed over the three time points is to (manually) build a *Longitudinal Results* table (Table 10.5). This is the same sort of results table that we assembled to comprehend ANOVA results. SPSS does not produce this table directly, but you can derive it from key figures in the output that we ordered SPSS to generate. To bring all of the critical figures together into one comprehensive table, assemble the *Longitudinal Results* table (Table 10.7): Draw the *Means* from the *Descriptive Statistics* table (Table 10.3) and the p values (Sig.) from the *Pairwise Comparisons* tables (Table 10.4, 10.5, and 10.6).

NOTE: Tables 10.4, 10.5, and 10.6 are the same table but with different circle placements to point out the pairs being compared along with their corresponding p values.

To comprehend the results of this 3-week study, we will discuss findings in the *Longitudinal Results* table, one row at a time.

The first comparison shows a decline in smoking from *Week*$_1$ (μ = 29.40) to *Week*$_2$ (μ = 28.60); this change is statistically significant (p = .010).

The next comparison shows a further decline in smoking from *Week*$_2$ (μ = 28.80) to *Week*$_3$ (μ = 28.60); however, this change is not statistically significant (p = .512).

Whereas the first two rows compare the scores at adjacent time points (*Week*$_1$: *Week*$_2$ and *Week*$_2$: *Week*$_3$), the last row compares the first measurement to the last to assess the overall performance of the program. This row compares *Week*$_1$ (μ = 29.40) to *Week*$_3$ (μ = 28.60), which is a statistically significant change in smoking rates (p = .013).

Table 10.7 Manually Built *Longitudinal Results* Table: *Means* Drawn From *Descriptive Statistics* (Table 10.3) and *p* Values (Sig.) Drawn From *Pairwise Comparisons* (Tables 10.4, 10.5, and 10.6).

Longitudinal Results	
Times	p
$\mu(Week_1) = 29.40 : \mu(Week_2) = 28.80$	.010*
$\mu(Week_2) = 28.80 : \mu(Week_3) = 28.60$	.512
$\mu(Week_1) = 29.40 : \mu(Week_3) = 28.60$	.013*

*Statistically significant difference detected between groups ($p \leq .05$).

The plot that we ordered clearly graphs these three findings (Figure 10.9). Notice the steep slope of the line between $Time_1$ and $Time_2$, indicating the statistically significant reduction in smoking. Also notice the less steep line between $Time_2$ and $Time_3$, indicating the insignificant drop in smoking between $Week_2$ and $Week_3$.

Figure 10.9 A graphical representation of the mean number of cigarettes smoked (Y-axis) at each of the three time points (X-axis).

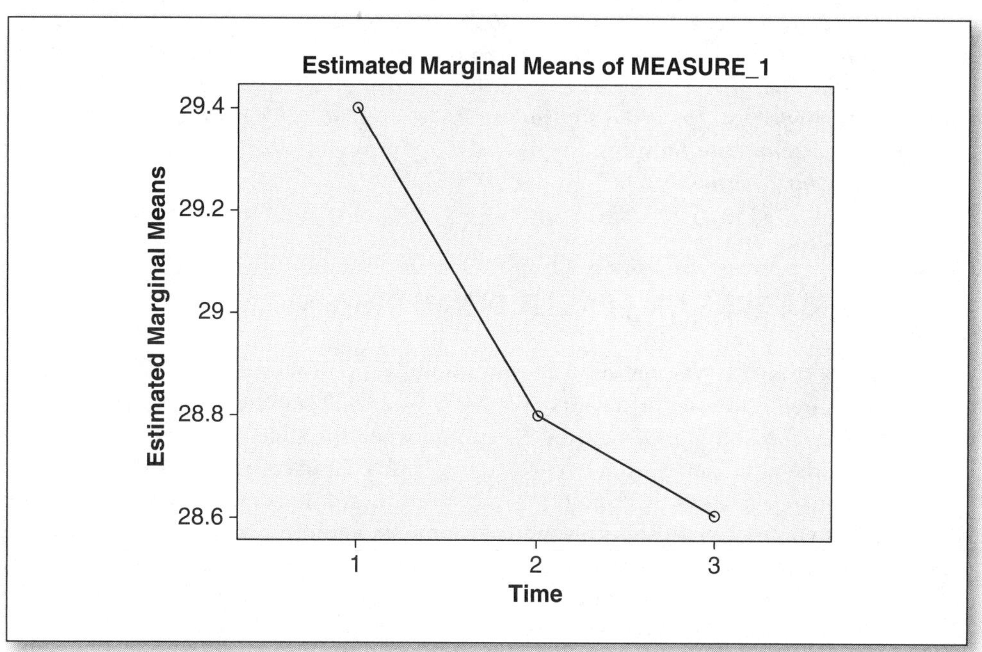

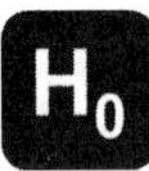

Hypothesis Resolution

H_0: The smoking cessation seminar is not effective in reducing smoking.

H_1: The smoking cessation seminar is effective in reducing smoking.

Since we detected a statistically significant reduction in mean daily smoking between $Week_1$ and $Week_2$, as well as between $Week_1$ and $Week_3$, we would reject H_0.

For the same reasons, we would not reject H_1.

Document Results

Documenting the results for the ANOVA repeated measures is similar to the paired *t* test; however, since more variables are involved, the results section is typically a bit longer:

> *We implemented a smoking cessation program involving 40 voluntary participants who were motivated to quit smoking. Each participant was issued a complimentary cigarette lighter equipped with technology to digitally record the date and time of each light. Based on the data gathered, we compared weekly average smoking figures at three time points: (1) the week before the program (baseline), (2) the week following our 1-hour smoking cessation workshop, and (3) one additional week. Participants showed a statistically significant 2% drop in mean daily cigarette smoking in the week following the workshop, down from 29.4 in week 1 to 28.8 in week 2 ($p = .01$, $\alpha = .05$). Although mean daily smoking continued to decrease from 28.8 in week 2 to 28.6 in week 3, this decrease of .2 is not statistically significant ($p = .512$, $\alpha = .05$). Over the course of this 3-week pilot study, participants achieved a significant 2.7% reduction in smoking ($p = .013$, $\alpha = .05$). Based on these findings, we intend to offer weekly workshops to facilitate further smoking reduction.*

VARIATIONS ON LONGITUDINAL DESIGN

Whereas the ANOVA repeated-measures statistic can assess measurements taken over three or more time points, the test is essentially oblivious to anything (treatment/interventions) that may be occurring in between the specified time points; it only computes the data gathered in each variable. This characteristic lends this test to a variety of research designs. Although the following examples demonstrate three unique longitudinal research designs, each involving data gathered over three time points ($Time_1$, $Time_2$, and $Time_3$), they would all be coded and processed exactly the same way—from a statistical processing standpoint, each design merely focuses on the measurement data gathered at each of the three time points.

Design A—Treatment Effect and Sustainability (O X O O)

This is the design that we used for the example in this chapter. Comparing $Time_1$ to $Time_2$ detects the initial effectiveness of the *Treatment*. Comparing $Time_2$ to $Time_3$ allows us to check for sustainability, answering the question, "At this point, does smoking go up/down/stabilize?" Finally, one could compare $Time_1$ to $Time_3$ to detect the overall effect of the treatment (Figure 10.10).

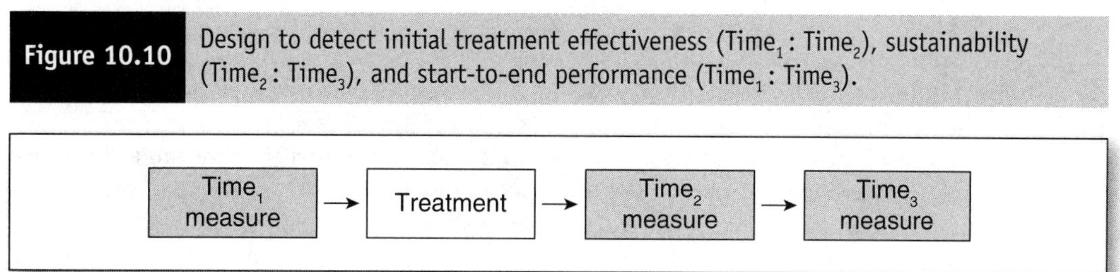

Figure 10.10 Design to detect initial treatment effectiveness ($Time_1$: $Time_2$), sustainability ($Time_2$: $Time_3$), and start-to-end performance ($Time_1$: $Time_3$).

NOTE: O = observation (measurement); X = treatment.

Design B—Incremental Monitoring (O X O X O)

This design involves ongoing treatment; repeated measures placed along the treatment timeline allows us to incrementally assess the effectiveness of the intervention (Figure 10.11).

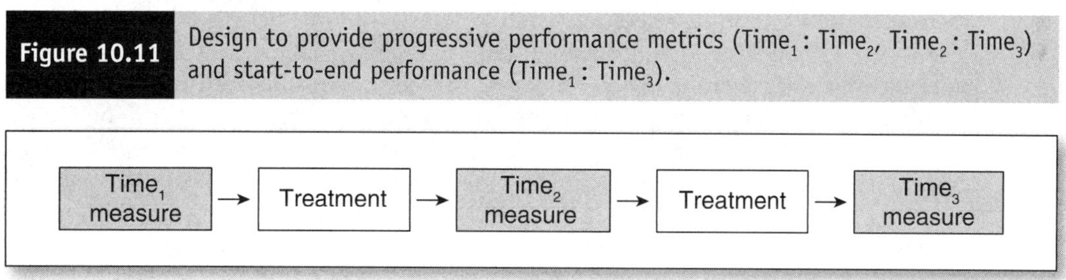

Figure 10.11 Design to provide progressive performance metrics ($Time_1$: $Time_2$, $Time_2$: $Time_3$) and start-to-end performance ($Time_1$: $Time_3$).

Design C—Stable Baseline and Treatment Effect (O O X O)

In cases where it is essential to establish a stable baseline, optimal results would render no statistically significant difference between $Time_1$ and $Time_2$, followed by the treatment, and last, the posttreatment data would be gathered at $Time_3$, wherein a statistically significant difference between measurements gathered at $Time_2$ and $Time_3$ would suggest the effectiveness of the treatment (Figure 10.12).

Figure 10.12 Design to detect stable baseline ($Time_1 : Time_2$) and treatment effectiveness ($Time_2 : Time_3$).

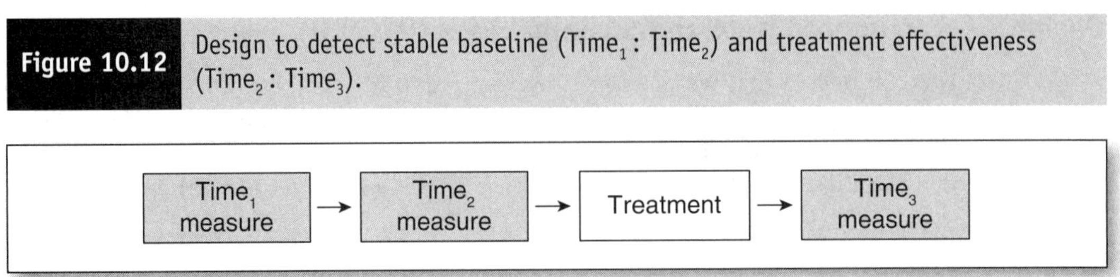

Despite the conceptual diversity of these designs, when it comes to the ANOVA repeated-measures coding and processing, SPSS would see all of them identically—as a data set simply consisting of three variables: *Time1, Time2,* and *Time3*.

As we have discussed, the ANOVA repeated-measures statistic is not limited to measurements taken over (only) three time points, gathered over 3 weeks. The ANOVA repeated-measures test can process data gathered from any number of time points spanning minutes, hours, days, weeks, months, or even years. Additionally, as shown in Designs A, B, and C, the ANOVA repeated-measures test can accommodate designs where treatments and measurements are placed anywhere they are needed.

As versatile as these designs are, one needs to adhere to the fundamental rule of consistency when it comes to gathering data that are to be analyzed with the ANOVA repeated-measures method: The same metric (e.g., survey, self-administered questionnaire, archival data, etc.) must be used consistently among the same participants.

GOOD COMMON SENSE

While the ANOVA repeated-measures statistic lends itself to tracking the progress of a variety of longitudinal models, it is important to remember that since the data are being gathered from a single group of subjects, these models are classified as quasi-experimental since there is no random assignment to two or more groups. Such models can be vulnerable to threats to internal validity.

Since this is a one-group design wherein measurements are taken over time, one must consider the historical threat to internal validity. Specifically speaking, changes taking place outside of the realm of the study (e.g., social events, political changes, changes in the personal lives of the participants, etc.) may act as confounding variables, bringing change(s) to the data that are being gathered over the course of a study. This is a particular vulnerability involving designs that span longer time periods.

If the data are being gathered via survey, as opposed to biometrics (e.g., pulse rate, blood count), the data can be vulnerable to test-retest reliability issues; upon (repeated) retesting, the participant's score may improve due to the participant becoming progressively more familiar and proficient at responding to the question(s). Naturally, as the number of measurement iterations increases, so increases the risk of test-retest reliability issues.

Additionally, studies that take place over extended periods of time are also vulnerable to participant attrition/mortality—over time, some participants may opt to drop out of the study, or the researcher may rule out participants who no longer meet the criteria for this study (e.g., a study focusing on pregnant women may specify ruling out the participant upon giving birth). When launching such a study, it is advised that you recruit a sufficient number of participants in anticipation of such (expected) attrition.

Key Concepts

- Time-series designs
    - Treatment effect and sustainability: O X O O
    - Incremental monitoring: O X O X O
    - Stable baseline and treatment effect: O O X O
- Mauchly's test of sphericity
- Confounds/threats to internal validity
    - History
    - Testing (test/retest)
    - Attrition/mortality

Practice Exercises

Exercise 10.1

Nursing students are given a list of 60 pills that they need to visually identify. Students are issued a deck of 60 flashcards with the picture of the pill on one side and the name of the pill on the other side. Before studying, students are instructed to record their baseline score (*Time1*)—the number of pills they correctly identify from the picture (0–60) on their first pass through the deck. After 30 minutes of studying the cards that they got wrong, the student is instructed to shuffle all of the cards and record their *Time2* identification score. Finally, the student studies the cards for 30 more minutes and performs one more self-quiz, rendering the *Time3* score.

Data set: **Ch 10 – Exercise 01A.sav**

Codebook

Variable: ID
Definition: Student ID
Type: Alphanumeric

Variable: Time1
Definition: Number of pills correctly identified on the first (baseline) attempt
Type: Continuous

Variable: Time2
Definition: Number of pills correctly identified on the second attempt
Type: Continuous

Variable: Time3
Definition: Number of pills correctly identified on the third attempt
Type: Continuous

a. Write the hypotheses.
b. Run the criteria of the pretest checklist (Mauchly's test of sphericity) and discuss your findings.
c. Run the ANOVA repeated measures and document your findings (means and Sig. [*p* value]), graphical plot, and hypothesis resolution.
d. Write an abstract under 200 words detailing a summary of the study, the ANOVA repeated-measures test results, hypothesis resolution, and implications of your findings.

Repeat this exercise using data set: **Ch 10 – Exercise 01B.sav.**

Exercise 10.2

Prior to a Heart Health presentation, you administer a survey asking participants to indicate how many times they used the stairs (as opposed to the elevator) in the past week. A week after the lecture, you resurvey the attendees. Finally, 2 weeks after the lecture, you resurvey the attendees (a third time).

Data set: **Ch 10 – Exercise 02A.sav**

Codebook

Variable: ID
Definition: Participant ID
Type: Alphanumeric

Variable: Time1
Definition: Number of times the steps were used in the week before the seminar
Type: Continuous

Variable: Time2
Definition: Number of times the steps were used in the week after the seminar
Type: Continuous

Variable: Time3
Definition: Number of times the steps were used in the week 2 weeks after the seminar
Type: Continuous

a. Write the hypotheses.
b. Run the criteria of the pretest checklist (Mauchly's test of sphericity) and discuss your findings.

c. Run the ANOVA repeated measures and document your findings (means and Sig. [*p* value]), graphical plot, and hypothesis resolution.

d. Write an abstract under 200 words detailing a summary of the study, the ANOVA repeated-measures test results, hypothesis resolution, and implications of your findings.

Repeat this exercise using data set: **Ch 10 – Exercise 02B.sav.**

Exercise 10.3

In an effort to reduce the medication dosage(s) needed to manage patients diagnosed with generalized anxiety disorder (GAD), meditation therapy was introduced as an ancillary method of relaxation. The treatment consists of a briefing on meditation, followed by a 30-minute guided meditation exercise. The nurse who was leading this training recorded the pulse rates of each participant at the conclusion of each of the three sessions.

Data set: **Ch 10 – Exercise 03A.sav**

Codebook

Variable: ID
Definition: Participant ID
Type: Alphanumeric

Variable: Session1
Definition: Pulse rate at the end of Session 1
Type: Continuous

Variable: Session2
Definition: Pulse rate at the end of Session 2
Type: Continuous

Variable: Session3
Definition: Pulse rate at the end of Session 3
Type: Continuous

a. Write the hypotheses.

b. Run the criteria of the pretest checklist (Mauchly's test of sphericity) and discuss your findings.

c. Run the ANOVA repeated measures and document your findings (means and Sig. [*p* value]), graphical plot, and hypothesis resolution.

d. Write an abstract under 200 words detailing a summary of the study, the ANOVA repeated-measures test results, hypothesis resolution, and implications of your findings.

Repeat this exercise using data set: **Ch 10 – Exercise 03B.sav.**

Exercise 10.4

The staff at a mental health clinic wants to determine if their current form of short-term therapy substantially reduces depression. Prior to the first treatment, each patient will be asked to complete the Acme Depression Inventory (ADI), which renders a score from 0 to 75 (0 = low depression . . . 75 = high depression). Patients will be asked to complete the same instrument at the conclusion of their appointment on Week 5 and at the end of their final appointment on Week 10.

Data set: **Ch 10 – Exercise 04A.sav**

Codebook

Variable: ID
Definition: Participant ID
Type: Alphanumeric

Variable: Baseline
Definition: Acme Depression Inventory score at baseline
Type: Continuous

Variable: Week05
Definition: Acme Depression Inventory score at Week 5
Type: Continuous

Variable: Week10
Definition: Acme Depression Inventory score at Week 10
Type: Continuous

a. Write the hypotheses.
b. Run the criteria of the pretest checklist (Mauchly's test of sphericity) and discuss your findings.
c. Run the ANOVA repeated measures and document your findings (means and Sig. [*p* value]), graphical plot, and hypothesis resolution.
d. Write an abstract under 200 words detailing a summary of the study, the ANOVA repeated-measures test results, hypothesis resolution, and implications of your findings.

Repeat this exercise using data set: **Ch 10 – Exercise 04B.sav.**

Exercise 10.5

In a clinical nursing course, each student is paired with a nurse who is an expert on setting up IVs. The students will make their (baseline) first attempt with no instruction; the preceptor will score the quality of the work on a 0–10 scale (0 = none of the steps in the procedure done correctly . . . 10 = all steps in the procedure done perfectly). Each student will do a total of four IV setups with feedback after each. After each attempt, the preceptor will record the score and give constructive feedback along with corresponding tutorials.

Data set: **Ch 10 – Exercise 05A.sav**

Codebook

Variable: ID
Definition: Student ID
Type: Alphanumeric

Variable: IV_1
Definition: Proficiency score of first IV setup
Type: Continuous

Variable: IV_2
Definition: Proficiency score of second IV setup
Type: Continuous

Variable: IV_3
Definition: Proficiency score of third IV setup
Type: Continuous

Variable: IV_4
Definition: Proficiency score of fourth IV setup
Type: Continuous

a. Write the hypotheses.

b. Run the criteria of the pretest checklist (Mauchly's test of sphericity) and discuss your findings.

c. Run the ANOVA repeated measures and document your findings (means and Sig. [*p* value]), graphical plot, and hypothesis resolution.

d. Write an abstract under 200 words detailing a summary of the study, the ANOVA repeated-measures test results, hypothesis resolution, and implications of your findings.

Repeat this exercise using data set: **Ch 10 – Exercise 05B.sav.**

Exercise 10.6

The administrators of a nursing school want to assess students' grades (in percent) over four academic terms.

Data set: **Ch 10 – Exercise 06A.sav**

Codebook

Variable: ID
Definition: Student ID
Type: Alphanumeric

Variable: Term_1
Definition: Mean academic score from first term
Type: Continuous

Variable: Term_2
Definition: Mean academic score from second term
Type: Continuous

Variable: Term_3
Definition: Mean academic score from third term
Type: Continuous

Variable: Term_4
Definition: Mean academic score from fourth term
Type: Continuous

a. Write the hypotheses.

b. Run the criteria of the pretest checklist (Mauchly's test of sphericity) and discuss your findings.

c. Run the ANOVA repeated measures and document your findings (means and Sig. [*p* value]), graphical plot, and hypothesis resolution.

d. Write an abstract under 200 words detailing a summary of the study, the ANOVA repeated-measures test results, hypothesis resolution, and implications of your findings.

Repeat this exercise using data set: **Ch 10 – Exercise 06B.sav.**

Exercise 10.7

Acme Brand allergy medicine claims that its product reduces allergy-related sneezing. To test this claim, you recruit a group of allergy patients who are not currently taking any medications for their allergies and ask them to count the number of times they sneeze per day. On Days 2 and 3, each participant takes the Acme allergy medicine in the morning as directed and records the number of sneezes for each day.

Data set: **Ch 10 – Exercise 07A.sav**

Codebook

Variable: ID
Definition: Participant ID
Type: Alphanumeric

Variable: Day1
Definition: Number of sneezes per day (baseline)
Type: Continuous

Variable: Day2
Definition: Number of sneezes per day (with medication)
Type: Continuous

Variable: Day3
Definition: Number of sneezes per day (with medication)
Type: Continuous

a. Write the hypotheses.

b. Run the criteria of the pretest checklist (Mauchly's test of sphericity) and discuss your findings.

c. Run the ANOVA repeated measures and document your findings (means and Sig. [*p* value]), graphical plot, and hypothesis resolution.

d. Write an abstract under 200 words detailing a summary of the study, the ANOVA repeated-measures test results, hypothesis resolution, and implications of your findings.

Repeat this exercise using data set: **Ch 10 – Exercise 07B.sav.**

Exercise 10.8

An herbalist interested in natural remedies wants to assess the effectiveness of an herbal tea in reducing fever. The investigator recruits a group of patients who have fever and records the temperature for each person. Next, each participant is given one cup of the tea. After 1 hour, the investigator takes each participant's temperature again, and one hour after that, a third temperature is taken.

Data set: **Ch 10 – Exercise 08A.sav**

Codebook

Variable: ID
Definition: Participant ID
Type: Alphanumeric

Variable: Time1
Definition: Body temperature before tea (baseline)
Type: Continuous

Variable: Time2
Definition: Body temperature 1 hour after tea
Type: Continuous

Variable: Time3
Definition: Body temperature 2 hours after tea
Type: Continuous

a. Write the hypotheses.

b. Run the criteria of the pretest checklist (Mauchly's test of sphericity) and discuss your findings.

c. Run the ANOVA repeated measures and document your findings (means and Sig. [*p* value]), graphical plot, and hypothesis resolution.

d. Write an abstract under 200 words detailing a summary of the study, the ANOVA repeated-measures test results, hypothesis resolution, and implications of your findings.

Repeat this exercise using data set: **Ch 10 – Exercise 08B.sav.**

Exercise 10.9

In an effort to discover ways to boost morale, the nurse manager wants to assess the effects that fresh gourmet coffee has on attitude. The nurses on each ward agree to partake in this study. At the beginning of their shift, each nurse is asked to complete the Acme Attitude Survey (AAS), a 10-question instrument that renders a score ranging from 0 to 10 (0 = very bad attitude . . . 10 = very good attitude). Next, the nurses are given free unlimited access to the coffee machine at each nursing station as they proceed with their nursing duties. Four hours later, the nurse manager administers the AAS to the nurses a second time, and finally, the nurses respond to the AAS at the end of the shift.

Data set: **Ch 10 – Exercise 09A.sav**

Codebook

Variable: ID
Definition: Participant ID
Type: Alphanumeric

Variable: Time1
Definition: Acme Attitude Survey score (baseline)
Type: Continuous

Variable: Time2
Definition: Acme Attitude Survey score (at midshift, with coffee)
Type: Continuous

Variable: Time3
Definition: Acme Attitude Survey score (at end of shift, with coffee)
Type: Continuous

a. Write the hypotheses.

b. Run the criteria of the pretest checklist (Mauchly's test of sphericity) and discuss your findings.

c. Run the ANOVA repeated measures and document your findings (means and Sig. [*p* value]), graphical plot, and hypothesis resolution.

d. Write an abstract under 200 words detailing a summary of the study, the ANOVA repeated-measures test results, hypothesis resolution, and implications of your findings.

Repeat this exercise using data set: **Ch 10 – Exercise 09B.sav.**

Exercise 10.10

In addition to providing dialysis to inpatients, Acme Hospital has an outpatient hemodialysis center. Outpatients are scheduled for treatment three times per week (Monday, Wednesday, and Friday or Tuesday, Thursday, and Saturday). The nurse manager of the center has identified patients with a history of missed appointments and has implemented an Adherence Coaching program, wherein a nurse on staff works with vulnerable patients to provide education, emotional support, and round-trip transportation assistance (transit tokens, taxi vouchers, shuttle service), along with phone calls to track progress, clear roadblocks, and provide positive emotional support. Weekly appointment keeping is tracked (0–3 appointments kept) over the course of the 2 weeks following the intervention.

Data set: **Ch 10 – Exercise 10A.sav**

Codebook

Variable: ID
Definition: Participant ID
Type: Alphanumeric

Variable: Baseline
Definition: Weekly appointments kept before Adherence Coaching
Type: Continuous

Variable: With_Coaching1
Definition: Weekly appointments kept with Adherence Coaching for first week of coaching
Type: Continuous

Variable: With_Coaching2
Definition: Weekly appointments kept with Adherence Coaching for second week of coaching
Type: Continuous

a. Write the hypotheses.

b. Run the criteria of the pretest checklist (Mauchly's test of sphericity) and discuss your findings.

c. Run the ANOVA repeated measures and document your findings (means and Sig. [*p* value]), graphical plot, and hypothesis resolution.

d. Write an abstract under 200 words detailing a summary of the study, the ANOVA repeated-measures test results, hypothesis resolution, and implications of your findings.

Repeat this exercise using data set: **Ch 10 – Exercise 10B.sav.**

PART V

Measuring Relationship Between Variables

These chapters compute statistics that describe the nature of the relationship(s) between variables.

Chapter 11: Correlation and Regression uses the **Pearson** statistic to assess the relationship between two continuous variables. Similarly, the **Spearman** statistic is generally used to assess the relationship between two ordered lists.

Chapter 12: Chi-Square assesses the relationship between categorical variables.

Chapter 13: Logistic Regression predicts the odds of a dichotomous outcome occurring (or not) based on data from continuous and/or categorical predictors.

CHAPTER 11

Correlation and Regression

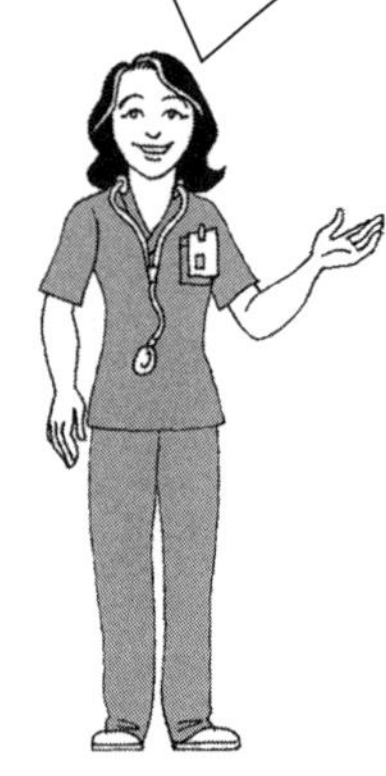

Correlation and **Regression** show the relationship between continuous variables.

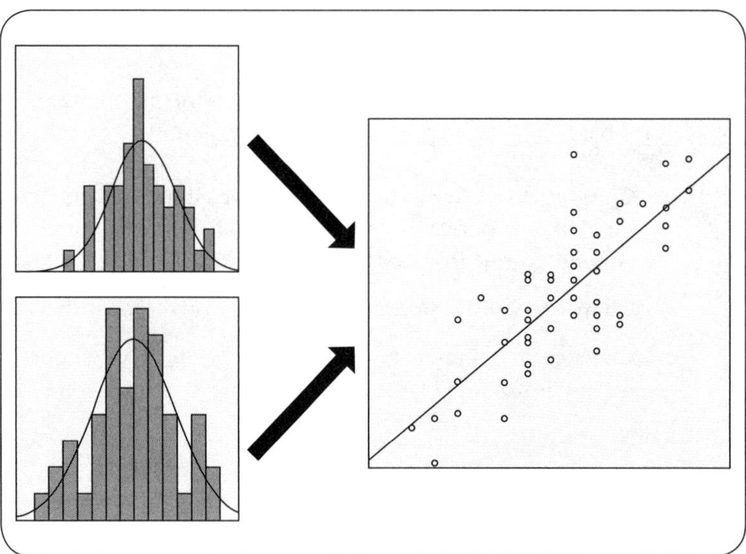

He who laughs most, learns best.

—John Cleese

LEARNING OBJECTIVES

Upon completing this chapter, you will be able to:

- Determine when it is appropriate to run Pearson regression and Spearman correlational analyses
- Interpret the direction and strength of a correlation
- Verify that the data meet the criteria for running regression and correlational analyses: normality, linearity, and homoscedasticity

- Order a regression analysis: correlation and scatterplot with regression line
- Interpret the test results
- Resolve the hypotheses
- Document the results in plain English
- Understand the criteria for causation: association/correlation, temporality, and nonspurious
- Differentiate between correlation and causation

TUTORIAL VIDEO

The videos for this chapter are **Ch 11 – Correlation and Regression – Pearson.mp4** and **Ch 11 – Correlation and Regression – Spearman.mp4.** These videos provide overviews of these tests, instructions for carrying out the pretest checklist, run, and interpreting the results of the tests using the data sets: **Ch 11 – Example 01 – Correlation and Regression.sav** (for Pearson) and **Ch 11 – Example 02 – Correlation and Regression.sav** (for Spearman).

OVERVIEW—PEARSON CORRELATION

Regression involves assessing the association (correlation) between two variables. Before proceeding, let us deconstruct the word *correlation:* The prefix *co* means *two*—hence, *correlation* is about *the relationship between two things. Regression* is about *assessing the correlation between two continuous variables.*

Correlation involving two variables, sometimes referred to as *bivariate correlation,* is notated using the lowercase *r* and has a value between −1 and +1. Correlations have two primary attributes: *direction* and *strength.*

Direction is indicated by the sign of the *r* value: + or −. Positive correlations ($r = 0 \ldots +1$) emerge when the two variables move in the same direction. For example, we would expect that low homework hours would correlate with low grades, just as we would expect that high homework hours would correlate with high grades. Negative correlations ($r = -1 \ldots 0$) emerge when the two variables move in different directions. For example, we would expect that high alcohol consumption would correlate with low grades, just as we would expect that low alcohol consumption would correlate with high grades (see Table 11.1).

Strength is indicated by the numeric value. A correlation wherein the *r* is close to 0 is considered weaker than those nearer to −1 or +1 (see Figure 11.1).

Table 11.1 Correlation Direction Summary.

Correlation (r) Direction Summary		
Correlation	**r**	**Variable Directions**
Positive	0 . . . +1	X↑ Y↑ or X↓ Y↓
Negative	−1 . . . 0	X↑ Y↓ or X↓ Y↑

Figure 11.1 Correlation strength.

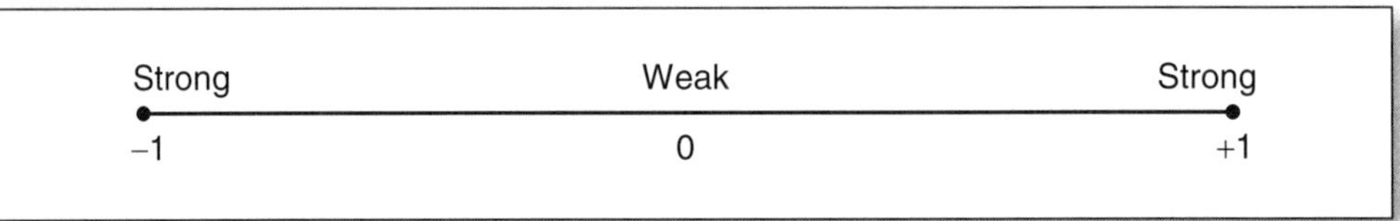

Continuing with the prior example, we would expect to find a strong positive correlation between homework hours and grade (e.g., $r = +.81$); conversely, we would expect to find a strong negative correlation between alcohol consumption and grade (e.g., $r = -.81$). However, we would not expect that a variable such as height would have much to do with academic performance, and hence we would expect to find a relatively weak correlation between *height* and *grade* (e.g., $r = +.02$ or $r = -.02$).

The concepts of correlation, direction, and strength will become clearer as we examine the test results, specifically upon inspecting the graph of the scatterplot with the regression line in the Results section.

This chapter covers *Pearson regression,* which is the most common, and *Spearman correlation,* which will be explained in Example 2 on page **254**.

Example 1—Pearson Regression

A nurse wants to discover if there is a correlation between the length of hospitalization and depression.

Research Question

Is there a statistically significant correlation between hospital length of stay and depression?

GROUPS

Bivariate regression/correlation involves only *one group,* but *two different continuous variables* are gathered for each participant: In this case, the variables are (1) *Length_of_stay* (number of days in hospital) and (2) *Depression.*

Notice that in correlation analysis, you can mix apples and oranges; *Length_of_stay* is a measure of *time,* whereas *Depression* is a measure of *mood.* The only constraints in this respect are that the two metrics must both be continuous variables, and of course, the comparison needs to inherently make sense—it is reasonable to consider the correlation between *Length_of_stay* and *Depression,* whereas it is implausible to assess the correlation between *Length_of_stay* and *Height,* even though *Height* is a continuous variable.

Procedure

The nurse managing this research will use the hospital census to identify the length of stay for each patient and will visit each patient to administer the Acme Depression Scale (ADS)—a 10-question survey that renders a score indicating the level of depression (0 = No depression . . . 70 = High depression). The nurse will then record the patient ID, length of stay, and ADS score for each patient.

Hypotheses

H_0: There is no correlation between length of stay and depression.

H_1: There is a correlation between length of stay and depression.

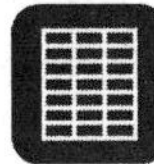

Data Set

Use the following data set: **Ch 11 – Example 01 – Correlation and Regression.sav.**

Codebook

Variable: Pt_ID
Definition: Patient identification code
Type: Alphanumeric

Variable: Length_of_stay
Definition: Total number of days hospitalized
Type: Continuous

Variable: Depression
Definition: Score on Acme Depression Scale
Type: Continuous

Pretest Checklist

Correlation and Regression Pretest Checklist

☑ 1. Normality*

☑ 2. Linearity**

☑ 3. Homoscedasticity**

*Run prior to correlation and regression test

**Results produced upon correlation and regression test run

The pretest criteria for running a correlation/regression involve checking the data for **(1) normality, (2) linearity,** and **(3) homoscedasticity** (pronounced *hoe-moe-skuh-daz-tis-city*).

Pretest Checklist Criterion 1—Normality

The two variables involved in the correlation/regression each need to be inspected for normality. To do this, generate separate histograms with normal curves for *Length_of_stay* and *Depression* (this is similar to the steps used to check for normality when using the *t* test and ANOVA).

For more details on this procedure, refer to Chapter 4—Descriptive Statistics; see the star (★) icon on page **58** and follow the procedure*: SPSS—Descriptive Statistics: Continuous Variables (Age);* instead of processing *Age,* load the two variables: *Length_of_stay* and *Depression*. Alternatively, the following steps will produce a histogram with a normal curve for *Length_of_stay* and *Depression:*

1. From the main screen, select *Analyze, Descriptive Statistics, Frequencies*; this will take you to the *Frequencies* menu.
2. On the *Frequencies* menu, move *Length_of_stay* and *Depression* from the left window to the right (*Variables*) window. This will order histograms for both variables at the same time.
3. Click on the *Charts* button; this will take you to the *Charts* menu.
4. Click on the *Histograms* button, and check the *Show normal curve on histogram* checkbox.
5. Click on the *Continue* button; this will return you to the *Frequencies* menu.
6. Click on the *OK* button, and the system will produce (two) histograms with normal curves for *Length_of_stay* and *Depression* (Figures 11.2 and 11.3).

Figure 11.2 Histogram with a normal curve for *Length_of_stay*.

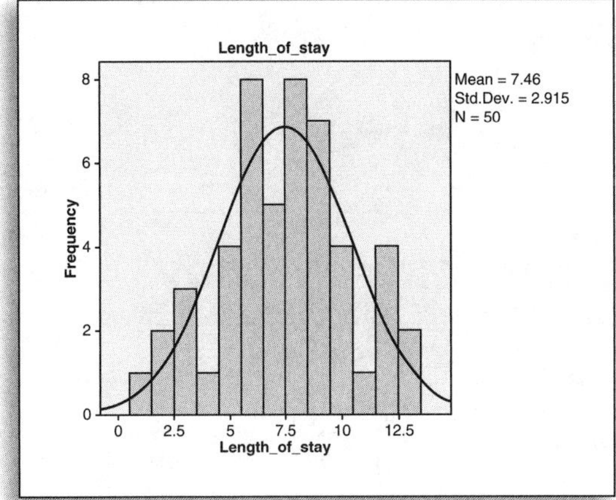

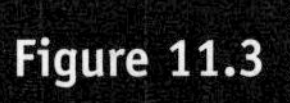

Figure 11.3 Histogram with a normal curve for *Depression*.

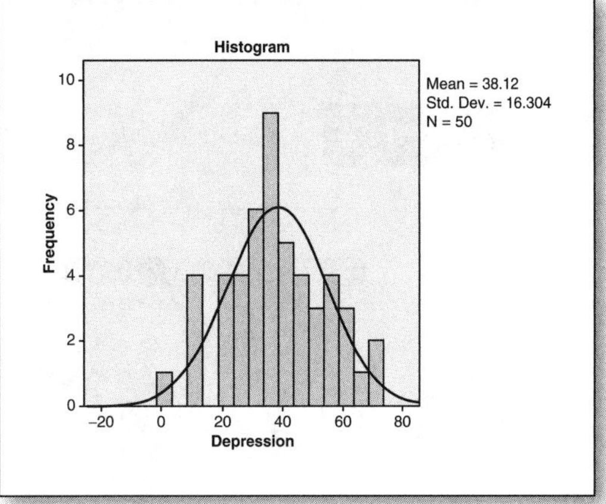

The curves on each histogram are reasonably symmetrically bell shaped; there is no notable skewing, and hence these criteria are satisfied.

The remaining two pretest criteria, **(2) linearity** and **(3) homoscedasticity,** are graphical in nature; they will be processed during the **Test Run** and finalized in the **Results** section.

Test Run

The test run for correlation and regression is a two-part process; first we will process the correlation table, which will render the correlation value (*r*) and the corresponding *p* value. Next, we will order a scatterplot, which will provide a clear graph showing the paired points from both variables plotted on an X,Y-axes along with the regression line, sometimes referred to as a *trend line*, which can be thought of as the average pathway through the points.

Correlation

1. To run a correlation, starting from the main screen, click on *Analyze, Correlate, Bivariate.* (Figure 11.4).

2. On the *Bivariate Correlations* menu (Figure 11.5), move the *Length_of_stay* and *Depression* variables from the left window to the right (*Variables*) window.

3. Click the *OK* button, and the correlation will process. For now, set aside the correlations table that is produced; we will interpret it in the Results section.

4. To order a scatterplot with a regression line, from the main menu, click on *Graph, Chart Builder* (Figure 11.6).

Figure 11.4 Accessing the *Correlation* menu: *Analyze, Correlate, Bivariate.*

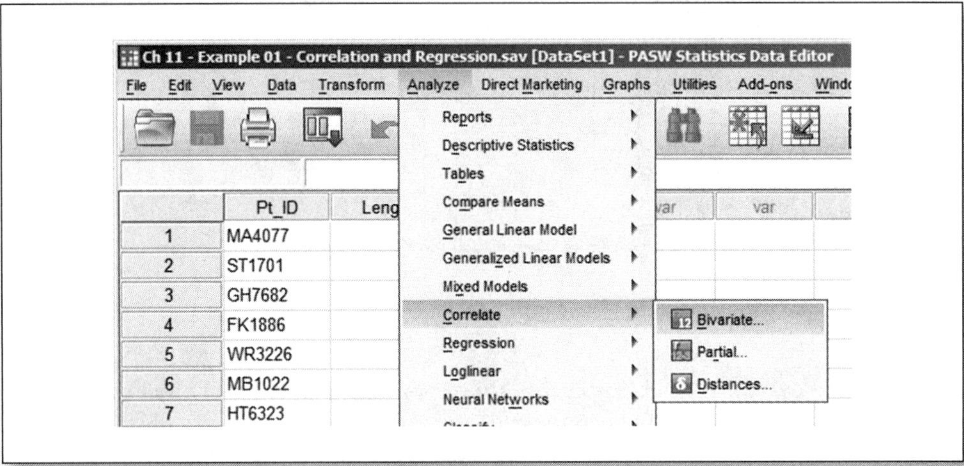

Figure 11.5 Accessing the *Correlation* menu: *Analyze, Correlate, Bivariate.*

Bivariate Correlations

Variables:
Length_of_stay
Depression

Options...
Bootstrap...

Correlation Coefficients
Pearson Kendall's tau-b Spearman

Test of Significance
Two-tailed One-tailed

Flag significant correlations

OK Paste Reset Cancel Help

Figure 11.6 Accessing the *Chart Builder* menu: *Graphics, Chart Builder.*

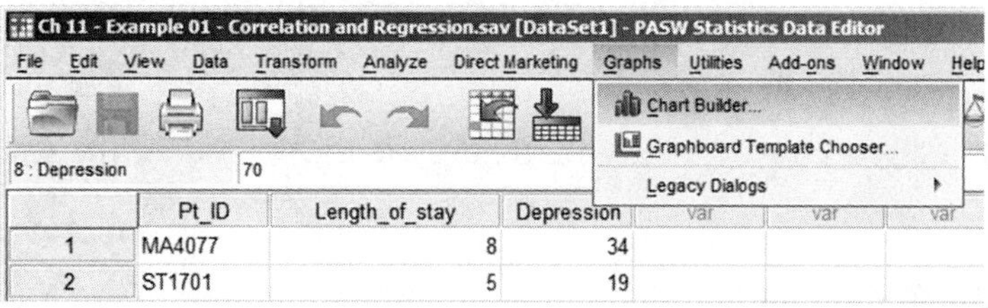

Regression (Scatterplot With Regression Line)

NOTE: SPSS graphics processing menus tend to differ across versions. If these instructions do not fit your version of the software, use the *Help* menu to guide you to order a scatterplot with the regression line. Indicate that you want the *Length_of_stay* variable on the X-axis and the *Depression* variable on the Y-axis.

5. In the *Choose from*: list, click on *Scatter/Dot* (Figure 11.7).

Figure 11.7 *Chart Builder* menu.

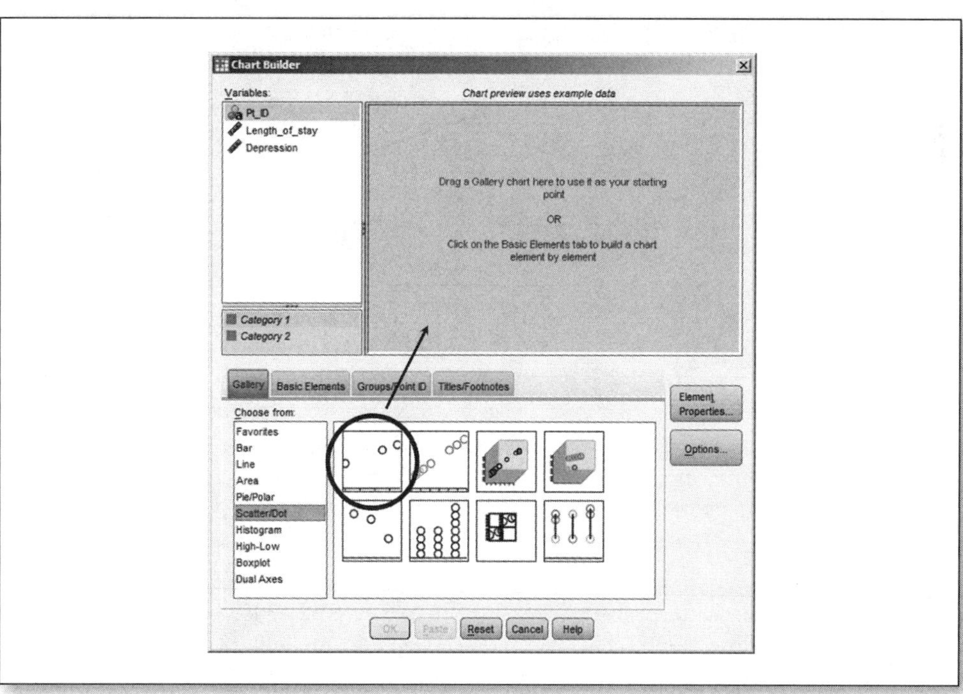

6. Double-click on the (circled) first choice, or click and drag this icon to the *Chart preview uses example data* window.
7. Click and drag *Length_of_stay* from the *Variables* window to the *X-Axis?* box (Figure 11.8).
8. Click and drag *Depression* from the *Variables* window to the *Y-Axis?* box.
9. Click on the *OK* button, and the system will produce the scatterplot.

Figure 11.8 *Chart Builder* menu—assign *Length_of_stay* to X-axis and *Depression* to Y-axis.

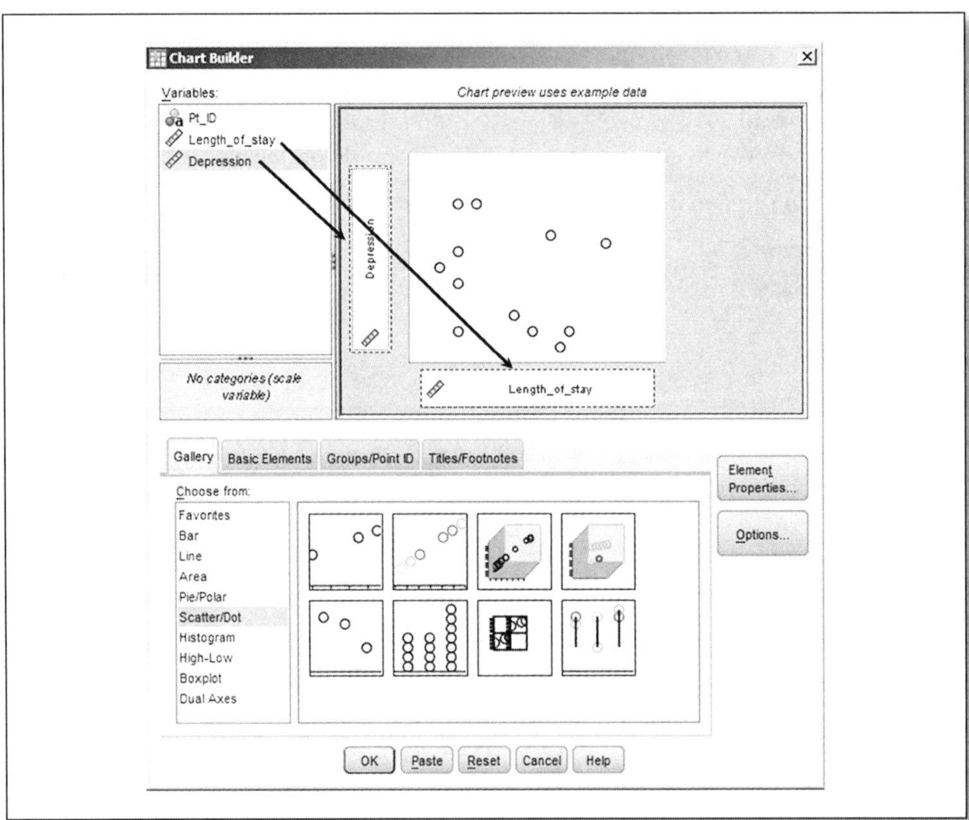

When the scatterplot emerges, you will need to order the regression line: In the Output window, double-click on the scatterplot. This will bring you to the *Chart Editor* (Figure 11.9).

Figure 11.9 *Chart Editor* menu—click on *Add Fit Line* to include the regression line on the scatterplot.

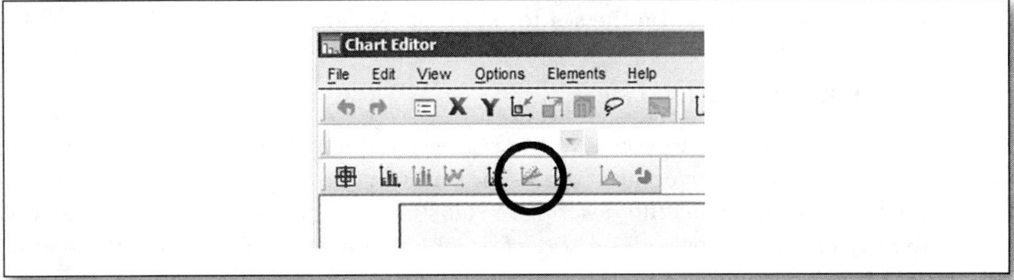

10. Click on the *Add Fit Line at Total* icon to include the regression line on the scatterplot.
11. When you see the regression line emerge on the scatterplot, close the *Chart Editor* and you will see that the regression line is now included on the scatterplot in the *Output* window.

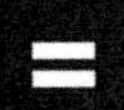

Results

In this section, we will begin by explaining the two elements on the scatterplot: (1) the points and (2) the regression line. Next, we will finalize the two remaining pretest criteria (linearity and homoscedasticity), and finally, we will discuss the overall meaning of the scatterplot and correlation findings.

Scatterplot Points

The coordinates of each point on the scatterplot are derived from the two variables: *Length_of_stay* and *Depression* for each record (individual).

Figure 11.10 Source data for scatterplot.

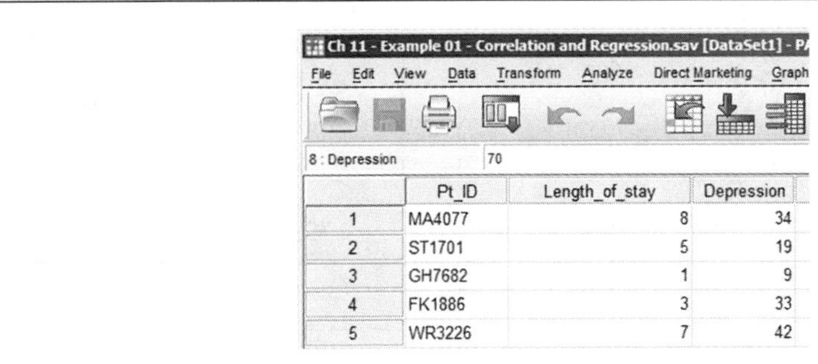

	Pt_ID	Length_of_stay	Depression
1	MA4077	8	34
2	ST1701	5	19
3	GH7682	1	9
4	FK1886	3	33
5	WR3226	7	42

The first record of the data set shows that patient MA4077 has been hospitalized for 8 days, and this patient scored 34 on the Acme Depression Index (Figure 11.10). When we ordered the histogram, we placed *Length_of_stay* on the X-axis and *Depression* on the Y-axis—hence, patient MA4077's point on the scatterplot is at coordinates (8, 34), patient ST1701's point on the scatterplot is at (5, 19), and so on.

Scatterplot Regression Line

The simplest way to conceive the regression line, without presenting the formula, is to think of it as the average straight-line pathway through the cloud of points, based on their positions. Just as the descriptive statistics provide a summary of a single variable, the regression line provides a sort of graphical summary of two variables—in this case, *Length_of_stay* and *Depression*.

Pretest Checklist Criterion 2—Linearity

The points on the scatterplot should form a relatively straight line (Figure 11.11); the regression line should take a middle-of-the-road path through the cloud of points. If the overall shape of the points departs into some other shape(s) that is not conducive to drawing a straight (regression) line through it (Figure 11.12), then this would constitute a violation of the linearity assumption.

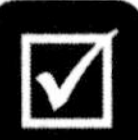

Pretest Checklist Criterion 3—Homoscedasticity

Homoscedasticity pertains to the density of the points along the regression line. The criterion of homoscedasticity is satisfied when the cloud of points is densest in the middle and tapers off at the ends (Figure 11.13) as opposed to the points being

Figure 11.11 Linearity satisfied.

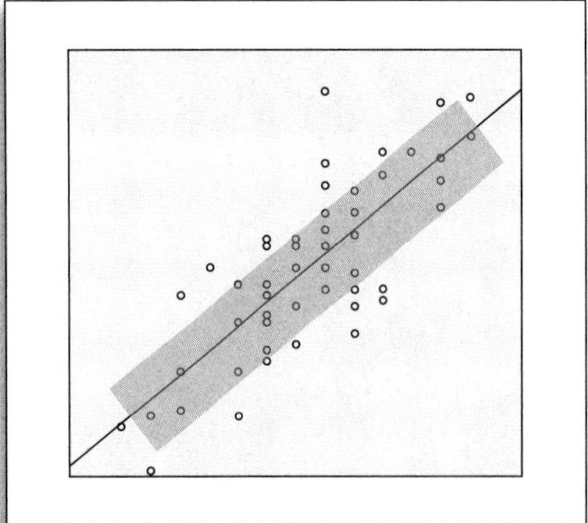

Figure 11.12 Linearity violated.

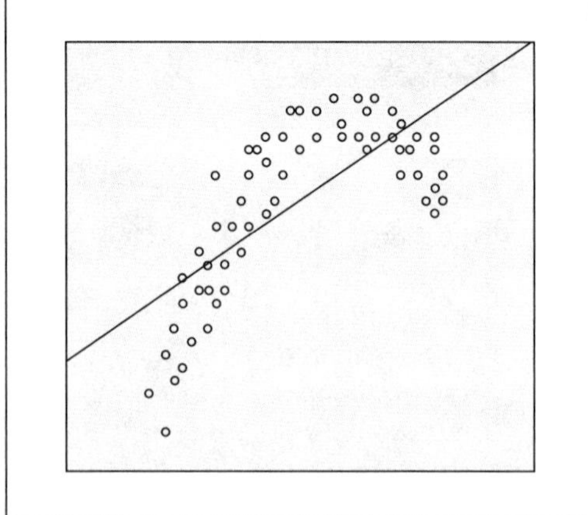

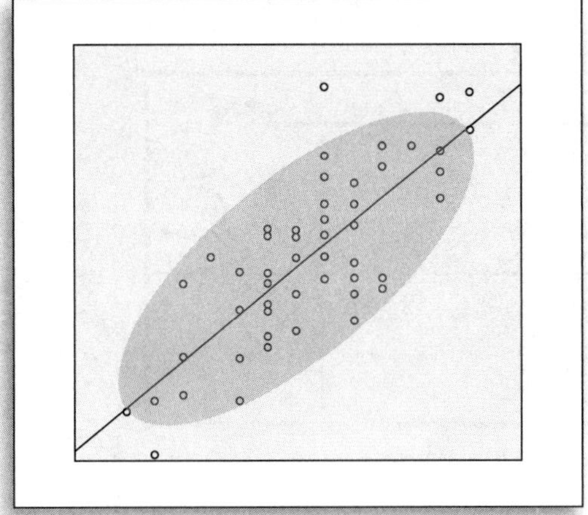

Figure 11.13 Homoscedasticity satisfied.

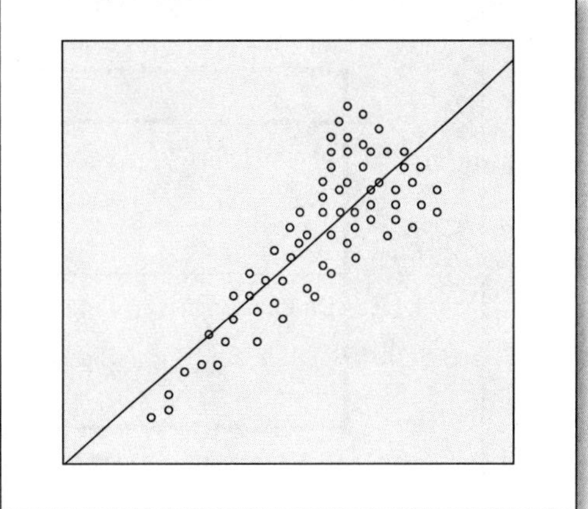

Figure 11.14 Homoscedasticity violated.

concentrated in some other way (Figure 11.14). The rationale for this distribution of points on the scatterplot follows the same notion as the shape of the normal curve of the histogram—the majority of the values are gathered around the mean, which accounts for the height of the normal bell-shaped curve on the histogram, whereas the tapered tails signify that there are considerably fewer very low and very high values. The positions of the points on the scatterplot are derived from the same data that rendered the normally distributed histograms for the two variables (Figures 11.2 and 11.3), so it follows that the middle of the cloud should contain considerably more points (and be denser) than the ends.

Correlation

Table 11.2 shows a positive correlation (r = .789) between *Length_of_stay* and *Depression*, with a (Sig.) p value of .000. As mentioned in Chapter 4, the p value never really goes to zero; in this case, p = .0000000000101841491265621. When the p value is less than .001, it is typically notated as "p < .001." Since the p value is less than the α level of .05, and the r is greater than zero, we would say that there is a statistically significant positive correlation (p < .001, α = .05) between *Length_of_stay* and *Depression*. The positive correlation (r = .789) pertains to the positive slope of the regression line.

Notice that the correlations table (Table 11.2) is double-redundant; there are two .789s and two .000s in the table. This is because the correlation between *Length_of_stay* and *Depression* is the same as the correlation between *Depression* and *Length_of_stay*. A larger image of the corresponding graph (scatterplot with regression line) is shown in Figure 11.15.

Table 11.2 Correlations Between *Length_of_stay* and *Depression*.

Correlations

		Length_of_stay	Depression
Length_of_stay	Pearson Correlation	1	.789**
	Sig. (2-tailed)		.000
	N	50	50
Depression	Pearson Correlation	.789**	1
	Sig. (2-tailed)	.000	
	N	50	50

**. Correlation is significant at the 0.01 level (2-tailed).

Figure 11.15 Scatterplot with regression line for the *Length_of_stay* : *Depression* correlation.

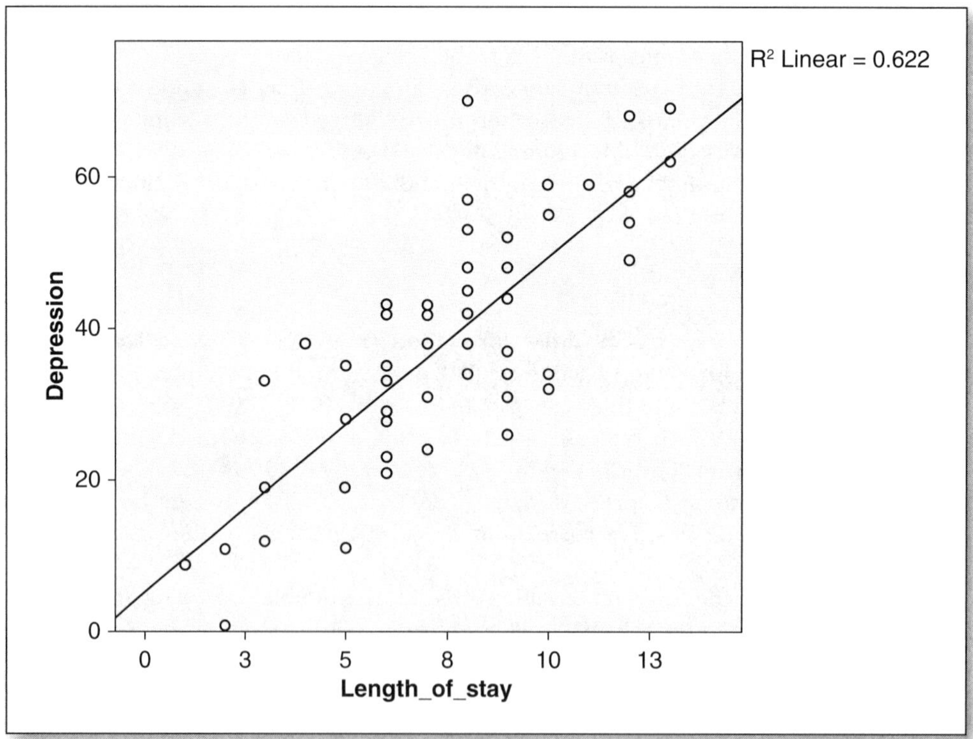

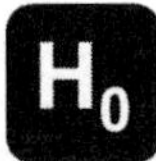

Hypothesis Resolution

H_0: There is no correlation between *Length_of_stay* and *Depression.*

H_1: There is a correlation between *Length_of_stay* and *Depression.*

Since the correlation calculation produced a *p* ($p < .001$) that is less than the specified .05 α level, we would say that there is a statistically significant (positive) correlation between length of stay and depression. As such, we would reject H_0 and not reject H_1.

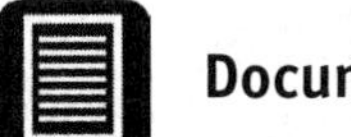

Document Results

Prior to documenting the results, it can be helpful to run descriptive statistics for the two variables involved in the correlation (the procedure for running descriptive statistics can be found at the ★ icon on page **58**; you can load *Length_of_stay* and *Depression* into the *Variables* window together) (Table 11.3).

Discussing the *n,* means, and standard deviations of each variable along with the regression results can add to the substance of the abstract:

*We were interested in discovering if there was a correlation between the length of hospitalization and depression. We derived the length of stay (*μ = *7.46,* SD = *2.9) of 50 patients from the hospital census and invited each patient to complete the Acme*

Table 11.3 Descriptive Statistics for *Length_of_stay* and *Depression.*

Statistics

		Length_of_stay	Depression
N	Valid	50	50
	Missing	0	0
Mean		7.46	38.12
Median		8.00	37.50
Mode		6[a]	34[a]
Std. Deviation		2.915	16.304
Variance		8.498	265.822
Range		12	69
Minimum		1	1
Maximum		13	70

a. Multiple modes exist. The smallest value is shown

Depression Scale (ADS)—a 10-question survey that renders a score indicating the level of depression (0 = No depression . . . 70 = High depression) (μ = 38.1, SD = *16.3). Correlation analysis revealed a strong positive correlation between these two variables (*r = *.789), which was statistically significant (*p < *.001,* α = *.05) suggesting that depression increases as the hospitalization advances.*

OVERVIEW—SPEARMAN CORRELATION

The Spearman correlation, formally referred to as *Spearman's rho* (pronounced *row*), can be thought of as a close cousin of the more commonly used Pearson regression; however, whereas the Pearson regression assesses the relationship between two continuous variables gathered from a data sample (e.g., height and weight), the Spearman correlation assesses the relationship between two rankings using the same –1 . . . +1 value range as the Pearson regression. The most common use of Spearman's rho is to determine how similarly two lists are sequenced.

For example, suppose you want to determine how similar a nurse and a patient are in terms of their favorite (to least favorite) nutritional supplement flavors. You could write the names of the flavors on the front of each card with the corresponding code number on the back (in this demonstration, the code numbers are shown on the front of each card for easy reference). In this case, the nurse and patient arrange their cards in identical order (Figure 11.16).

Figure 11.16 Two lists ranked identically produces a Spearman's rho of +1.

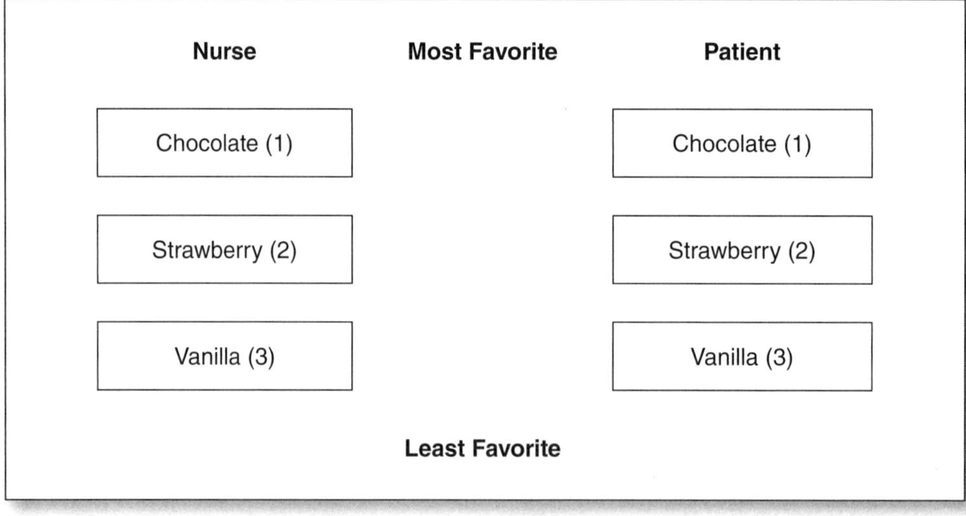

Since the nurse and the patient arranged their cards in exactly the same order, this would produce a Spearman rho of +1, signifying a perfectly positive correlation between the two prioritized lists.

If instead, the patient would have sorted the flavors: *Vanilla, Strawberry, Chocolate* (3, 2, 1) and compared that to the nurse's sequence: *Chocolate, Strawberry, Vanilla* (1, 2, 3), these two rankings would be exactly opposite of each other, which would produce a Spearman rho of −1, signifying a (perfectly) negative correlation between the two lists (Figure 11.17).

Figure 11.17 Two lists ranked oppositely produces a Spearman's rho of −1.

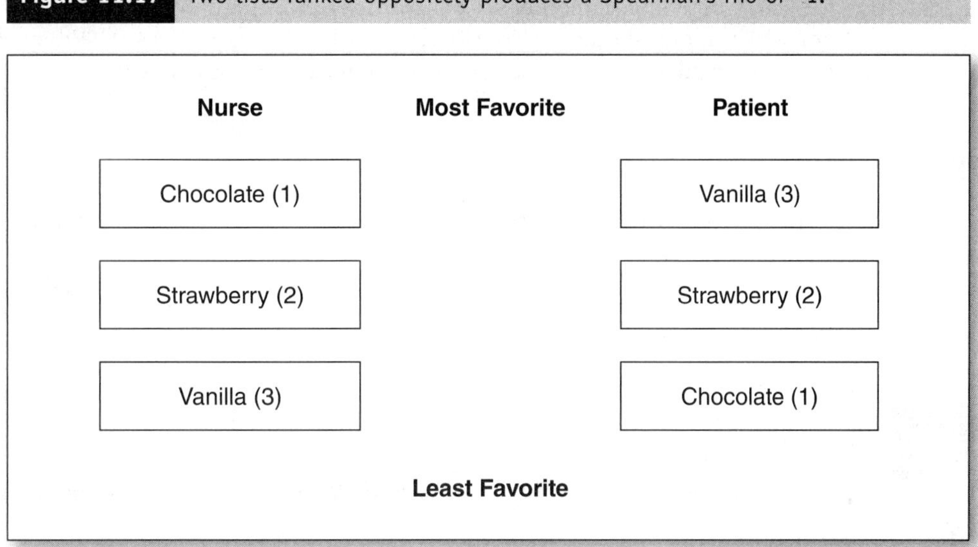

In this concise example, three items were used; however, there is no limit to the number of items that can constitute these lists. As you might expect, a variety of rankings of the items are possible, producing Spearman rho values anywhere between −1 and +1. As with the Pearson correlation, the corresponding p value indicates if there is (or is not) a statistically significant difference between the (two) rankings.

Example 2—Spearman Correlation

A patient is referred to confer with a dietician to collaboratively build a (more) healthful eating plan. Part of this process involves ascertaining the patient's food preferences.

Research Question

Is there a statistically significant correlation between the dietician's recommended food ranking and the patient's current food preferences?

Groups

Unlike the Pearson regression, which gathers two continuous variables from each sample, the Spearman correlation gathers a sequence of ranked data from each of the two participants—in this case, food rankings from the dietician and the patient.

Procedure

At the initial consultation meeting, the dietician issues the patient five cards and asks the patient to arrange them in order of preference, with the most favorite food at the top. The dietician will then use another set of cards to demonstrate the recommended diet in terms of which foods should be considered best (to worst) choices. The dietician will record the two card sequences and compare them using Spearman's rho.

Hypotheses

H_0: There is no correlation between the dietician's recommended food ranking and the patient's food preferences.

H_1: There is a correlation between the dietician's recommended food ranking and the patient's food preferences.

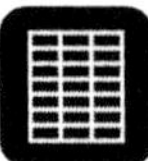

Data Set

Use the following data set: **Ch 11 – Example 02 – Correlation and Regression.sav.**

Codebook

Variable:	Dietician
Definition:	Dietician's recommended food ranking (1 = Vegetables, 2 = Fish, 3 = Poultry, 4 = Beef, 5 = Pork)
Type:	Continuous
Variable:	Patient
Definition:	Patient's food preferences (1 = Vegetables, 2 = Fish, 3 = Poultry, 4 = Beef, 5 = Pork)
Type:	Continuous

Per the specified procedure, the cards rankings for the dietician (1, 2, 3, 4, 5) and the patient (2, 1, 3, 4, 5) (Figure 11.18) have been recorded and entered into the SPSS database; on the main *Data View* screen, click on the *Value Labels* icon to toggle between the numeric values and the corresponding assigned value labels.

Figure 11.18 Food rankings for dietician and patient.

Dietician	Most Favorite	Patient
Vegetables (1)		Fish (2)
Fish (2)		Vegetables (1)
Poultry (3)		Poultry (3)
Beef (4)		Beef (4)
Pork (5)		Pork (5)
	Least Favorite	

Pretest Checklist

The Spearman's rho is a nonparametric (pronounced *non-pair-uh-metric*) test, meaning that the data are not expected to be normally distributed, and hence the pretest criteria for the Pearson regression (normality, linearity, and homoscedasticity) are not pertinent when it comes to running Spearman's correlation. Since each item is only present once per variable, a bar chart, or histogram with a normal curve, would render all the bars at the same height, signifying one entry per value, which would be unrevealing.

The only real pretest criterion for Spearman's rho is to be certain that both lists consist of the same items—in this case, both the dietician and the patient ranked the same five food items, each in their own way.

Test Run

The test run for Spearman test involves the same order menu and results table as the Pearson correlation.

1. Click on *Analyze, Correlate, Bivariate* (Figure 11.19); this will take you to the *Bivariate Correlations* menu (Figure 11.20).

Figure 11.19 Accessing the *Correlation* menu: *Analyze, Correlate, Bivariate.*

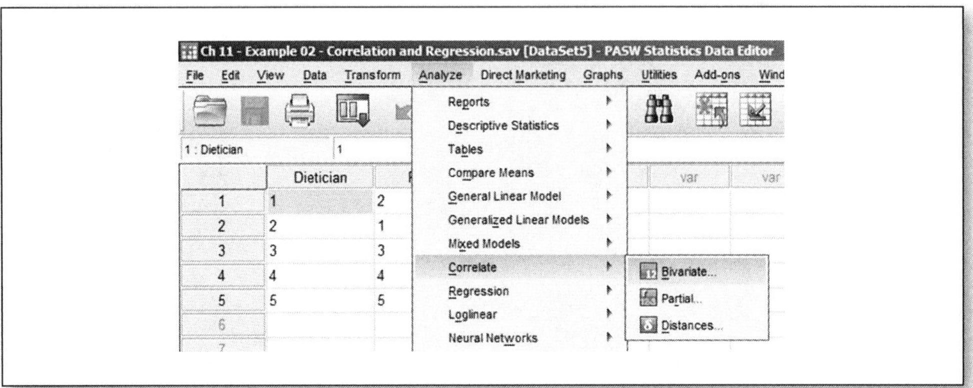

2. On the *Bivariate Correlations* menu (Figure 11.20), move both variables (*Dietician* and *Patient*) from the left window to the right *Variables* window.

3. On the *Correlation Coefficients* options, uncheck ☐ *Pearson* and check ☑ *Spearman*.

4. Click *OK*, and the regression will run.

Figure 11.20 On the bivariate *Correlations* table, move the two variables into the right Variables window, then uncheck ☐ *Pearson* and check ☑ *Spearman*.

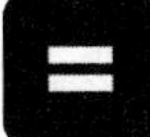

Results

The results are presented in a single *Correlations* table (Table 11.4) indicating a Spearman rho of .900 with a corresponding *p* (Sig.) value of .037. This indicates a significant positive correlation in the ranking of the two food lists. In other words, there is a strong similarity in the order of the foods on these two lists.

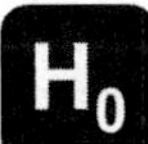

Hypothesis Resolution

The Spearman rho is .900, indicating a positive correlation between the two lists; since the *p* value of .037 is less than the specified .05 α level, we would say that there is a statistically significant (positive) correlation between the food rankings of the dietician and the patient. As such, we would reject H_0 and not reject H_1.

Document Results

To work collaboratively with the patient in building a palatable healthy eating plan, as part of the initial encounter, the dietician asks the patient to sequence five food cards from favorite to least favorite without prompting. The dietician compared the patient's food preference (Fish, Vegetables, Poultry, Beef, Pork) to the recommended optimal nutrition for this patient (Vegetables, Fish, Poultry, Beef, Pork); Spearman's rho produced a statistically significant ($p = .037$, $\alpha = .05$) positive correlation of .900 indicating a strong concurrence between the two lists, suggesting that it should be fairly plausible to assemble a healthy dietary plan that is suitable to this patient's tastes.

Table 11.4 Correlations Table Showing the Spearman's Rho of .900 and Corresponding Statistically Significant *p* (Sig.) Value of .037.

Correlations

			Dietician	Patient
Spearman's rho	Dietician	Correlation Coefficient	1.000	.900*
		Sig. (2-tailed)	.	.037
		N	5	5
	Patient	Correlation Coefficient	.900*	1.000
		Sig. (2-tailed)	.037	.
		N	5	5

*. Correlation is significant at the 0.05 level (2-tailed).

ALTERNATE USE FOR SPEARMAN CORRELATION

The Spearman statistic is a viable alternative to the Pearson statistic when there is one or more substantial violation of the (Pearson) pretest criteria (normality, linearity, homoscedasticity).

Correlation vs. Causation

Correlation only means that two variables appear to move in a predictable direction with respect to each other (e.g., when one goes up, the other goes up; when one goes down, the other goes down; or when one goes up, the other goes down), but keep in mind, this is not necessarily due to *causation,* which would involve the change in one variable *causing* the change in the other. To make the leap from *correlation* to *causation,* three criteria must be met: (1) association/correlation, (2) temporality (meaning timing), and (3) nonspurious (meaning authentic) (Table 11.5).

Admittedly, the criteria to claim causation are strict, but without this rigor, numerous spurious (bogus) correlations could be wrongly attributed to causality, leading to inappropriate conclusions and potentially misguided interventions.

For example, one might find a positive correlation between chocolate milk consumption and automobile theft—as chocolate milk sales go up, so do car thefts. Instead of concluding that chocolate milk causes people to steal cars or that car theft causes one to crave chocolate milk, anyone reasonable would continue his or her investigation and

Table 11.5 Three Criteria for Satisfying Causality: Association/Correlation, Temporality, Nonspurious.

Causality Criteria		
Criteria	**Rule**	**Example**
1. **Association/ correlation**	Variable A and variable B must be empirically related; there must be a (scientific) logical relationship between A and B.	Taking a dose of aspirin lowers fever.
2. **Temporality**	A (cause [independent variable]) precedes B (effect [dependent variable]).	The person took aspirin, and *then* the fever went down, not the other way around.
3. **Nonspurious**	The relationship between A and B is not caused by other variable(s).	The drop in fever is not due to the room getting colder, submerging the person in an ice bath, or other factors.

probably discover that *population* may be a variable worth consideration: In a town with a population of 2,000, we would find low chocolate milk sales and few car thefts, whereas in a city with a population of 2,000,000, chocolate milk sales and car thefts would both be considerably higher. In this case, we would be free to notice the positive correlation between chocolate milk consumption and car theft, but the causal criteria between these two variables clearly breaks down at all three levels.

GOOD COMMON SENSE

Reflecting back on the Pearson regression example, even though a statistically significant, strong positive correlation was found between *Length_of_stay* and *Depression,* it is presumptuous to simply claim that the length of hospitalization (and nothing else) *caused* the depression. There may be an underlying, unaccounted-for factor that would not necessarily be revealed by correlational analysis. Such a factor may be responsible for affecting mood, which, in turn, may have affected the depression score. For example, an adverse factor (e.g., household stress, financial problem, adverse social issue, etc.) may predominately account for the patient's level of depression; conversely, deprivation of a pleasurable factor may degrade one's mood (e.g., missing the joys of being at home, missed socialization, and missing other positive activities).

Alternatively, an overarching factor may affect both the length of the hospitalization and depression, such as a preexisting (depressive) mood disorder, longstanding sense of (learned) helplessness, and so forth.

The point is that correlation, no matter what the r or the p, is just that—an overall *correlation;* try to avoid jumping to conclusions regarding *causation.*

Key Concepts

- Pearson regression (r)
- Correlation
  - Strength
  - Direction
- Normality
- Linearity
- Homoscedasticity
- Bivariate correlation
- Scatterplot
- Regression
- Spearman correlation (rho)
- Correlation vs. causation

Practice Exercises

NOTE: Exercises 11.1 to 11.8 involve continuous data; use the Pearson statistic for these. Exercises 11.9 and 11.10 involve ordinal data; as such, use the Spearman's rho statistic.

Exercise 11.1

A nurse working in the Fitness Center wants to determine the effect that walking rigorously has on weight loss and recruits participants for a weeklong study. At the start and end of the week, each participant will record his or her weight, which will render the total amount of weight lost in the week. During the week, each participant will wear a pedometer, which will count the total number of steps taken that week.

Data set: **Ch 11 – Exercise 01A.sav**

Codebook

Variable:	ID
Definition:	Participant ID (first and last initials)
Type:	Alphanumeric
Variable:	Steps
Definition:	Number of steps walked in a week
Type:	Continuous
Variable:	Weight_loss
Definition:	Number of pounds lost in a week
Type:	Continuous

NOTE: In Data Set A, Record 3, notice that the weight loss (Weight_loss) is −1.00; this indicates that the participant gained 1 pound. Data Set B, Record 16 also signifies a half-pound weight gain for that participant.

a. Write the hypotheses.
b. Run the criteria of the pretest checklist (normality [for both variables], linearity, homoscedasticity) and discuss your findings.
c. Run the bivariate correlation, scatterplot with regression line, and descriptive statistics for both variables and document your findings (r and Sig. [p value], ns, means, standard deviations) and hypothesis resolution.
d. Write an abstract under 200 words detailing a summary of the study, the bivariate correlation, hypothesis resolution, and implications of your findings.

Repeat this exercise using data set: **Ch 11 – Exercise 01B.sav.**

Exercise 11.2

Per concerns that calorie consumption per meal is typically higher when dining out than meals at home, a dietician wants to discover if there is a correlation between age and number of meals eaten outside the home. The dietician recruits participants and administers a two-question survey: (1) How old are you? and (2) How many times do you eat out (meals not eaten at home) in an average week?

Data set: **Ch 11 – Exercise 02A.sav**

Variable: ID
Definition: Participant ID (first and last initials)
Type: Alphanumeric

Variable: Age
Definition: Participant's age
Type: Continuous

Variable: Meals_out
Definition: Number of meals out participant eats per week
Type: Continuous

a. Write the hypotheses.
b. Run the criteria of the pretest checklist (normality [for both variables], linearity, homoscedasticity) and discuss your findings.
c. Run the bivariate correlation, scatterplot with regression line, and descriptive statistics for both variables and document your findings (r and Sig. [p value], ns, means, standard deviations) and hypothesis resolution.
d. Write an abstract under 200 words detailing a summary of the study, the bivariate correlation, hypothesis resolution, and implications of your findings.

Repeat this exercise using data set: **Ch 11 – Exercise 02B.sav.**

Exercise 11.3

A nurse observes that fear of needles is not limited to pediatric patients. In order to determine if there is a connection between age and fear of needles, prior to giving injections, the nurse administers the Acme Needle Phobia Scale (0 = No fear of needles . . . 50 = High fear of needles) to a group of patients.

Data set: **Ch 11 – Exercise 03A.sav**

Variable: ID
Definition: Participant ID
Type: Alphanumeric

Variable: Age
Definition: Participant's age
Type: Continuous

Variable: Needle_phobia
Definition: Score on Acme Needle Phobia Scale
Type: Continuous

a. Write the hypotheses.

b. Run the criteria of the pretest checklist (normality [for both variables], linearity, homoscedasticity) and discuss your findings.

c. Run the bivariate correlation, scatterplot with regression line, and descriptive statistics for both variables and document your findings (*r* and Sig. [*p* value], *ns*, means, standard deviations) and hypothesis resolution.

d. Write an abstract under 200 words detailing a summary of the study, the bivariate correlation, hypothesis resolution, and implications of your findings.

Repeat this exercise using data set: **Ch 11 – Exercise 03B.sav.**

Exercise 11.4

A nurse manager wants to determine if reaction time changes over the duration of the shift. Nurses who volunteer for this study will be asked to take part in a reaction time test, wherein they will push a button as soon as they see a light change from red to blue. Shift time (number of minutes the nurse has been on duty) and reaction time (measured in milliseconds) will be recorded for each test.

NOTE: 1 millisecond (ms) = 1/1000th of a second.

Data set: **Ch 11 – Exercise 04A.sav**

Variable: Time_on_duty
Definition: Time on duty (in minutes)
Type: Continuous

Variable: Reaction_time
Definition: Reaction time (in milliseconds)
Type: Continuous

a. Write the hypotheses.

b. Run the criteria of the pretest checklist (normality [for both variables], linearity, homoscedasticity) and discuss your findings.

c. Run the bivariate correlation, scatterplot with regression line, and descriptive statistics for both variables and document your findings (*r* and Sig. [*p* value], *ns*, means, standard deviations) and hypothesis resolution.

d. Write an abstract under 200 words detailing a summary of the study, the bivariate correlation, hypothesis resolution, and implications of your findings.

Repeat this exercise using data set: **Ch 11 – Exercise 04B.sav.**

Exercise 11.5

A nurse working in audiology wants to discover if there is a correlation between age and the highest frequency (in Hz) that can be heard. For each patient, the nurse records the age and the highest frequency that he or she can hear reliably.

Data set: **Ch 11 – Exercise 05A.sav**

Variable: ID
Definition: Participant ID
Type: Alphanumeric

Variable: Age
Definition: Age
Type: Continuous

Variable: Frequency
Definition: Frequency (in Hertz [Hz])
Type: Continuous

a. Write the hypotheses.
b. Run the criteria of the pretest checklist (normality [for both variables], linearity, homoscedasticity) and discuss your findings.
c. Run the bivariate correlation, scatterplot with regression line, and descriptive statistics for both variables and document your findings (*r* and Sig. [*p* value], *n*s, means, standard deviations) and hypothesis resolution.
d. Write an abstract under 200 words detailing a summary of the study, the bivariate correlation, hypothesis resolution, and implications of your findings.

Repeat this exercise using data set: **Ch 11 – Exercise 05B.sav.**

Exercise 11.6

The nurse manager who is conducting chart reviews wants to determine if the number of patients a nurse has is related to charting mistakes (errors and omissions) during a shift.

Data set: **Ch 11 – Exercise 06A.sav**

Variable: Patients
Definition: Number of patients assigned to the nurse on a shift
Type: Continuous

Variable: Chart_errors
Definition: Nurse's errors and omissions found in medical records for the specified shift
Type: Continuous

a. Write the hypotheses.
b. Run the criteria of the pretest checklist (normality [for both variables], linearity, homoscedasticity) and discuss your findings.
c. Run the bivariate correlation, scatterplot with regression line, and descriptive statistics for both variables and document your findings (*r* and Sig. [*p* value], *n*s, means, standard deviations) and hypothesis resolution.
d. Write an abstract under 200 words detailing a summary of the study, the bivariate correlation, hypothesis resolution, and implications of your findings.

Repeat this exercise using data set: **Ch 11 – Exercise 06B.sav.**

Exercise 11.7

An obstetrics nurse wants to determine if there is a correlation between prenatal care and birth weight. After delivery, the nurse gathers the total number of prenatal appointments kept by the mother and the infant's birth weight.

Data set: **Ch 11 – Exercise 07A.sav**

Variable: ID
Definition: Participant ID
Type: Alphaunmeric

Variable: Prenatal_appts
Definition: Number of prenatal appointments kept
Type: Continuous

Variable: Birth_weight
Definition: Infant's birth weight (in ounces)
Type: Continuous

a. Write the hypotheses.
b. Run the criteria of the pretest checklist (normality [for both variables], linearity, homoscedasticity) and discuss your findings.
c. Run the bivariate correlation, scatterplot with regression line, and descriptive statistics for both variables and document your findings (*r* and Sig. [*p* value], *n*s, means, standard deviations) and hypothesis resolution.

d. Write an abstract under 200 words detailing a summary of th correlation, hypothesis resolution, and implications of your fir

Repeat this exercise using data set: **Ch 11 – Exercise 07B.sav.**

Exercise 11.8

To determine the effectiveness of a drug designed to increase hemoglobin oxygenation, a nu identifies a cohort of patients who are taking this drug reliably and records the day number (that each patient has been taking the drug) and the corresponding O_2 level.

Data set: **Ch 11 – Exercise 08A.sav**

Variable:	Participant
Definition:	Participant number
Type:	Continuous
Variable:	Day
Definition:	Number of days the patient has been taking the drug
Type:	Continuous
Variable:	Oxygenation
Definition:	Oxygen saturation level
Type:	Continuous

a. Write the hypotheses.

b. Run the criteria of the pretest checklist (normality [for both variables], linearity, homoscedasticity) and discuss your findings.

c. Run the bivariate correlation, scatterplot with regression line, and descriptive statistics for both variables and document your findings (*r* and Sig. [*p* value], *n*s, means, standard deviations) and hypothesis resolution.

d. Write an abstract under 200 words detailing a summary of the study, the bivariate correlation, hypothesis resolution, and implications of your findings.

Repeat this exercise using data set: **Ch 11 – Exercise 08B.sav.**

NOTE: Exercises 11.9 and 11.10 involve ordinal data; as such, use the Spearman's rho statistic.

Exercise 11.9

To determine the accuracy of nurses' presumption of patients' priorities during hospitalizations, a patient is asked to identify his or her priorities, while separately, the nurse sequences the same list, attempting to anticipate the patient's unique needs. To quantify the nurse's ability to anticipate the patient's priorities, the data from each list are analyzed using Spearman's rho.

Data set: **Ch 11 – Exercise 09A.sav**

Variable:	Nurse
Definition:	Expected patient priorities (1 = Quiet at night, 2 = Punctual pain Rx, 3 = Prompt response time to nurse call, 4 = Quality of food, 5 = Spiritual support, 6 = Internet access)
Type:	Categorical
Variable:	Patient
Definition:	Patient's priorities in hospital (1 = Quiet at night, 2 = Punctual pain Rx, 3 = Prompt response time to nurse call, 4 = Quality of food, 5 = Spiritual support, 6 = Internet access)
Type:	Categorical

a. Write the hypotheses.

b. Verify the pretest checklist (both independently ranking the same set of items).

c. Run the bivariate correlation for Spearman's rho, and document your findings (Spearman rho and Sig. [*p* value]) and hypothesis resolution.

d. Write an abstract under 200 words detailing a summary of the study, the bivariate correlation, hypothesis resolution, and implications of your findings.

Repeat this exercise using data set: **Ch 11 – Exercise 09B.sav.**

Exercise 11.10

A nurse working individually with patients to enhance healthy living practices begins by asking patients to rank five cards to determine the activities that patients are most amenable to. The patient's ranking is then compared to the nurse's optimal ranking (exercise 30 minutes per day, reduce caloric intake, quit smoking, sleep 8 hours per night, eliminate alcohol consumption). To quantify the concurrence between the recommended plan and the patient's action preferences, the data from each list are analyzed using Spearman's rho.

Data set: **Ch 11 – Exercise 10A.sav**

Variable:	Nurse
Definition:	Recommended healthy practices (1 = Exercise 30 minutes per day, 2 = Reduce caloric intake, 3 = Quit smoking, 4 = Sleep 8 hours per night, 5 = Eliminate alcohol consumption)
Type:	Categorical
Variable:	Patient
Definition:	Recommended healthy practices (1 = 30 minutes of exercise per day, 2 = Reduce caloric intake, 3 = Quit smoking, 4 = Sleep 8 hours per night, 5 = Eliminate alcohol consumption)
Type:	Categorical

a. Write the hypotheses.

b. Verify the pretest checklist (both independently ranking the same set of items).

c. Run the bivariate correlation for Spearman's rho, and document your findings (Spearman rho and Sig. [*p* value]) and hypothesis resolution.

d. Write an abstract under 200 words detailing a summary of the study, the bivariate correlation, hypothesis resolution, and implications of your findings.

Repeat this exercise using data set: **Ch 11 – Exercise 10B.sav.**

CHAPTER 12

Chi-Square

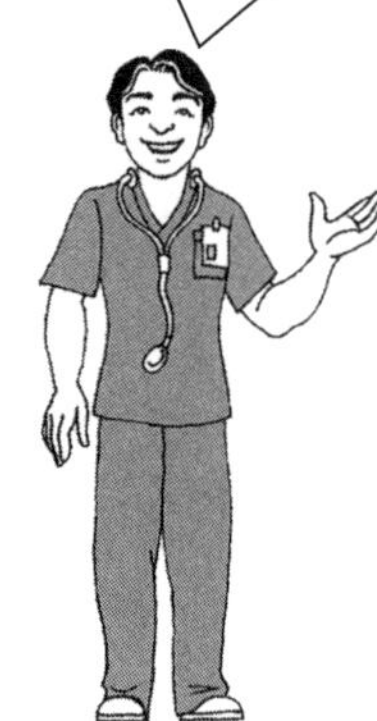
Chi-Square shows the relationship between categorical variables.

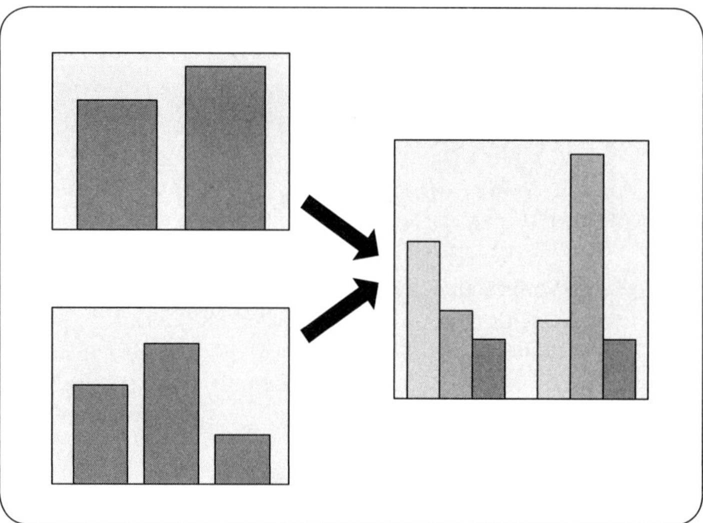

Some people are passionate about aisles, others about window seats.

—Terry Jones

LEARNING OBJECTIVES

Upon completing this chapter, you will be able to:

- Determine when it is appropriate to run a chi-square test
- Identify dichotomous and polychotomous variables
- Verify that the data meet the criteria for running a chi-square test: $n \geq 5$ per cell
- Order a chi-square test: table and bar chart
- Interpret the test results
- Resolve the hypotheses
- Document the results in plain English
- Calculate the % formula

TUTORIAL VIDEO

The tutorial video for this chapter is **Ch 12 – Chi-Square.mp4.** This video provides an overview of chi-square, followed by the SPSS procedures for processing the pretest checklist, ordering the statistical run, and interpreting the results of this test using the data set: **Ch 12 – Example 01 – Chi-Square.sav.**

OVERVIEW—CHI-SQUARE

As we have seen, variables can be *continuous,* such as temperature, distance, weight, bank account balance, mood score, and height. Alternatively, variables may be *categorical,* such as gender, race, religion, blood type, and marital status.

A categorical variable may consist of any number of categories. Variables that contain two categories are referred to as *dichotomous* (pronounced *die-cot-uh-muss*), such as

- Gender: female/male
- Voter status: registered/not registered
- Opinion: yes/no
- Attendance: present/absent
- Dwelling: house/apartment
- Grade: pass/fail

A categorical variable that contains more than two categories is referred to as polychotomous (pronounced *poly-cot-uh-muss*) such as

- Appointment status: on time/late/canceled/no-show/rescheduled
- Marital status: single/married/separated/divorced/widowed
- Organ donor: no/all organs/selective organ(s)
- Visual aids: none/glasses/contact lenses/surgical correction
- Transportation: train/plane/car/bus/taxi/motorcycle/bicycle/walk
- Blood type: A+/A–/B+/B–/AB+/AB–/O+/O–

The statistical function for comparing categorical variables to each other is the chi-square (*chi* is pronounced *k-eye*), sometimes written as χ^2 (χ is the Greek letter chi). The chi-square does not need you to specify how many categories are in each variable; chi-square automatically handles any mix of dichotomous and polychotomous variables.

The chi-square organizes the data from the categorical variables into a grid, compares the categories to each other, and computes a *p* value. If the chi-square produces a *p* value that is less than or equal to α (.05), then this indicates that there is a statistically significant difference among the categories; alternatively, a *p* value greater than α (.05) indicates that no statistically significant differences among the categories exist.

Chi-square can be used to answer questions involving categorical variables, such as, Is *Gender* (Female/Male) correlated with emergency department (ED) entry method (walk-in/ambulance/doctor referral)? In other words, *Do females and males tend to arrive at the ED in the same manner, or are there differences (e.g., walk-ins tend to be female patients, males tend to be brought in by ambulance more so than females, etc.)?*

If the p value is less than or equal to α (.05), then we would say that there is a statistically significant difference between females and males in terms of how they arrive for emergency care. Alternatively, if the p value is greater than the α (.05), then we would say that there is no statistically significant difference between the genders when it comes to how they arrive for emergency care (e.g., the same proportion of females and males arrive via walk-in, ambulance, and doctor referral).

To recap, chi-square can be used to compare categorical variables with the same number of categories in each variable, such as *Gender* (*Female/Male*) to *Opinion* (*Yes/No*), which would render a 2 × 2 chi-square table. Chi-square can also analyze categorical variables that have different category counts without having to specify any additional processing parameters, such as *Gender* (Female/Male) to *Blood type* (*A+/A−/B+/B−/AB+/AB−/O+/O−*); this chi-square test would produce a 2 × 8 or an 8 × 2 chi-square table, depending on how you choose to load the variables into rows and columns—either way, the analysis would produce equivalent results.

Example

The nurse manager of the emergency department wants to determine if gender (female/male) is associated with how patients arrive at the ED (via walk-in/ambulance/doctor referral).

Research Question

Is gender associated with how a patient arrives at the emergency department?

Groups

When it comes to chi-square, it is not so much a matter of *groups* as *categories* within the variables. This inquiry involves two categorical variables: *Gender,* which has two categories (*Female/Male*), and *ED_entry,* which has three categories (*Walk-in/Ambulance/Doctor referral*); notice that *Gender* is dichotomous and *ED_entry* is polychotomous:

- Gender: Female, Male
- ED_entry: Walk-in, Ambulance, Doctor referral

Procedure

The nurse manager will review the emergency department triage records for the prior day, gathering two variables for each patient: *Gender* (*Female/Male*) and *ED entry* method (*Walk-in/Ambulance/Doctor referral*).

Hypotheses

H_0: There is no correlation between gender and ED entry method.

H_1: There is a correlation between gender and ED entry method.

Data Set

Use the following data set: **Ch 12 – Example 01 – Chi-Square.sav.**

Codebook

Variable:	Gender
Definition:	Gender
Type:	Categorical (1 = Female, 2 = Male)
Variable:	ED_entry
Definition:	ED arrival method (1 = Walk-in, 2 = Ambulance, 3 = Doctor referral)
Type:	Categorical

Pretest Checklist

Chi-Square Pretest Checklist

☑ 1. $n \geq 5$ per cell minimum*

*Results produced upon chi-square test run

Pretest Checklist Criterion 1—$n \geq 5$ per Cell Minimum

The chi-square will organize the categorical data from the variables into a table. It is easy to anticipate the dimensions of the table simply by multiplying the number of categories in each variable. In this case, *Gender* has two categories (Female/Male), and *ED_entry* has three categories (Walk-in/Ambulance/Doctor referral); hence, the chi-square table will consist of (2 × 3 =) 6 cells (Table 12.1).

The pretest checklist rule for chi-square states that each cell should have at least 5 entries; initially, one might anticipate that the total *n* for this study should be 30 (6 cells × 5 entries per cell = 30). Actually, the total *n* will need to be more than 30, since a total *n* of 30 would presume that participants' responses will fill the 6 cells evenly (5 per cell). Since this is implausible, we should consider 30 as the ***minimum*** total *n;* we will require a total *n* of more than 30.

The chi-square report will show the counts for each cell. This pretest criteria will be processed during the **Test Run** and finalized in the **Results** section.

Table 12.1 Chi-Square Table Basic Structure for Gender and ED_entry Contains Six Cells.

	Walk-in	*Ambulance*	*Doctor Referral*
Female			
Male			

Test Run

1. From the main screen, click on *Analyze, Descriptive Statistics, Crosstabs* (Figure 12.1); this will bring you to the *Crosstabs* menu (Figure 12.2).

Figure 12.1 Run the chi-square analysis; click on *Analyze, Descriptive Statistics, Crosstabs*.

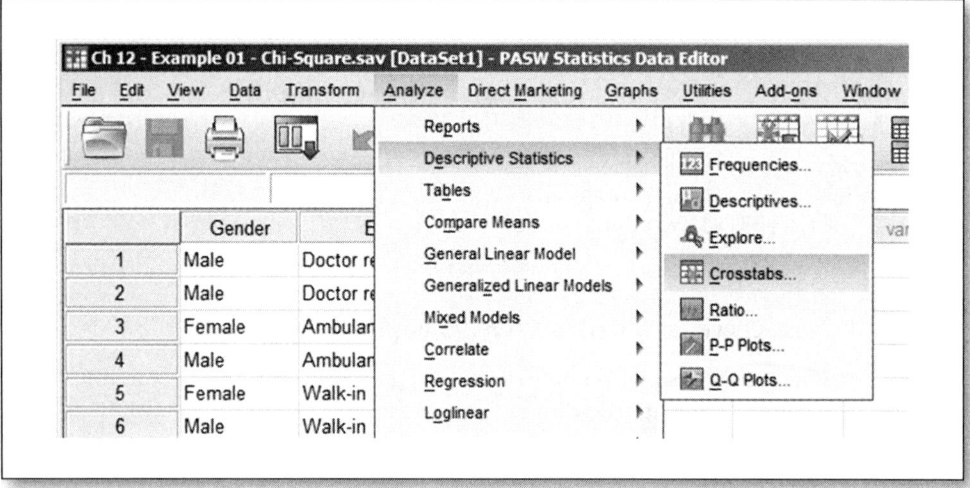

2. On the *Crosstabs* menu, move *Gender* from the left window to the *Row(s)* window, and move *ED_entry* from the left window to the *Column(s)* window.
3. Check the ☑ *Display clustered bar charts* checkbox.
4. Click on the *Statistics* button; this will take you to the *Crosstabs: Statistics* menu (Figure 12.3).

Figure 12.2 Load *Gender* into *Row(s)* and *ED_entry* into *Column(s)* windows and check *Display clustered bar charts.*

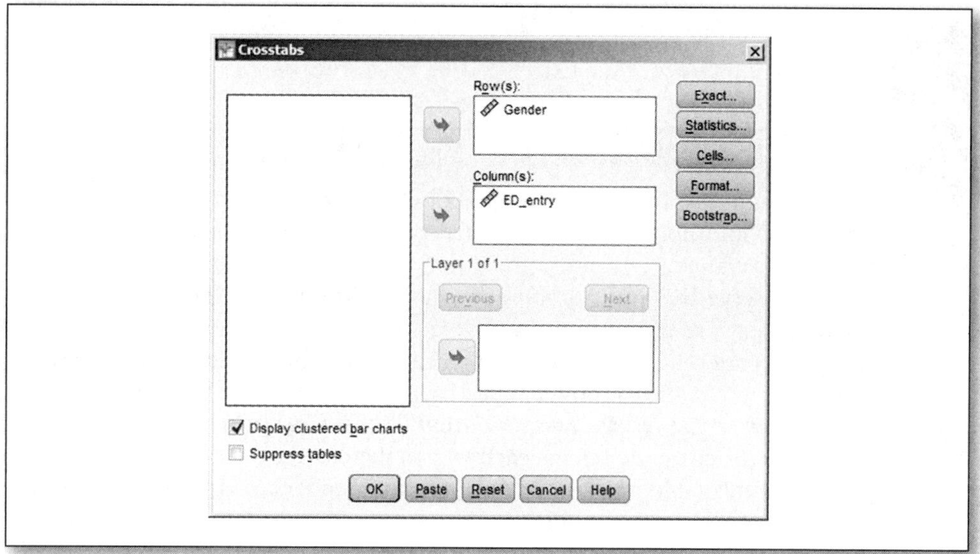

Figure 12.3 *Crosstabs: Statistics* menu: check the *Chi-square* checkbox.

Crosstabs: Statistics

Chi-square
Correlations

Nominal
Contingency coefficient
Phi and Cramer's V
Lambda
Uncertainty coefficient

Ordinal
Gamma
Somers' d
Kendall's tau-b
Kendall's tau-c

Nominal by Interval
Eta

Kappa
Risk
McNemar

Cochran's and Mantel-Haenszel statistics
Test common odds ratio equals: 1

Continue
Cancel
Help

5. Check the ☑ *Chi-square* checkbox.
6. Click on the *Continue* button. This will take you back to the *Crosstabs* menu.
7. Click the *OK* button, and the chi-square will process.

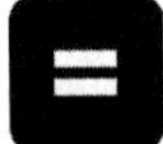

Results

Pretest Checklist Criterion 1—$n \geq 5$ per Cell Minimum

We begin by inspecting the (six) circled cells in the *Crosstabulation* table (Table 12.2) and note that each cell has a count (n) of at least 5; hence, the pretest criterion is satisfied.

Next, observe the Sig. (p) value in the *Chi-Square Tests* table (Table 12.3) on the Pearson chi-square row; it indicates a Sig. (p) value of .009; since this is less than the specified .05 α level, we conclude that there is a statistically significant difference among genders when it comes to how they arrive at the emergency department.

The *Gender * ED_entry Crosstabulation* (Table 12.2) provides clear results detailing how many of each gender arrive each way to the emergency department; even a cursory overview of this table helps us to see that the numbers for females look very different from those of males. The differences among these figures are confirmed by the .009 p value (Table 12.3), but to get a more intuitive grasp of these (numerical) data, inspect the corresponding bar chart (Figure 12.4).

The better you can conceptualize the data, the better prepared you will be to write a cogent Results section detailing your findings. In addition to discussing that the p value indicates a statistically significant difference in ED entry among the genders, the bar chart can help provide additional meaning to the discussion. You may include a narrative explaining that the differences detected in this sample show that females tend to be *Walk-ins* whereas the majority of males are brought in by ambulance, which is graphically evident in the *Bar Chart* (Figure 12.4).

Table 12.2 Gender * ED_entry Crosstabulation.

Gender * ED_entry Crosstabulation

Count

		ED_entry			
		Walk-in	Ambulance	Doctor referral	Total
Gender	Female	16	9	6	31
	Male	8	25	6	39
Total		24	34	12	70

Table 12.3 Chi-Square Tests Results: Sig. (p) = .009.

Chi-Square Tests

	Value	df	Asymp. Sig. (2-sided)
Pearson Chi-Square	9.405[a]	2	.009
Likelihood Ratio	9.637	2	.008
Linear-by-Linear Association	2.584	1	.108
N of Valid Cases	70		

a. 0 cells (.0%) have expected count less than 5. The minimum expected count is 5.31.

Figure 12.4 Chi-square *Bar Chart—Row(s): Gender*, and *Column(s): ED_entry*.

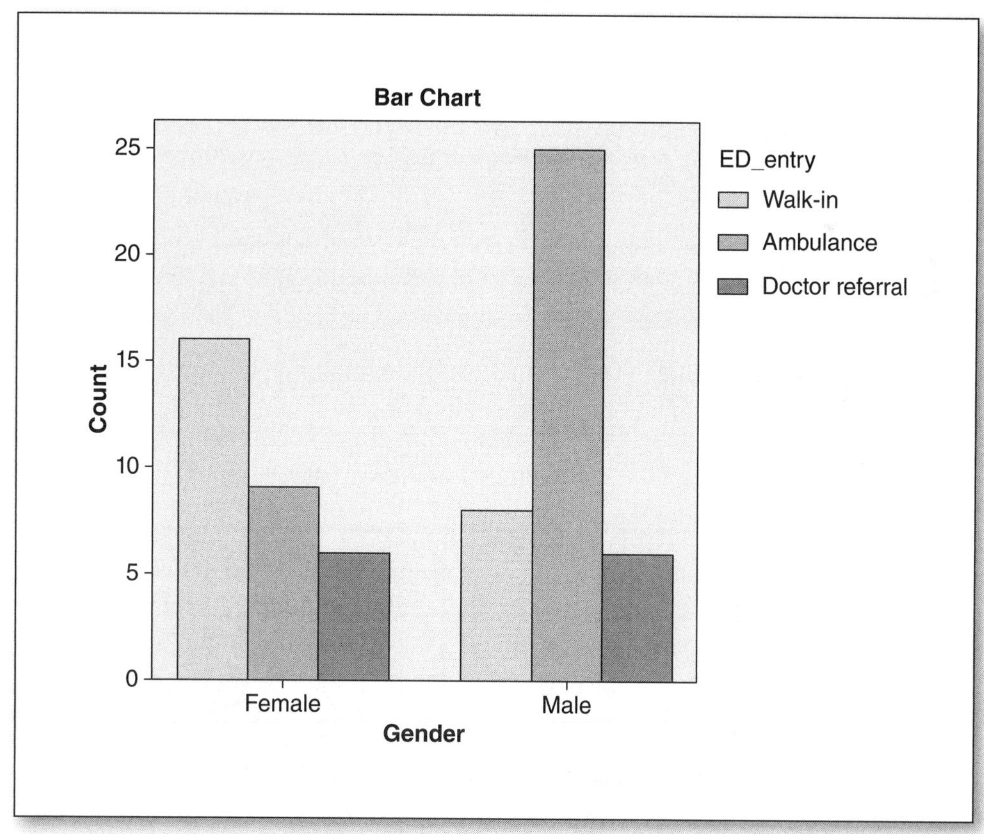

It can be useful to run the chi-square test a second time; swapping the variables (rows/columns) will reconfigure the presentation of the chi-square results, which may offer a different perspective (Figure 12.5).

This will produce the same statistical results as the initial run; notice that the *Chi-Square Tests* tables (Table 12.3 and Table 12.5) are identical, but exchanging the

Figure 12.5 Load *ED_entry* into *Row(s)* and *Gender* into *Column(s)* windows and check *Display clustered bar charts.*

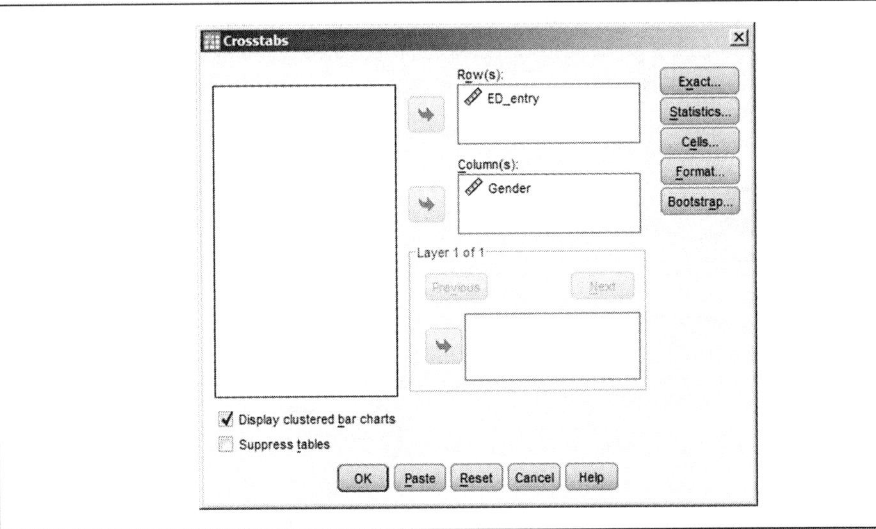

Table 12.4 ED_entry * Gender Crosstabulation.

ED_entry * Gender Crosstabulation

Count

		Gender		Total
		Female	Male	
ED_entry	Walk-in	16	8	24
	Ambulance	9	25	34
	Doctor referral	6	6	12
Total		31	39	70

Table 12.5 Chi-Square Tests Results: Sig. (p) = .009.

Chi-Square Tests

	Value	df	Asymp. Sig. (2-sided)
Pearson Chi-Square	9.405[a]	2	.009
Likelihood Ratio	9.637	2	.008
Linear-by-Linear Association	2.584	1	.108
N of Valid Cases	70		

a. 0 cells (.0%) have expected count less than 5. The minimum expected count is 5.31.

Figure 12.6 Chi-square *Bar Chart—Row(s): ED_entry* and *Column(s): Gender.*

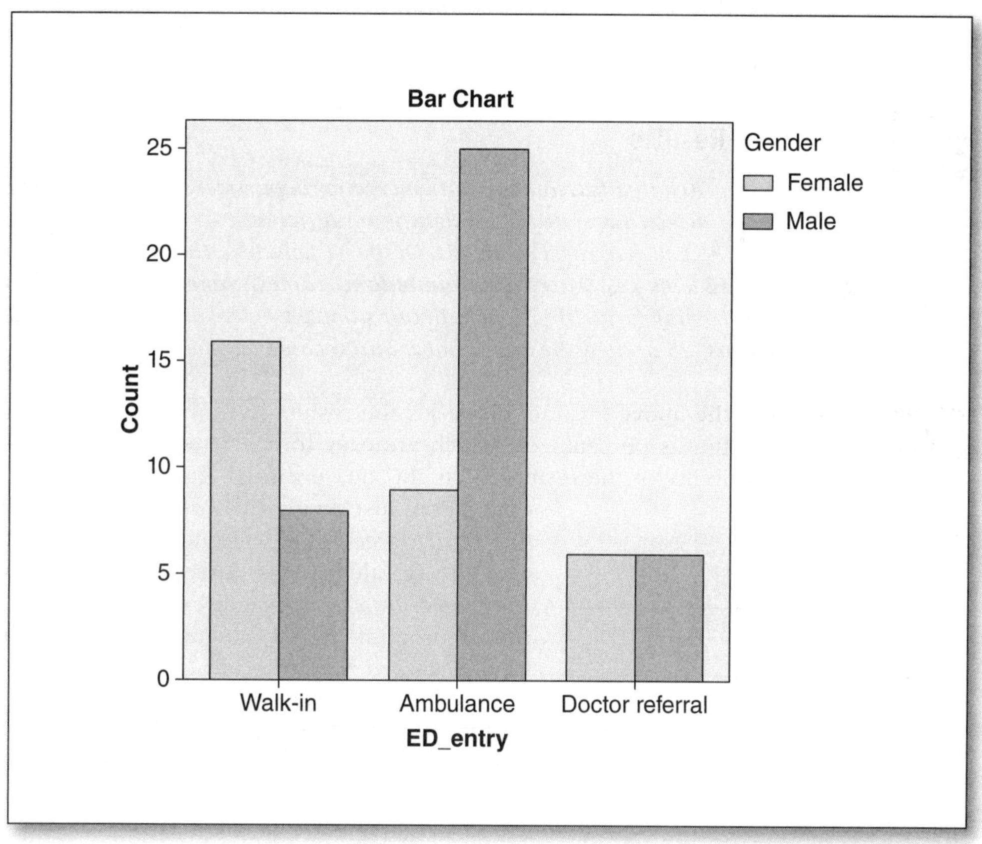

variables in this way arranges the data differently in the Crosstabulation table (Table 12.4) and corresponding bar chart (Figure 12.6), which may offer further insights when interpreting and documenting the results.

The better you can conceptualize the data, the better prepared you will be to write a cogent Results section detailing your findings. In addition to discussing that the *p* value indicates a statistically significant difference in ED entry types among the Genders, the bar chart(s) can help provide additional meaning to the discussion. You may include a narrative explaining that the differences detected in this sample show that in this emergency department, the majority of walk-ins tend to be female, whereas the majority of those brought in by ambulance tend to be male.

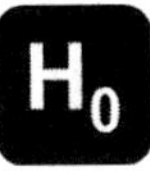

Hypothesis Resolution

H_0: There is no correlation between gender and ED entry method.

H_1: There is a correlation between gender and ED entry method.

The chi-square produced a *p* of .009, which is less than the specified .05 α level, indicating that there is a statistically significant difference between the genders with respect to how they arrive at the emergency department. As such, we would reject H_0 and not reject H_1.

Document Results

Among the 70 patients treated in our emergency department (ED) over a 24-hour period, we detected a statistically significant difference (p = .009, α = .05) with respect to how they arrived at the ED. Of the 31 female patients, most arrived via walk-in (16 walk-ins, 9 arrivals by ambulance, and 6 came via doctor referrals), whereas the majority of the 34 men in our sample were brought in by ambulance (8 walk-ins, 25 arrivals by ambulance, and 6 came via doctor referrals).

Whereas the above abstract discusses the results in terms of the *n*s, this could also be written as percentages, which are easy to calculate and can enhance the comprehensibility of the results. With chi-square results, percentages are a simple calculation; just divide the *Part* (smaller number) by the *Total* (larger number) and multiply by 100. For example, to calculate the *percentage of males brought in by ambulance,* use the following values: **Part = 25** (males brought in by ambulance), **Total = 34** (total number of males) (Table 12.6).

Table 12.6 % Formula.

% Formula
% = **Part ÷ Total × 100**
% = 25 ÷ 34 × 100
% = .7352 × 100
% = 73.52

Consider this documentation variation; the bracketed portions below are included to clarify the percentage calculations but would not typically be included in the write-up:

An assessment of a 24-hour timeframe revealed that our emergency department tended to 70 patients (44% [31 ÷70 = .4429] females and 56% [39 ÷ 70 = .5571] males); 67% [16 ÷ 24 = .6666] of the females were walk-in patients, whereas 73% [25 ÷ 34 = .7352] of men were brought in by ambulance. Chi-square analysis revealed a statistically significant difference (p = .009, α = .05) between genders when it comes to emergency room entry.

GOOD COMMON SENSE

You may find it useful to order the chi-square crosstabulation data with the percentages included instead of (just) the *ns*. To try this, go to the *Crosstabs* menu (Figure 12.2) and click on the *Cells* button. This will take you to the *Crosstabs: Cell Display* menu (Figure 12.7), where you can order *Percentages* for *Row, Column,* and *Total.*

Figure 12.7 *Crosstabs: Cell Display* for percentages, check selections.

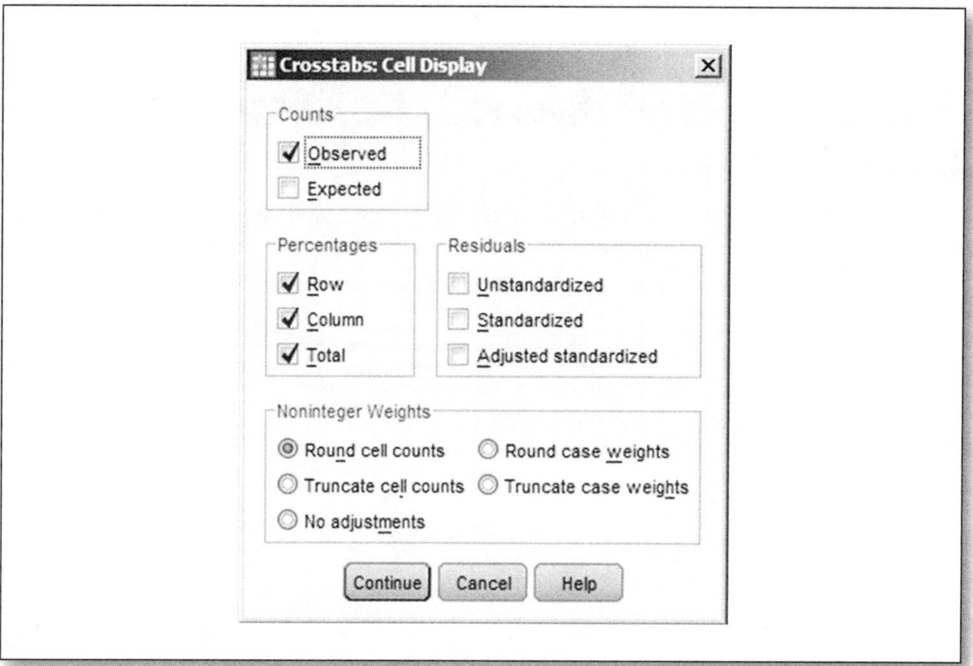

Occasionally, a continuous variable can be converted to a categorical variable, thereby facilitating chi-square analyses. For example, *Age* is a continuous variable (ranging from 0–100), but *Age* could be reduced to two categories: 1 = *Minor* and 2 = *Adult*. SPSS includes an easy-to-use *Recode* feature that helps automate such processes.

Recoding would leave the continuous variable *Age* as is, but based on the *Age*, we could generate values for a new categorical variable, *AgeClass* (1 = *Pediatric*, 2 = *Adult*), using the following criteria:

If *Age* is less than 18, then *AgeClass* = 1.

If *Age* is 18 or greater, then *AgeClass* = 2.

The procedure for recoding variables in this way is detailed in Chapter 14 (see the ★ icon on page **339**).

Key Concepts

- Continuous
- Categorical variables
  - Dichotomous
  - Polychotomous
- Chi-square (χ^2)
- Pretest checklist ($n \geq 5$ per cell)
- Overall n actually required
- Crosstabs
- Percentage calculation

Practice Exercises

Exercise 12.1

The clinicians at Acme Health Clinic want to determine how useful the flu shot is in their community. A nurse approaches patients as they exit the clinic; those who are willing to partake in this study are asked to sign an informed consent document and complete the following card:

Flu Shot Survey

1. Did you receive a flu shot today?

   ☐ Yes

   ☐ No

2. Phone number or email ID: ______________________

A member of our staff will contact you in 90 days to ask if you've contracted the flu this season. Please drop this card in the collection box. Thank you for your participation.

FOR ADMINISTRATIVE USE ONLY

☐ *Got sick with flu*

☐ *Did not get sick with flu*

After 90 days, the nurse administering this study will contact each participant to ask if he or she contracted the flu, and mark the bottom of each card accordingly.

Data set: **Ch 12 – Exercise 01A.sav**

Codebook

Variable:	Flu_shot
Definition:	Patient's flu shot status
Type:	Categorical (1 = Had flu shot, 2 = Did not have flu shot)
Variable:	Flu_sick
Definition:	Patient's (flu) health status
Type:	Categorical (1 = Got sick with flu, 2 = Did not get sick with flu)

HINT: For better clarity on the bar chart, on the *Crosstabs* menu, load *Flu_sick* into *Row(s)* and *Flu_shot* into *Column(s)*. Also, on the *Crosstabs/Cells* menu, consider selecting *Percentages*: ☑ *Row*.

a. Write the hypotheses.
b. Run the criteria of the pretest checklist (*n* is at least 5 per cell in the Crosstabs) and discuss your findings.
c. Run the chi-square test and document your findings (*n*s and/or percentages, Sig. [*p* value]) and hypothesis resolution.
d. Write an abstract under 200 words detailing a summary of the study, the chi-square test results, hypothesis resolution, and implications of your findings.

Repeat this exercise using data set: **Ch 12 – Exercise 01B.sav.**

Exercise 12.2

To determine if the media used to ask a sensitive health-related question (Have you ever used an illegal drug?) has any bearing on the response, you recruit willing participants and randomly assign them to one of three groups: Those in Group 1 will be asked the question via face-to-face interview, those in Group 2 will respond using a standard pencil-and-paper mail-in survey, and those in Group 3 will be directed to an online survey; no names or identifying information will be gathered.

Data set: **Ch 12 – Exercise 02A.sav**

Codebook

Variable:	Media
Definition:	Media used to respond to drug use survey
Type:	Categorical (1 = Face-to-face interview, 2 = Mail-in, 3 = Online survey)
Variable:	Drug
Definition:	Has patient used illegal drugs?
Type:	Categorical (1 = Yes, 2 = No)

HINT: For better clarity on the bar chart, on the *Crosstabs* menu, load *Media* into *Row(s)* and *Drug* into *Column(s)*. Also, on the *Crosstabs/Cells* menu, consider selecting *Percentages:* ☑ *Row*.

a. Write the hypotheses.
b. Run the criteria of the pretest checklist (n is at least 5 per cell in the Crosstabs) and discuss your findings.
c. Run the chi-square test and document your findings (ns and/or percentages, Sig. [p value]).
d. Write an abstract under 200 words detailing a summary of the study, the chi-square test results, hypothesis resolution, and implications of your findings.

Repeat this exercise using data set: **Ch 12 – Exercise 02B.sav.**

Exercise 12.3

On the day of a blood drive, a nurse asked each adult entering the building if he or she is willing to donate blood. Those who agreed to donate were escorted to a donor room; others were thanked courteously. The nurse recorded the responses on a log:

Gender	Blood Donor
☐ Female ☐ Male	☐ Yes ☐ No
☐ Female ☐ Male	☐ Yes ☐ No
☐ Female ☐ Male	☐ Yes ☐ No
☐ Female ☐ Male	☐ Yes ☐ No
☐ Female ☐ Male	☐ Yes ☐ No

At the end of the day, the data were processed to determine if gender was associated with willingness to donate blood.

Data set: **Ch 12 – Exercise 03A.sav**

Codebook

Variable: Gender
Definition: Gender
Type: Categorical (1 = Female, 2 = Male)

Variable: Blood_donor
Definition: Is the person willing to donate blood?
Type: Categorical (1 = Yes, 2 = No)

HINT: For better clarity on the bar chart, on the *Crosstabs* menu, load *Gender* into *Row(s)* and *Blood_donor* into *Column(s)*. Also, on the *Crosstabs/Cells* menu, consider selecting *Percentages:* ☑ *Row*.

a. Write the hypotheses.
b. Run the criteria of the pretest checklist (n is at least 5 per cell in the Crosstabs) and discuss your findings.
c. Run the chi-square test and document your findings (ns and/or percentages, Sig. [p value]).
d. Write an abstract under 200 words detailing a summary of the study, the chi-square test results, hypothesis resolution, and implications of your findings.

Repeat this exercise using data set: **Ch 12 – Exercise 03B.sav.**

Exercise 12.4

A nurse involved in community health wanted to determine if gender was associated with cigarette smoking. The nurse spent the day handing out survey cards in the waiting room:

Smoking Survey

1. Do you smoke cigarettes?

☐ Yes

☐ No

2. What is your gender?

☐ Female

☐ Male

Please drop this card in the collection box.

Thank you for your participation.

Data set: **Ch 12 – Exercise 04A.sav**

Codebook

Variable: Smoker
Definition: Do you smoke cigarettes?
Type: Categorical (1 = Yes, 2 = No)

Variable: Gender
Definition: Gender
Type: Categorical (1 = Female, 2 = Male)

HINT: For better clarity on the bar chart, on the *Crosstabs* menu, load *Gender* into *Row(s)* and *Smoker* into *Column(s)*. Also, on the *Crosstabs/Cells* menu, consider selecting *Percentages:* ☑ *Row*.

a. Write the hypotheses.
b. Run the criteria of the pretest checklist (*n* is at least 5 per cell in the Crosstabs) and discuss your findings.
c. Run the chi-square test and document your findings (*ns* and/or percentages, Sig. [*p* value]).
d. Write an abstract under 200 words detailing a summary of the study, the chi-square test results, hypothesis resolution, and implications of your findings.

Repeat this exercise using data set: **Ch 12 – Exercise 04B.sav.**

Exercise 12.5

To determine if race is associated with taking vitamins, the nurse researcher provided the following survey card to willing volunteers:

Vitamin Survey

1. Do you take one or more vitamins regularly?

☐ Yes
☐ No

2. What is your race?

☐ African American
☐ Asian
☐ Caucasian
☐ Latino
☐ Native American
☐ Other

Please drop this card in the collection box.
Thank you for your participation.

Data set: **Ch 12 – Exercise 05A.sav**

Codebook

Variable: Vitamin
Definition: Takes vitamin(s)
Type: Categorical (1 = Yes, 2 = No)

Variable: Race
Definition: Race
Type: Categorical (1 = African American, 2 = Asian, 3 = Caucasian, 4 = Latino, 5 = Native American, 6 = Other)

HINT: For better clarity on the bar chart, on the *Crosstabs* menu, load *Race* into *Row(s)* and *Vitamin* into *Column(s)*. Also, on the *Crosstabs/Cells* menu, consider selecting *Percentages:* ☑ *Row*.

a. Write the hypotheses.
b. Run the criteria of the pretest checklist (n is at least 5 per cell in the Crosstabs) and discuss your findings.
c. Run the chi-square test and document your findings (ns and/or percentages, Sig. [p value]).
d. Write an abstract under 200 words detailing a summary of the study, the chi-square test results, hypothesis resolution, and implications of your findings.

Repeat this exercise using data set: **Ch 12 – Exercise 05B.sav.**

Exercise 12.6

To better comprehend the distribution of female-to-male nursing ratios among local hospitals, (deidentified) data were gathered from four facilities indicating the gender of each nurse on staff.

Data set: **Ch 12 – Exercise 06A.sav**

Codebook

Variable: Facility
Definition: Facility name
Type: Categorical (1 = Northport Health Clinic, 2 = Eastview Memorial Hospital, 3 = Southside Community Hospital, 4 = Westbridge Wellness Center)

Variable: Gender
Definition: Nurse's gender
Type: Categorical (1 = Female, 2 = Male)

HINT: For better clarity on the bar chart, on the *Crosstabs* menu, load *Facility* into *Row(s)* and *Gender* into *Column(s)*. Also, on the *Crosstabs/Cells* menu, consider selecting *Percentages:* ☑ *Row*.

a. Write the hypotheses.
b. Run the criteria of the pretest checklist (n is at least 5 per cell in the Crosstabs) and discuss your findings.

c. Run the chi-square test and document your findings (*n*s and/or percentages, Sig. [*p* value]).

d. Write an abstract under 200 words detailing a summary of the study, the chi-square test results, hypothesis resolution, and implications of your findings.

Repeat this exercise using data set: **Ch 12 – Exercise 06B.sav.**

Exercise 12.7

A nurse manager gathered data from the last 24 hours to determine if the triage levels in the emergency department are (proportionately) the same across day and night shifts.

Data set: **Ch 12 – Exercise 07A.sav**

Codebook

Variable:	Shift
Definition:	Time of shift
Type:	Categorical (1 = 7:00 a.m.–7:00 p.m., 2 = 7:00 p.m.–7:00 a.m.)

Variable:	Triage
Definition:	Triage level
Type:	Categorical (1 = first priority, 2 = second priority, 3 = third priority)

HINT: For better clarity on the bar chart, on the *Crosstabs* menu, load *Shift* into *Row(s)* and *Triage* into *Column(s)*. Also, on the *Crosstabs/Cells* menu, consider selecting *Percentages:* ☑ *Row*.

a. Write the hypotheses.

b. Run the criteria of the pretest checklist (*n* is at least 5 per cell in the Crosstabs) and discuss your findings.

c. Run the chi-square test and document your findings (*n*s and/or percentages, Sig. [*p* value]).

d. Write an abstract under 200 words detailing a summary of the study, the chi-square test results, hypothesis resolution, and implications of your findings.

Repeat this exercise using data set: **Ch 12 – Exercise 07B.sav.**

Exercise 12.8

A nurse working primarily with psychiatric patients wants to determine if patients with some diagnoses are more medication adherent than others. The patients who opt to participate agree to report their medication adherence.

Data set: **Ch 12 – Exercise 08A.sav**

Codebook

Variable:	Diagnosis
Definition:	Psychiatric diagnosis
Type:	Categorical (1 = Major depressive disorder, 2 = Bipolar, 3 = Schizophrenia)
Variable:	Rx_adherent
Definition:	Is patient adherent with medication dosages?
Type:	Categorical (1 = Yes, 2 = No)

HINT: For better clarity on the bar chart, on the *Crosstabs* menu, load *Diagnosis* into *Row(s)* and *Rx_adherent* into *Column(s)*. Also, on the *Crosstabs/Cells* menu, consider selecting *Percentages:* ☑ *Row*.

a. Write the hypotheses.
b. Run the criteria of the pretest checklist (n is at least 5 per cell in the Crosstabs) and discuss your findings.
c. Run the chi-square test and document your findings (*ns* and/or percentages, Sig. [p value]).
d. Write an abstract under 200 words detailing a summary of the study, the chi-square test results, hypothesis resolution, and implications of your findings.

Repeat this exercise using data set: **Ch 12 – Exercise 08B.sav.**

Exercise 12.9

A nurse wants to determine if the patient's disease has any bearing on his or her willingness to partake in a peer support group. The nurse offers all patients with a diagnosis of cancer, HIV, diabetes, or hypertension information regarding the appropriate group and asks if the patient wishes to attend a meeting.

Data set: **Ch 12 – Exercise 09A.sav**

Codebook

Variable:	Diagnosis
Definition:	Medical diagnosis
Type:	Categorical (1 = Cancer, 2 = HIV, 3 = Diabetes, 4 = Hypertension)
Variable:	Support_group
Definition:	Does patient opt to attend support group?
Type:	Categorical (1 = Yes, 2 = No)

HINT: For better clarity on the bar chart, on the *Crosstabs* menu, load *Diagnosis* into *Row(s)* and *Support_group* into *Column(s)*. Also, on the *Crosstabs/Cells* menu, consider selecting *Percentages:* ☑ *Row*.

a. Write the hypotheses.
b. Run the criteria of the pretest checklist (*n* is at least 5 per cell in the Crosstabs) and discuss your findings.
c. Run the chi-square test and document your findings (*n*s and/or percentages, Sig. [*p* value]).
d. Write an abstract under 200 words detailing a summary of the study, the chi-square test results, hypothesis resolution, and implications of your findings.

Repeat this exercise using data set: **Ch 12 – Exercise 09B.sav.**

Exercise 12.10

A nurse administrator wants to determine if there is a difference in day and night shift nurses when it comes to completing all clinical recertification/continuing professional educational courses on time.

Data set: **Ch 12 – Exercise 10A.sav**

Codebook

Variable:	Shift
Definition:	Day or night shift
Type:	Categorical (1 = Day, 2 = Night)
Variable:	Recertification
Definition:	Did the nurse complete all required courses on time?
Type:	Categorical (1 = Complete, 2 = Incomplete)

HINT: For better clarity on the bar chart, on the *Crosstabs* menu, load *Shift* into *Row(s)* and *Recertification* into *Column(s)*. Also, on the *Crosstabs/Cells* menu, consider selecting *Percentages:* ☑ *Row*.

a. Write the hypotheses.
b. Run the criteria of the pretest checklist (*n* is at least 5 per cell in the Crosstabs) and discuss your findings.
c. Run the chi-square test and document your findings (*n*s and/or percentages, Sig. [*p* value]).
d. Write an abstract under 200 words detailing a summary of the study, the chi-square test results, hypothesis resolution, and implications of your findings.

Repeat this exercise using data set: **Ch 12 – Exercise 10B.sav.**

CHAPTER 13

Logistic Regression

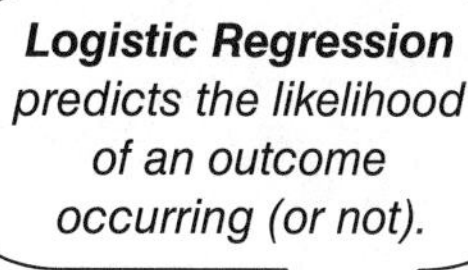

Logistic Regression predicts the likelihood of an outcome occurring (or not).

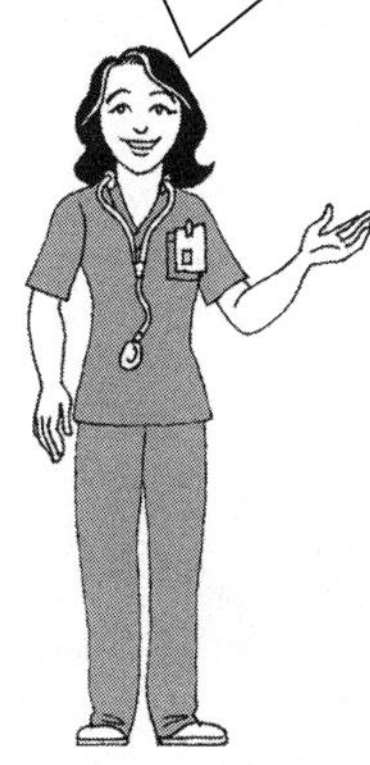

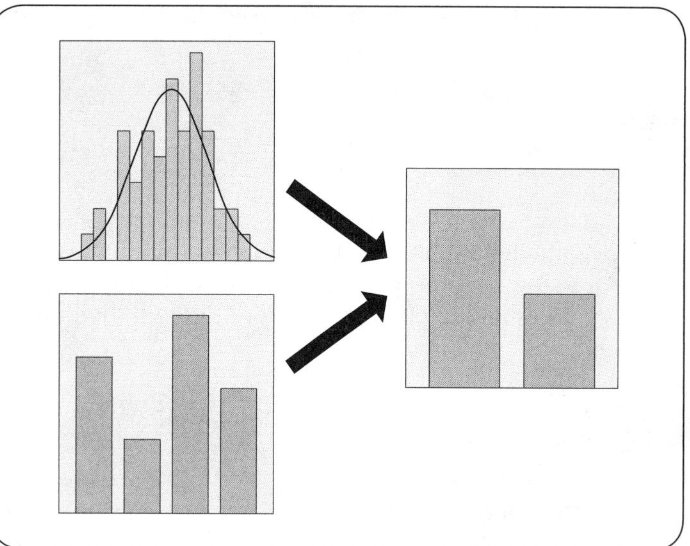

The right choices over time greatly improve your odds of a long and healthy life.

—Tom Rath

LEARNING OBJECTIVES

Upon completing this chapter, you will be able to:

- Determine when it is appropriate to run a logistic regression analysis
- Verify that the data meet the criteria for logistic regression processing: sample size, normality, and multicollinearity

(Continued)

(Continued)

- Order a logistic regression test
- Comprehend the R^2 statistic
- Label and derive results from the *Variables in the Equation* table
- Selectively process findings to respond to a variety of research questions
- Understand the rationale for recoding categorical variables
- Resolve the hypotheses
- Document the results in plain English
- Comprehend the fundamental principle of multiple regression (R^2)

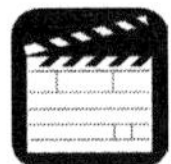

VIDEO

The tutorial video for this chapter is **Ch 13 – Logistic Regression.mp4.** This video provides an overview of the logistic regression statistic, followed by the SPSS procedures for processing the pretest checklist, ordering the statistical run, and interpreting the results of this test using the data set: **Ch 13 – Example 01 – Logistic Regression.sav.**

OVERVIEW—LOGISTIC REGRESSION

In health science, there are interventions, experiments, and general happenstances that produce dichotomous results, wherein one of two possible outcomes occurs. For example, resuscitation could be thought of as having one of two possible outcomes—the patient either does or does not survive. Other examples that could be considered as having dichotomous outcomes involve did/did not have an adverse drug reaction, did/did not develop a nosocomial infection, did/did not adhere to prescribed medication regime, did/did not have surgical complications, and does/does not have fever.

In addition to including the outcome variable (e.g., still smoking/quit smoking) in a logistic regression model, it also includes (predictor) variables (e.g., age, income, baseline daily smoking, gender, race); these are variables that are reasonably thought to be associated with the outcome variable. The logistic regression processor assesses the relationships among the variables to provide a model that describes the (predictive) factors associated with the observed outcome.

While the logistic regression model insists on a dichotomous (two-category) outcome variable, you may have surmised from this example that this statistic is liberal in terms of the types of predictor variables that can be included. Logistic regression accommodates continuous predictor variables (e.g., age, income, baseline daily smoking), categorical predictor variables (e.g., gender, race), or any combinations(s) thereof.

The findings from a logistic regression model can provide insights as to the outcome of a current investigation, or in some cases, the findings may serve as a viable predictive model, anticipating the outcome of a future similar circumstance.

Example

A nurse has conducted a smoking cessation workshop for a wide variety of patients who wish to quit smoking. At the conclusion of the series, instead of simply calculating the percentage of the participants who quit smoking, logistic regression is used to better comprehend the characteristics of those who succeeded.

Research Question

What influences do (predictive) variables such as age, income, baseline mean number of cigarettes smoked daily, gender, and race have when it comes to quitting (or not quitting) smoking?

Groups

In this example, all of the members are included in a single group—everyone receives the same smoking cessation intervention.

Procedure

As a public service, the Acme Health Center advertises and offers a free 90-day smoking cessation program, consisting of nurse-facilitated psychoeducational meetings, peer support from those who have been smoke free for more than 1 year, and multimedia resources designed to promote smoking cessation.

At the conclusion of the intervention, each participant is requested to respond to a self-administered anonymous *Smoking Cessation Survey* card (Figure 13.1).

Hypotheses

Considering that this is the first run of this intervention, we have no plausible basis for presuming that any of the predictors will produce statistically significant findings (e.g., females will quit more frequently than males, those with higher income will have a better chance at quitting than those with lower income, etc.). Naturally, such hypotheses could be drafted; however, for this initial run, we will take a less specific exploratory approach:

H_0: Age, income, baseline smoking, gender, and race do not influence one's success in a smoking cessation intervention.

H_1: Age, income, baseline smoking, gender, or race influence one's success in a smoking cessation intervention.

Figure 13.1 *Smoking Cessation Survey* card, anonymously completed by each participant at the conclusion of the intervention.

Smoking Cessation Survey

1. What is your age? __________
2. What is your annual (gross) income? __________
3. Prior to this intervention, how many cigarettes did you smoke in an average day? __________
4. What is your gender?

   ☐ Female ☐ Male
5. What is your race?

   ☐ African American ☐ Asian ☐ Caucasian ☐ Latino ☐ Other
6. What is your current smoking status?

   ☐ Still smoking ☐ Quit smoking

Please drop this card into the survey box.

Thank you for your participation.

Data Set

Use the following data set: **Ch 13 – Example 01 – Logistic Regression.sav.**

Codebook

Variable: Gender
Definition: Predictor: Gender
Type: Categorical
0 = Female [← *REFERENCE*]
1 = Male

Variable: Race
Definition: Predictor: Race
Type: Categorical
0 = African American [← *REFERENCE*]
1 = Asian
2 = Caucasian
3 = Latino
4 = Other

Variable: Age
Definition: Predictor: Age
Type: Continuous

Variable: Income
Definition: Predictor: Annual gross income (in dollars)
Type: Continuous

Variable: Cigarettes
Definition: Predictor: Baseline mean number of cigarettes smoked daily
Type: Continuous

Variable: Smoking_status
Definition: Outcome: Smoking status at conclusion of smoking cessation intervention
Type: Categorical
0 = Still smoking
1 = Quit smoking [← *BASIS FOR MODEL*]

This codebook includes six variables: The five predictor variables consist of two categorical variables (*Gender* and *Race*) and three continuous variables (*Age, Income,* and *Cigarettes*). The (one) outcome variable is a dichotomous categorical variable (*Smoking_status*).

For the most part, this codebook resembles the others presented throughout this text; in fact, there are no modifications to the way that the continuous variables (*Age, Income,* and *Cigarettes*) are presented, but in preparation for logistic regression processing, notice that some of the attributes for the categorical variables are different:

- The values for each categorical variable are arranged vertically to facilitate better visual clarity.
- The numbering of the categorical values begins with 0 instead of 1.
- For each of the categorical predictor variables (*Gender* and *Race*), the first category (0) is identified as the *REFERENCE* category; this will be explained in further detail in the Results section.
- For the outcome variable (*Smoking_status*), the last category (1 = *Quit smoking*) is identified as the *BASIS* for this logistic regression model; this will be explained in further detail in the Results section.

Pretest Checklist

Logistic Regression Pretest Checklist

☑ 1. *n* quota*

☑ 2. Normality*

☑ 3. Multicollinearity*

*Run prior to logistic regression test

Three pretest criteria need to be assessed to better ensure the robustness of the findings: **(1) *n* quota, (2) normality,** and **(3) multicollinearity.**

Pretest Checklist Criterion 1—*n* Quota

Considering that the logistic regression statistic is unique in that it accommodates both continuous and categorical predictor variables, there are several steps involved in determining the minimum required sample size.

First, determine the minimum *n:*

1. Count the total number of continuous predictor variables (*Age, Income, Cigarettes*) = **3**.
2. Count the number of categories contained within each categorical variable (*Gender* and *Race*) and subtract 1 from each:
   - *Gender* has 2 categories (*Female, Male*): 2 − 1 = **1.**
   - *Race* has 5 categories (*African American, Asian, Caucasian, Latino, Other*): 5 − 1 = **4.**
3. Add the (**bold**) figures together: **3** + **1** + **4** = **8.**
4. Multiply that sum by 10: **8** × 10 = 80. The minimum *n* required to run this logistic regression is 80.

You may find it clearer to organize the variables in a table (Table 13.1).

- For each continuous variable, *n* = 10.
- For each categorical variable, *n* = (number of categories − 1) × 10.

Table 13.1 Assess the Variables to Determine the Minimum *n* Required to Run a Robust Logistic Regression (in This Case, *n* = 80).

Variable	Type	Categorical (Categories − 1) × 10	Continuous 10
Age	Continuous		10
Income	Continuous		10
Cigarettes	Continuous		10
Gender	Categorical	10	
Race	Categorical	40	
Total *n* quota = 80		**50**	**30**

Proceed by verifying that the data set contains the minimum required *n* (80):

5. On the SPSS main menu, click on *Analyze, Descriptive Statistics, Frequency* (Figure 13.2).

Figure 13.2 To determine the *n* of the data set, click on *Analyze, Descriptive Statistics, Frequencies.*

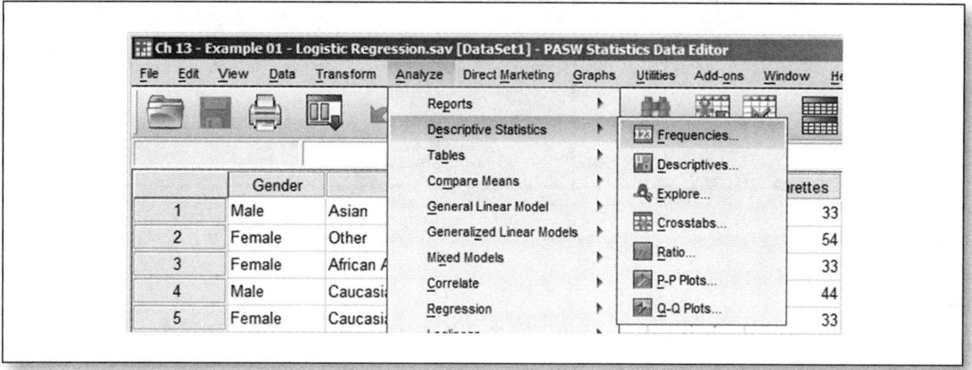

6. Move the outcome variable (*Smoking_Status*) into the *Variable(s)* window (Figure 13.3).

Figure 13.3 On the *Frequencies* menu, move the outcome variable (*Smoking_status*) into the *Variable(s)* window.

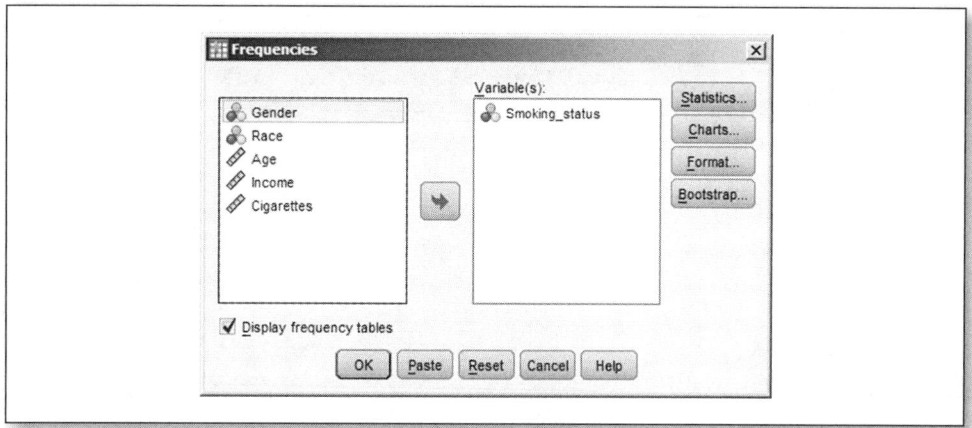

7. Click on *OK*.

The *Smoking_status* table shows a *Total Frequency* (n) of 218, which is greater than the minimum required ($n = 80$); hence, this pretest criterion is satisfied (Table 13.2).

Table 13.2 Descriptive Statistics for Smoking Status: Total (n) = 218.

Smoking_status

		Frequency	Percent	Valid Percent	Cumulative Percent
Valid	Still smoking	111	50.9	50.9	50.9
	Quit smoking	107	49.1	49.1	100.0
	Total	218	100.0	100.0	

Pretest Checklist Criterion 2—Normality

Each of the (three) continuous variables should be normally distributed. This will involve ordering histograms with normal curves and inspecting each for normality. The procedure for ordering these charts is detailed on page **58**; at the ★ icon, move *Age, Income, Cigarettes* into the *Variable(s)* window (Figure 13.4).

Figure 13.4 To order histograms with normal curves for the continuous variables, click on *Analyze, Descriptive Statistics, Frequencies.*

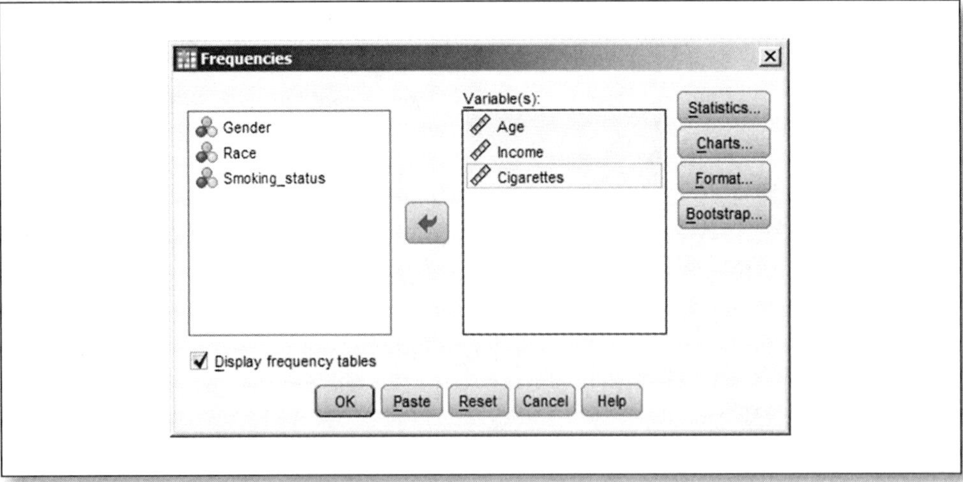

The histograms with normal curves for *Age, Income,* and *Cigarettes* (Figures 13.5, 13.6, and 13.7) are normally distributed; hence, this criterion is satisfied.

Figure 13.5 Histogram for *Age.*

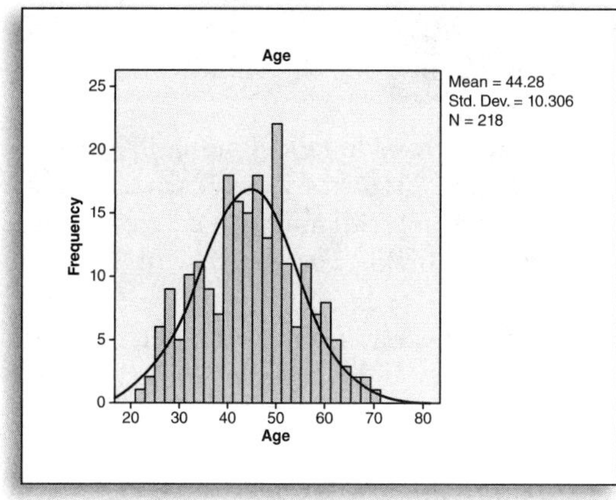

Figure 13.6 Histogram for *Income.*

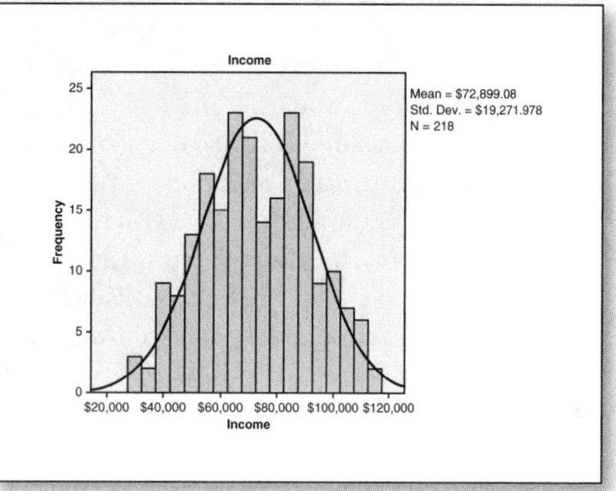

Figure 13.7 Histogram for *Cigarettes.*

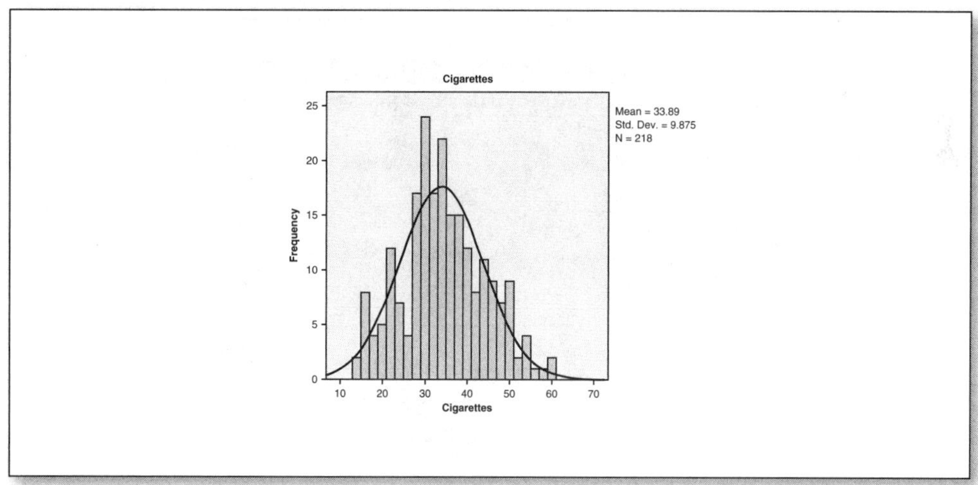

Pretest Checklist Criterion 3—Multicollinearity

The term *multicollinearity* describes two continuous variables that are very highly correlated. Loading two such variables into a logistic regression model essentially constitutes double-loading the processor; *checking that we do not have multicollinearity* assures us that each continuous variable that we intend to load into the logistic regression model is (statistically) unique. As a rule, variables that have a (Pearson) correlation that is either less than −.9 or greater than +.9 are considered too highly correlated, which would constitute multicollinearity. In such instances, one of the variables should be eliminated from the model—presumably the one that has less utility (e.g., conceptually less critical, more costly/inconvenient to gather). We will use the ±.9 cutoff to assess for multicollinearity, but this threshold is not set in stone; some statisticians set the cutoff at ±.7 or ±.8.

It is possible to construct a perfectly viable logistic regression model primarily consisting of categorical variables. If there are 0 or 1 continuous predictor variables in the logistic regression model, then you do not need to be concerned with multicollinearity—there would be no (other) continuous variable(s) to be too highly correlated with. In such cases, you can simply skip this step.

Considering that there are three continuous predictor variables in this model, we need to check for multicollinearity; we will run a correlational analysis involving all (three) continuous variables:

1. On the main screen, click on *Analyze, Correlate, Bivariate* (Figure 13.8).

Figure 13.8 Check for multicollinearity; click on *Analyze, Correlate, Bivariate.*

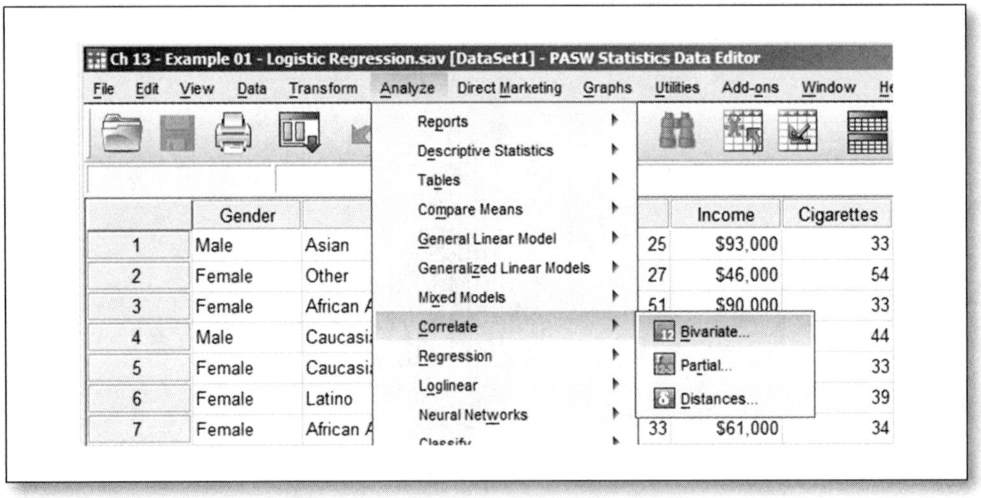

2. On the *Bivariate Correlations* menu (Figure 13.9), move the continuous variables (*Age, Income, Cigarettes*) into the *Variables* window.
3. Click on *OK*.

Figure 13.9 *Bivariate Correlation* menu—load *Age, Income,* and *Cigarettes* into *Variables* window.

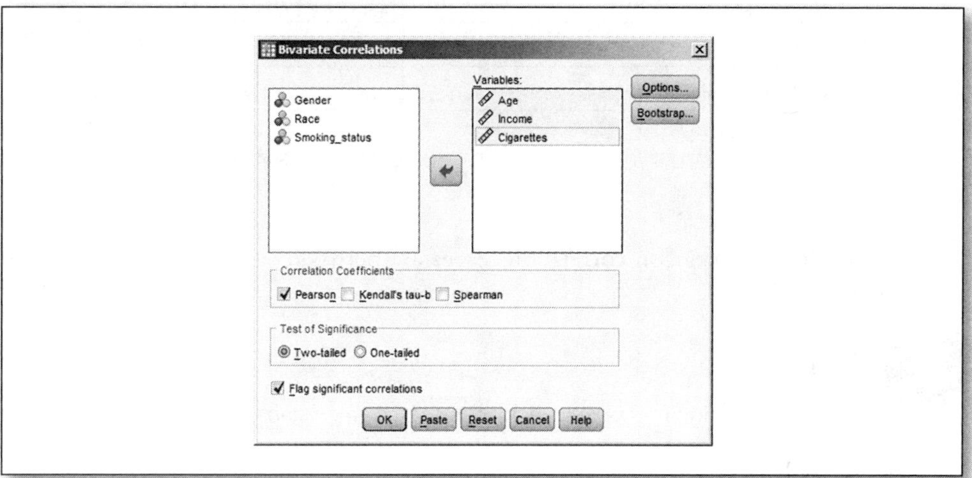

The *Correlations* table indicates the correlations between each pair of continuous variables (Table 13.3). For further clarity, these correlations are summarized in Table 13.4.

Table 13.3 *Correlations* Table Shows the Pearson Correlations for Each Pair of Continuous Variables (Age : Income, Age : Cigarettes, Income : Cigarettes).

Correlations

		Age	Income	Cigarettes
Age	Pearson Correlation	1	.073	-.250**
	Sig. (2-tailed)		.284	.000
	N	218	218	218
Income	Pearson Correlation	.073	1	-.095
	Sig. (2-tailed)	.284		.161
	N	218	218	218
Cigarettes	Pearson Correlation	-.250**	-.095	1
	Sig. (2-tailed)	.000	.161	
	N	218	218	218

**. Correlation is significant at the 0.01 level (2-tailed).

Table 13.4 Summary Correlation Table.

Pair	Pearson
Age : Income	.073
Age : Cigarettes	−.250
Income : Cigarettes	−.095

Each of the Pearson correlation scores are between −.9 and +.9; hence, this criterion is satisfied.

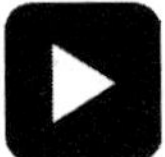

Test Run

1. On the main SPSS menu, click on *Analyze, Regression, Binary Logistic* (Figure 13.10).

Figure 13.10 To run a logistic regression, click on *Analyze, Regression, Binary Logistic.*

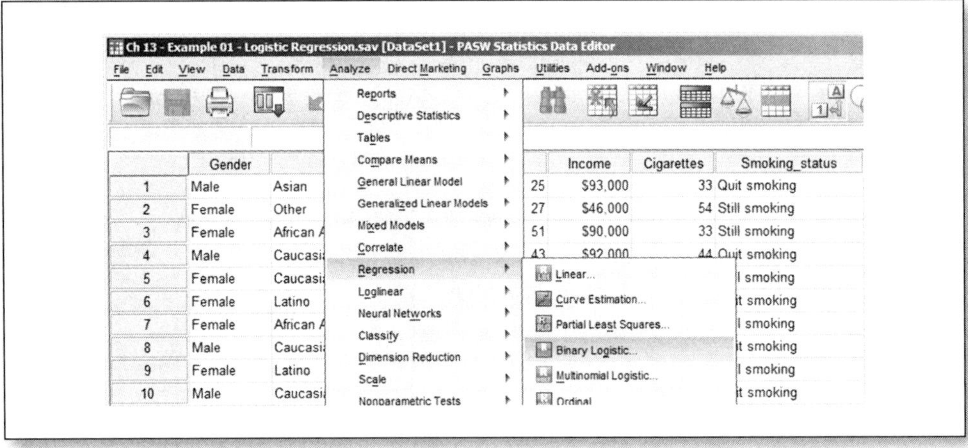

2. On the *Logistic Regression* menu (Figure 13.11), move the outcome variable *(Smoking_status)* into the *Dependent box.*

3. Move the predictor variables (*Gender, Race, Age, Income, Cigarettes*) into the *Covariates* window.

Figure 13.11 *Logistic Regression* menu—move outcome variable into the *Dependent* box and predictor variables into the *Covariates* window.

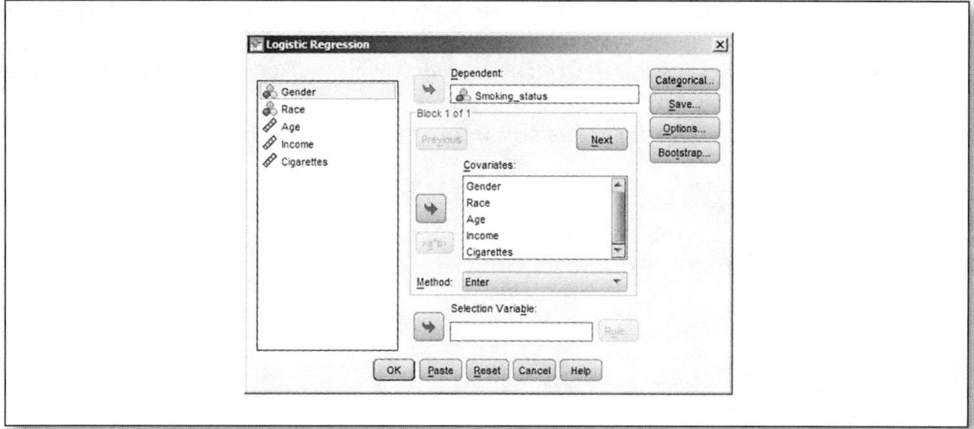

4. Next, identify the categorical variables: Click on *Categorical*.
5. On the *Logistic Regression: Define Categorical Variables* menu, move the two categorical variables (*Gender* and *Race*) into the *Categorical Covariates* window (Figure 13.12).

Figure 13.12 *Logistic Regression: Define Categorical Variables* menu—move categorical predictor variables into the *Categorical Variables* window.

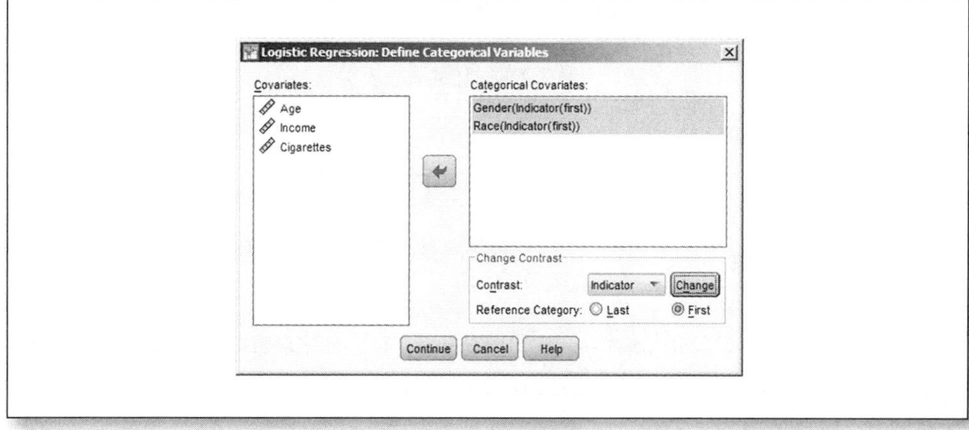

6. In this example, the first category within each categorical variable will be designated as the *Reference Category;* as such, select (highlight) the two variables in the *Categorical Covariates* window.
7. For the *Reference Category,* click on ⊙ *First,* and click on *Change.*

NOTE: The notion of the *Reference Category* will be discussed in the Results section.

8. Click on *Continue*—this will return you to the *Logistic Regression* menu.
9. Click on *Options.*
10. On the *Logistic Regression Options* menu, check ☑ *CI for exp(B).* Use the default value of 95% (Figure 13.13).

Figure 13.13 *Logistic Regression Options* menu—select the *CI for exp(B)* (confidence interval), using the default value of 95%.

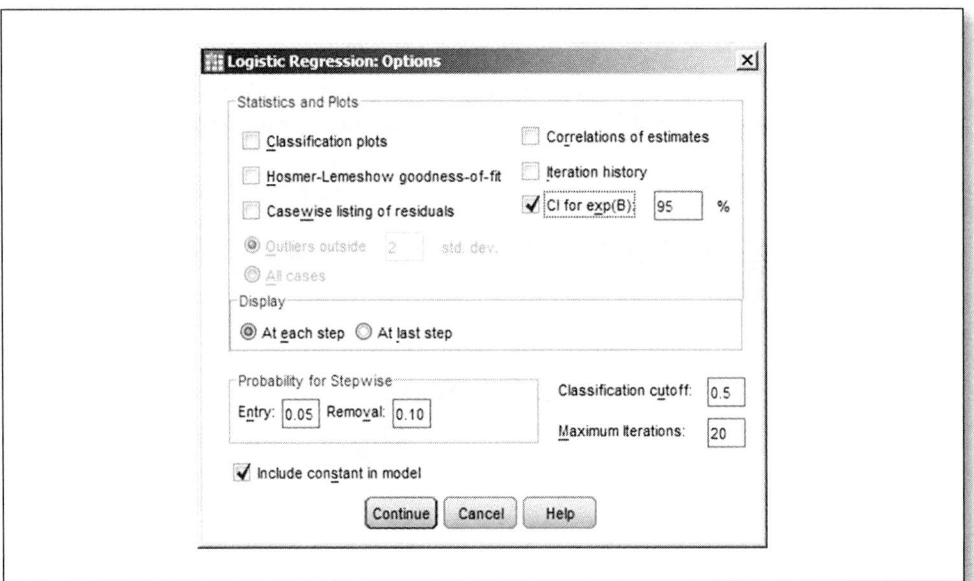

11. Click on *Continue*—this will return you to the *Logistic Regression* menu.
12. Click on *OK.*

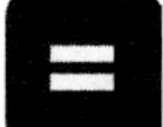

Results

Examine the first row of the *Omnibus Tests of Model Coefficients* table (Table 13.5); the Sig. (p) is .000, which is less than .05; this indicates that somewhere in the model, at least one of the predictor variables is statistically significant with respect to predicting the outcome variable (did/did not quit smoking). If this Sig. (p) is greater than .05, then this would indicate that the overall model is statistically insignificant, meaning that none of the predictors strongly predict the outcome variable. To discover *which* predictor variable(s) statistically significantly predict the outcome variable, we will look to the *Variables in the Equation* table and identify the rows where Sig. (p) is less than or equal to .05.

Table 13.5 Omnibus Tests of Model Coefficients Table Shows a Sig. (p) < .05—Hence, at Least One Predictor in the Model Is Statistically Significant.

Omnibus Tests of Model Coefficients

		Chi-square	df	Sig.
Step 1	Step	129.192	8	.000
	Block	129.192	8	.000
	Model	129.192	8	.000

Comprehending R^2

Prior to investigating the *Variables in the Equation* table, we will take a short diversion to discuss the R^2 statistic. The R^2 is regularly used in multiple regression, which is different from logistic regression; while both can process continuous and categorical predictors, the outcome variable in multiple regression is *continuous,* whereas the outcome variable in logistic regression is *categorical*—specifically, dichotomous.

The R^2 is used to express the extent to which the predictors account for the variability observed in the outcome variable. For example, suppose a multiple regression model produces $R^2 = .321$; we would document it as such: *This model accounts for 32.1% of the variability observed in the outcome variable.* The remaining 67.9% (100% – 32.1% = 67.9%) is (statistically) referred to as "error." In this context, the term *error* does not necessarily imply that someone made a mistake; rather, it simply means that while the predictor variables in the model account for 32.1% of the variability observed in the outcome variable, we do not (yet) know what *other* predictors account for the remaining 67.9% of the variability observed in the outcome variable.

Table 13.6 *Model Summary* Table Shows Nagelkerke $R^2 = .596$.

Model Summary

Step	-2 Log likelihood	Cox & Snell R Square	Nagelkerke R Square
1	172.947[a]	.447	.596

a. Estimation terminated at iteration number 6 because parameter estimates changed by less than .001.

Currently, there is no perfect R^2 equation for logistic regression; hence, this statistic is commonly referred to as a "pseudo-R^2." In Table 13.6, notice that the Cox & Snell $R^2 = .447$, whereas the Nagelkerke $R^2 = .596$; clearly, these results are quite different. Typically, the Nagelkerke R^2 is considered the better option, but there remains some debate regarding the wisdom of reporting the R^2 for logistic regression. If this statistic were to be included in the documentation, it could be phrased as such: *The Nagelkerke* R^2 *indicates that this model accounts for 59.6% of the variability in smoking cessation.*

The essential findings of the logistic regression are found in the *Variables in the Equation* table (Table 13.7).

Table 13.7 Unedited *Variables in the Equation* Table.

Variables in the Equation

		B	S.E.	Wald	df	Sig.	Exp(B)	95% C.I.for EXP(B) Lower	Upper
Step 1[a]	Gender(1)	3.101	.483	41.269	1	.000	22.223	8.628	57.241
	Race			9.873	4	.043			
	Race(1)	.913	.917	.990	1	.320	2.492	.413	15.043
	Race(2)	.218	.615	.125	1	.723	1.243	.372	4.150
	Race(3)	.504	.601	.704	1	.402	1.656	.510	5.376
	Race(4)	2.082	.721	8.335	1	.004	8.022	1.951	32.973
	Age	.101	.023	19.505	1	.000	1.107	1.058	1.158
	Income	.000	.000	1.138	1	.286	1.000	1.000	1.000
	Cigarettes	-.056	.023	5.904	1	.015	.946	.904	.989
	Constant	-3.720	1.528	5.926	1	.015	.024		

a. Variable(s) entered on step 1: Gender, Race, Age, Income, Cigarettes.

Notice that the numeric values are presented for the categorical variables but not the assigned text labels. In preparation for the documentation process, it is recommended that you manually include the text value labels for each categorical variable:

1. Copy the *Variables in the Equation* table from SPSS into the word processor.
2. Refer to the codebook (see the ★ icon on page **294**), and manually type in the text value labels that correspond to each categorical variable (you will need to adjust the column sizes of the table).
3. If a separate codebook document is not provided, these categorical labels can be derived from viewing the *Values* assigned to each categorical variable on the *Variable View* screen.
4. The **[BRACKETED BOLD]** text in Table 13.8 was typed in manually.

Table 13.8 Edited *Variables in the Equation* Table.

Variables in the Equation

		B	S.E.	Wald	df	Sig.	Exp(B)	95% C.I.for EXP(B)	
								Lower	Upper
Step 1[a]	Gender(1) **[0 = Female, 1 = Male]**	3.101	.483	41.269	1	.000	22.223	8.628	57.241
	Race **[0 = African American]**			9.873	4	.043			
	Race(1) **[1 = Asian]**	.913	.917	.990	1	.320	2.492	.413	15.043
	Race(2) **[2 = Caucasian]**	.218	.615	.125	1	.723	1.243	.372	4.150
	Race(3) **[3 = Latino]**	.504	.601	.704	1	.402	1.656	.510	5.376
	Race(4) **[4 = Other]**	2.082	.721	8.335	1	.004	8.022	1.951	32.973
	Age	.101	.023	19.505	1	.000	1.107	1.058	1.158
	Income	.000	.000	1.138	1	.286	1.000	1.000	1.000
	Cigarettes	-.056	.023	5.904	1	.015	.946	.904	.989
	Constant	-3.720	1.528	5.926	1	.015	.024		

a. Variable(s) entered on step 1: Gender, Race, Age, Income, Cigarettes.

NOTE: **[BRACKETED BOLD]** text manually typed in to clearly label categorical variables.

Notice that the confidence interval [*95% C.I. for EXP(B)*] is included in Table 13.8. The first row (*Gender*) indicates a lower CI of 8.628 and an upper CI of 57.241, pertaining to the Exp(B) of 22.233. This is saying that for the odds ratio pertaining to *Gender*, 95% of the values are expected to be between 8.628 and 57.241. Confidence intervals are traditionally included in logistic regression documentation for statistically significant predictors.

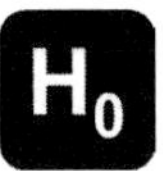

HYPOTHESIS RESOLUTION

The *Omnibus Tests of Model Coefficients* table indicates a Sig. (*p*) value of .000; since this is less than the .05 α level, this indicates that at least one of the (predictor) variables is statistically significant; hence, we reject H_0 and accept H_1.

REJECT: H_0: Age, income, baseline smoking, gender, and race do not influence one's success in a smoking cessation intervention.

ACCEPT: H_1: Age, income, baseline smoking, gender, and race influence one's success in a smoking cessation intervention.

The next step is to identify and document the specific predictor variable(s) that produced statistically significant results.

DOCUMENTING RESULTS

Documentation Overview

Considering that the logistic regression statistic accommodates an assortment of variables—(1) dichotomous outcome variable, (2) categorical predictor variables, and (3) continuous predictor variables—the documentation procedure will be presented in three parts:

- Part 1: Comprehending the outcome variable
- Part 2: Documenting categorical predictors
- Part 3: Documenting continuous predictors

Additionally, the logistic regression model is versatile in terms of its capacity to produce a variety of results. As such, this documentation section consists of three models:

- Model 1: Initial results
- Model 2: Selective results
- Model 3: Redefining a reference category

Model 1: Initial Results

Documenting Results Part 1: Outcome Variable

Consider this excerpt from the codebook detailing the dichotomous outcome variable:

Outcome variable: Smoking_status

0 = Still smoking (FAILED)

1 = Quit smoking (SUCCEEDED) **[← *BASIS FOR MODEL*]**

Although it may sound a bit redundant, since the intended goal of this intervention was to have patients successfully *Quit smoking,* we will want to discuss the results in terms of the characteristics of those who successfully *Quit smoking,* as opposed to those who are *Still smoking;* hence, the label *Quit smoking* is assigned a value of 1 in the outcome variable *Smoking_status.* This will serve as the (semantic) basis for this model. As you will see in Parts 2 and 3, the results in the *Variables in the Equation* table pertain to those who *Quit smoking.*

Table 13.9 Labeled *Variables in the Equation* Table, Focusing on Categorical Variables.

Variables in the Equation

		B	S.E.	Wald	df	Sig.	Exp(B)	95% C.I.for EXP(B)	
								Lower	Upper
Step 1[a]	Gender(1) **[0 = Female, 1 = Male]**	3.101	.483	41.269	1	.000	22.223	8.628	57.241
	Race **[0 = African American]**			9.873	4	.043			
	Race(1) **[1 = Asian]**	.913	.917	.990	1	.320	2.492	.413	15.043
	Race(2) **[2 = Caucasian]**	.218	.615	.125	1	.723	1.243	.372	4.150
	Race(3) **[3 = Latino]**	.504	.601	.704	1	.402	1.656	.510	5.376
	Race(4) **[4 = Other]**	2.082	.721	8.335	1	.004	8.022	1.951	32.973
	Age	.101	.023	19.505	1	.000	1.107	1.058	1.158
	Income	.000	.000	1.138	1	.286	1.000	1.000	1.000
	Cigarettes	-.056	.023	5.904	1	.015	.946	.904	.989
	Constant	-3.720	1.528	5.926	1	.015	.024		

a. Variable(s) entered on step 1: Gender, Race, Age, Income, Cigarettes.

Documenting Results Part 2: Categorical Predictors

We will begin by documenting the results from all of the values in each categorical variable regardless of the Sig. (p) value to thoroughly demonstrate how to translate the data on this table into appropriately written results. After that process, as expected, we will narrow our discussion to only those variables that are statistically significant (where $p \leq .05$).

This model contains two categorical predictor variables: *Gender* and *Race.* We will begin by interpreting and documenting the *Gender* variable.

For *Gender, Female* is coded as 0, establishing it as the *reference category* for *Gender.* As such, all of the results for *Gender* will be expressed as comparisons to *Females.* Referring to the data in the first column (which contains the variable names) and the figures in the *Exp(B)* column, we document the results as such:

- Males have 22.223 times the odds of quitting smoking compared to females (95% CI 8.63, 57.24) (meaning that the men in this study succeeded in quitting smoking significantly more frequently than women).

Alternatively, this could be rephrased as follows:

- The odds of quitting smoking are 22.223 times higher for males compared to females (95% CI 8.63, 57.24).

For *Race,* the categories are arranged alphabetically; hence, *African American* is coded as 0, establishing it as the reference category for *Race*. As such, all of the results for *Race* will be expressed as comparisons to *African Americans.*

- Asians have 2.492 times the odds of quitting smoking compared to African Americans (95% CI.41, 15.04).
- Caucasians have 1.243 times the odds of quitting smoking compared to African Americans (95% CI.37, 4.15).
- Latinos have 1.656 times the odds of quitting smoking compared to African Americans (95% CI.51, 5.38).
- Others have 8.022 times the odds of quitting smoking compared to African Americans (95% CI 1.95, 32.97).

You may include the corresponding p (Sig.) values, flagging those where $p \leq .05$. Alternatively, you may wish to provide detailed discussion of only those categories wherein $p \leq .05$ (*Other*) and briefly mention the others as statistically insignificant (*Asians, Caucasians, Latinos*). These findings will be carried forward when we draft the abstract.

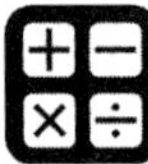

Categorical Documentation Option: Alternate Write-Up if Exp(B) Is Less Than 1

In the above table, *Gender* produced *Exp(B) = 22.223,* which is greater than 1. Suppose instead of *22.223,* it was .456. When *Exp(B)* is less than 1 for a categorical predictor, the semantics of the write-up may seem a bit awkward (see ORIGINAL documentation phrasing below). One option that may help to clarify the documentation is to "flip" the sentence. This involves calculating the reciprocal of *Exp(B),* which is simply **1** ÷ Exp(B); this would be **1 ÷ .456** = **2.193,** and swapping the variable labels in the sentence.

- ORIGINAL: *Males have .456 times the odds of quitting smoking compared to females.*
- FLIPPED: *Females have 2.193 times the odds of quitting smoking compared to males.*

Documenting Results Part 3: Continuous Predictors

Next, we will document the results produced by the three continuous predictors (*Age, Income, Cigarettes*) in Table 13.10.

Table 13.10 Labeled *Variables in the Equation* Table, Focusing on Continuous Variables.

Variables in the Equation

		B	S.E.	Wald	df	Sig.	Exp(B)	95% C.I.for EXP(B)	
								Lower	Upper
Step 1[a]	Gender(1) **[0 = Female, 1 = Male]**	3.101	.483	41.269	1	.000	22.223	8.628	57.241
	Race **[0 = African American]**			9.873	4	.043			
	Race(1) **[1 = Asian]**	.913	.917	.990	1	.320	2.492	.413	15.043
	Race(2) **[2 = Caucasian]**	.218	.615	.125	1	.723	1.243	.372	4.150
	Race(3) **[3 = Latino]**	.504	.601	.704	1	.402	1.656	.510	5.376
	Race(4) **[4 = Other]**	2.082	.721	8.335	1	.004	8.022	1.951	32.973
	Age	.101	.023	19.505	1	.000	1.107	1.058	1.158
	Income	.000	.000	1.138	1	.286	1.000	1.000	1.000
	Cigarettes	-.056	.023	5.904	1	.015	.946	.904	.989
	Constant	-3.720	1.528	5.926	1	.015	.024		

a. Variable(s) entered on step 1: Gender, Race, Age, Income, Cigarettes.

Continuous variables are best expressed in terms of odds percentages. There are two possible outcomes and documentation procedures for continuous predictors: Either *Exp(B)* is less than 1 or *Exp(B)* is greater than 1:

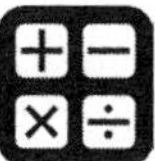

Documenting Continuous Variable Results if Exp(B) Is Less Than 1

If Exp(B) < 1, then the percentage = (1 − Exp(B)) × 100.

For *Cigarettes*, Exp(B) = .946; since this is less than 1, this indicates a *decrease*. We compute (1 − .946) × 100 = 5.4; hence, the write-up would be as follows:

- *For every additional cigarette smoked per day, the odds of quitting smoking decreases by 5.4% (95% CI .90, .99).*

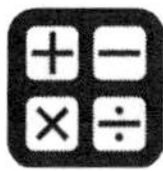

Documenting Continuous Variable Results if Exp(B) Is Greater Than 1

If Exp(B) > 1, then the percentage = (Exp(B) − 1) × 100.

For *Age, Exp(B)* = 1.107; since this is greater than 1, this indicates an *increase*. We compute (1.107 − 1) × 100 = 10.7; hence, the write-up would be as follows:

- *For every additional year of age, the odds of quitting smoking increases by 10.7% (95% CI 1.06, 1.16).*

Documenting Continuous Variable Results if Exp(B) Equals 1

For *Income, Exp(B)* = 1.000, indicating that *Income* produced 1:1 odds in terms of Income predicting the likelihood that a participant will quit smoking. In other words, about the same number of people with high income as low income quit smoking—the odds of quitting smoking are the same regardless of high/low income. As expected, the Sig. (*p*) value for *Income* is .286; since this is greater than the .05 α level, *Income* is considered statistically insignificant when it comes to predicting the likelihood that a participant will successfully quit smoking.

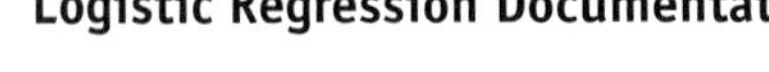

Logistic Regression Documentation Summary

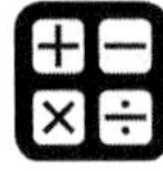

Categorical Predictors

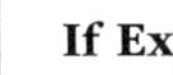

If Exp(B) > 1, then odds ratio = Exp(B).
The comparison category is **more likely** than the reference category to predict the outcome variable (basis for model).

If Exp(B) < 1, then odds ratio can be expressed as 1 ÷ Exp(B) and flip the variables.
The comparison category is **less likely** than the reference category to predict the outcome variable (basis for model).

Continuous Predictors

If Exp(B) > 1, then percentage = (Exp(B) − 1) × 100.
The comparison category **increases** in relation to the outcome variable (basis for model).

If Exp(B) < 1, then percentage = (1 − Exp(B)) × 100.
The comparison category **decreases** in relation to the outcome variable (basis for model).

Abstract for Model 1: Initial Results

You may include the corresponding p (Sig.) values, flagging those where $p \leq .05$. Alternatively, you may wish to provide detailed discussion of only those categories wherein $p \leq .05$ and briefly mention the others as statistically insignificant:

As a public service, the Acme Health Center advertises and offers a free 90-day smoking cessation program, consisting of nurse-facilitated psychoeducational meetings, peer support from those who have been smoke free for more than 1 year, and multimedia resources designed to promote smoking cessation.

At the conclusion of the intervention, each participant (n = *218) responded to a self-administered anonymous Smoking Cessation Survey card, which gathered data on gender, race, age, income, baseline mean number of cigarettes smoked per day, and current smoking status (still smoking/quit smoking).*

*To better comprehend the factors associated with successfully quitting smoking, we conducted a logistic regression analysis. We discovered that males had 22.223 times the odds of quitting smoking compared to females (*p *< .001) (95% CI 8.63, 57.24). Those who indicated that their race designation was "Other" had 8.022 times the odds of quitting smoking compared to African Americans (*p *= .004) (95% CI 1.95, 32.97). Older participants were more likely to quit than those who were younger; for every additional year of age, the odds of quitting smoking increased by 10.7% (*p *< .001) (95% CI 1.06, 1.16). We also discovered that baseline smoking was an influential factor; for every additional cigarette smoked per day, the odds of quitting smoking decreased by 5.4% (*p *= .015) (95% CI .90, .99). Income was not found to be a viable predictor when it comes to predicting who successfully quit smoking (*p *= .286) (95% CI 1.00, 1.00).*

Considering the volume of results produced by a logistic regression analysis in light of the relative brevity of an abstract (usually about 200 words), not every possible statistic was discussed. In a more comprehensive Results section, other statistical findings could be included (e.g., overall percentage of those who quit smoking, descriptive statistics for each categorical and continuous variable, discussion of statistically insignificant predictors).

Model 2: Selective Results

In the initial model, the results reflected the overall findings from both *Genders* (*Female* and *Male*); it was found that the men in this group were substantially more successful in quitting smoking than women. Such an observation may lead one to ponder: *Among the males (only), what were the significant predictors when it comes to successfully quitting smoking?* Statistically, this question is asking, *What would the results of this logistic regression look like if the females were removed from the picture?* This would be akin to recruiting only males to partake in this intervention.

Fortunately, we do not need to repeat this study as a *men-only* intervention to address this question; instead, we can access the existing database, using the *Select Cases* function to process only those records (rows of data) pertaining to males (*Gender* = 1).

1. On the main screen, click on the *Select Cases* icon.
2. On the *Select Cases* menu, click on ⊙ *If condition is satisfied.*
3. Click on *If.*
4. On the *Select Cases: If* menu, enter *Gender = 1* (Figure 13.14).

Figure 13.14 Selecting cases where *Gender* = 1 (Male).

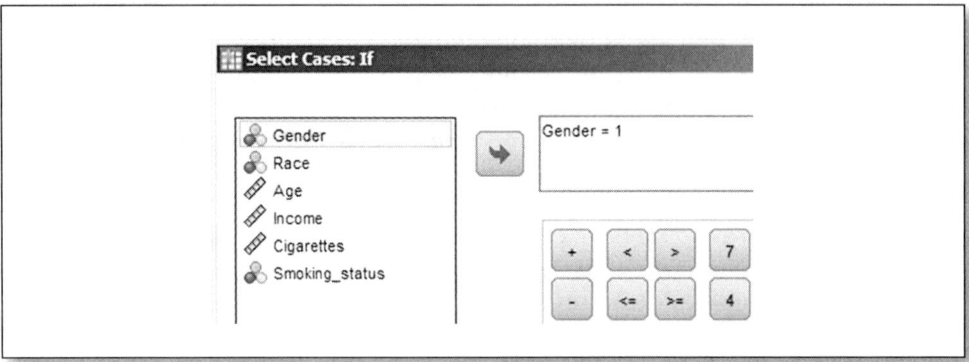

5. Click on *Continue* (this will return you to the *Select Cases* menu).
6. On the *Select Cases* menu, click on *OK*.
7. Now that only *Males* are selected, proceed to rerun the logistic regression analysis using each of the steps detailed in this chapter, as if all of the records were in play.

This analysis produces a table (Table 13.11) pertaining to the data gathered from the *Males* only. As expected, these findings are quite different compared to the initial run, which involved both genders.

Table 13.11 Labeled *Variables in the Equation* Table, for *Males*.

Variables in the Equation

		B	S.E.	Wald	df	Sig.	Exp(B)	95% C.I.for EXP(B) Lower	Upper
Step 1[a]	Race **[0 = African American]**			5.976	3	.113			
	Race(1) **[1 = Asian]**	2.395	13243.109	.000	1	1.000	10.967	.000	.
	Race(2) **[2 = Caucasian]**	-17.739	8095.370	.000	1	.998	.000	.000	.
	Race(3) **[3 = Latino]**	-20.050	8095.370	.000	1	.998	.000	.000	.
	Age	.163	.057	8.053	1	.005	1.176	1.052	1.316
	Income	.000	.000	.330	1	.566	1.000	1.000	1.000
	Cigarettes	-.151	.053	8.147	1	.004	.860	.775	.954
	Constant	18.863	8095.371	.000	1	.998	1.557E8		

a. Variable(s) entered on step 1: Race, Age, Income, Cigarettes.

First, notice that even if you attempted to load *Gender* as a variable, it was eliminated from the process since (now) *Gender* contains only one (selected) value: 1, signifying *Males* (only). Since all of the values for *Gender* = 1, technically, *Gender* ceases to be a *variable* because it does not vary; it is constantly 1, and hence, it is considered a constant. In this process, a constant has no predictive capacity since it is constantly 1 no matter what is happening among the other variables. As such, *Gender* is appropriately eliminated from the table.

Next, notice that *Race(4)* is missing. This is because there are no *Males* who specified their *Race* as category 4 (*Other*). For proof, run descriptive statistics (with a bar chart) for the *Race* variable, and notice that *Other* is absent.

As for documenting the results, although we may notice that *Asians* have 10.967 times the odds of quitting smoking compared to *African Americans,* we see that this finding is considered statistically insignificant (p = 1.000).

Abstract for Model 2: Selective Results

*Assessing only the male participants, we discovered that those who were older were more likely to quit than those who were younger; for every additional year of age, the odds of quitting smoking increased by 17.6% (*p *= .005) (95% CI 1.05, 1.32). We also discovered that baseline smoking was an influential factor; for every additional cigarette smoked per day, the odds of quitting smoking decreased by 14% (*p *= .004) (95% CI .77, .95).*

Model 3: Redefining a Reference Category

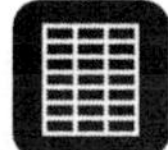

Data Set

Use the following data set: **Ch 13 – Example 02 – Logistic Regression.sav.**

In the prior two models, the reference category for *Race* has been *African American,* which produced statistics that compared all of the other racial categories to *African Americans* in terms of quitting smoking. This designation was merely due to the alphabetical arrangement of the categories—*African Americans* just happen to occupy the

Table 13.12 To Set *Other* as the New Reference Category, Recode *Other* From 4 to 0 and Recode *African American* From 0 to 4.

*Recoding Race Reference (Swap **African American** With **Other**)*	
Race	**Race_0**
0 = African American [← *REFERENCE*] 1 = Asian 2 = Caucasian 3 = Latino **4 = Other**	**0 = Other [← *REFERENCE*]** 1 = Asian 2 = Caucasian 3 = Latino **4 = African American**

first position. There may be instances where you want to designate a different category as the reference category for a variable. For this example, we will change the original coding so that *Other* becomes the new reference category for *Race*. One way to do this involves changing the categorical coding of *Other* from 4 to 0 and recode *African American* from 0 to 4.

The current database (**Ch 13 – Example 02 – Logistic Regression.sav**) is the same as the original, except the variable *Race* (which was initially coded as 0 = *African American* and 4 = *Other*) has been recoded to create *Race_O,* wherein 0 = *Other* and 4 = *African American* (Table 3.12). With *Other* now serving as the reference category for *Race_O,* all racial results will be presented as comparisons to *Other.*

As a side note, the Recode process was used to create *Race_O,* wherein all of the 0s were replaced with 4s, all of the 4s were replaced with 0s, and all of the other numbers (1, 2, 3) were kept as is. Finally, the value labels for *Race_O* were (manually) edited accordingly: 0 was changed to *Other,* and 4 was changed to *African American.*

The step-by-step instructions for this recoding procedure are detailed in Chapter 14, on page **343** at the ★ icon.

Table 13.13 Labeled *Variables in the Equation* Table, With *Other* Set to Reference Category in *Race_O.*

Variables in the Equation

		B	S.E.	Wald	df	Sig.	Exp(B)	95% C.I.for EXP(B)	
								Lower	Upper
Step 1[a]	Gender(1) **[0 = Female, 1 = Male]**	3.101	.483	41.269	1	.000	22.223	8.628	57.241
	Race_O **[0 = Other]**			9.873	4	.043			
	Race_O(1) **[1 = Asian]**	-1.169	.956	1.495	1	.221	.311	.048	2.024
	Race_O(2) **[2 = Caucasian]**	-1.864	.716	6.779	1	.009	.155	.038	.631
	Race_O(3) **[3 = Latino]**	-1.578	.624	6.399	1	.011	.206	.061	.701
	Race_O(4) **[4 = African American]**	-2.082	.721	8.335	1	.004	.125	.030	.512
	Age	.101	.023	19.505	1	.000	1.107	1.058	1.158
	Income	.000	.000	1.138	1	.286	1.000	1.000	1.000
	Cigarettes	-.056	.023	5.904	1	.015	.946	.904	.989
	Constant	-1.637	1.446	1.283	1	.257	.194		

a. Variable(s) entered on step 1: Gender, Race_O, Age, Income, Cigarettes.

Notice that the figures for *Race* are different from the initial results, since the reference category is now *Other* instead of *African American*. Additionally, notice that all of the other figures match the results in the initial run. The point is, recoding a variable only changes the presentation of the data contained within that variable.

As expected, a new write-up for *Race_O* is warranted:

Abstract for Model 3: Redefining a Reference Category

In terms of race, Caucasians have .155 times the odds of quitting smoking compared to those who identify their race as Other (p = .009) (95% CI.04, .63). Latinos were found to have .206 times the odds of quitting smoking compared to those who identify their race as Other (p = .011) (95% CI .06, .70), and African Americans have .125 times the odds of quitting compared to Other (p = .015) (95% CI .03, .51).

Alternatively, since these odds ratios are less than 1, the reading may be clearer if the semantics were flipped and the reciprocals [1 ÷ Exp(B)] were presented:

Those who identified their race as Other had 6.45 times the odds of quitting smoking compared to Caucasians (p = .009) (95% CI .04, .63), and Other (race category) had 4.85 times the odds of quitting smoking compared to Latinos (p = .011) (95% CI .06, .70). Additionally, Other had 8 times the odds of quitting smoking compared to African Americans (p = .015) (95% CI .03, .51).

Multiple Regression (R^2)—An Overview

Whereas logistic regression provides odds ratios to determine the influences that continuous and categorical predictors have on a *dichotomous* outcome variable, multiple regression (R^2) can be used to comprehend the influences of predictor variables when the outcome variable is *continuous*.

In the example processed in this chapter, the outcome variable, *Smoking_status,* is a dichotomous variable; the two categories are *Still smoking* and *Quit smoking,* but suppose instead of this dichotomous coding, *Smoking_status* had been coded as a continuous variable, wherein *Smoking_status* would now contain the average number of cigarettes that each participant smokes per day at the conclusion of the intervention. In this case, 0 would indicate that the participant has successfully quit smoking. Whereas logistic regression produces results in the form of odds ratios, the multiple regression identifies the predictors that have a statistically significant correlation to the outcome variable and expresses the results in terms of percentages. The following is a sample of how such results would be documented:

We recruited 218 smokers to participate in a smoking cessation intervention. Initially, we gathered data detailing each participant's gender, race, age, income, and average number of cigarettes smoked per day. At the conclusion of the treatment, we measured the (new) average number of cigarettes smoked per day (0 = quit smoking).

Multiple regression analysis revealed an overall R^2 of .40 (α = .05), wherein gender accounts for 30% of the variability observed in the outcome variable (posttreatment smoking), race accounts for an additional 7%, and baseline smoking rate accounts for 3%.

In this (hypothetical) example, notice that *age* and *income* are not mentioned; this is because the regression processor determined that they are not statistically significantly correlated to the outcome variable (posttreatment smoking). Also notice that the overall R^2 only accounts for 40% of the variability observed in the outcome variable, so the question stands: *What about the other 60% (100 – 40 = 60)?* The answer to that is *error*. In this context, "error" does not imply that somebody made a mistake; rather, this model is saying that three of the predictor variables (gender, race, and baseline smoking rate) account for 40% of the variability observed in the outcome variable, leaving 60% unaccounted for. Basically, this is saying that other predictors pertain to the outcome variable, which are not included in this model. If this study were to be repeated, we might consider retaining the three statistically significant predictors (gender, race, and baseline smoking rate), dropping the statistically insignificant predictors (age and income), and include some other, hopefully more relevant, predictor variables to increase the overall R^2.

GOOD COMMON SENSE

Logistic regression is a sophisticated type of analytic procedure that enables one to gain a deeper understanding of the relationships among the variables in terms of predicting a dichotomous outcome. In some cases, the findings from a logistic regression model can be used to predict/anticipate the likelihood of an outcome.

Despite the detailed findings produced by logistic regression, keep in mind that the model pertains to *a group of people*—it does not describe or predict the outcome of any one individual. In the same way that descriptive statistics can be used to compute the mean age of people in a sample, knowing that mean age (e.g., 25) does not empower you to point to any one person in the sample (or population) and confidently proclaim, "You are 25 years old." Keep in mind that this same principle also applies to more advanced processes, such as logistic regression.

Key Concepts

- Logistic regression
- Pretest checklist:
  - Sample size
  - Normality
  - Multicollinearity
- R^2 statistic
- Categorical variable labeling
- Selectively processing
- Categorical recoding principles
- Hypothesis resolution
- Documenting results
- Multiple regression overview
- Good common sense

Practice Exercises

Exercise 13.1

A public health nurse has conducted a survey of people in the community to better comprehend the effectiveness of the flu shot this season using the following survey instrument:

Flu Survey

1. Gender: ☐ Female ☐ Male
2. How old are you? _____
3. Did you have a flu shot this season? ☐ No ☐ Yes
4. Do you have any chronic disease(s)? ☐ No ☐ Yes
5. Have you been sick with the flu this season? ☐ No ☐ Yes

Data set: **Ch 13 – Exercise 01A.sav**

Codebook

Variable: Flu_sick
Definition: Outcome variable: Did this person get sick with the flu this season?
Type: Categorical (0 = Got the flu, 1 = No flu)

Variable: Gender
Definition: Predictor variable: Gender
Type: Categorical (0 = Female, 1 = Male)

Variable: Flu_shot
Definition: Predictor variable: Did person have a flu shot this season?
Type: Categorical (0 = Got a flu shot, 1 = Did not get a flu shot)

Variable: Chronic_disease
Definition: Predictor variable: Does the person have chronic disease(s)?
Type: Categorical (0 = Has chronic disease(s), 1 = No chronic disease(s))

Variable: Age
Definition: Predictor variable: Age
Type: Continuous

a. Write the hypotheses.
b. Run each criterion of the pretest checklist (sample size, normality, multicollinearity) and discuss your findings.
c. Run the logistic regression analysis and document your findings (odds ratios and Sig. [*p* value], hypotheses resolution).
d. Write an abstract under 200 words detailing a summary of the study, the logistic regression analysis results, hypothesis resolution, and implications of your findings.

Repeat this exercise using data set: **Ch 13 – Exercise 01B.sav.**

NOTE: This data set (**Ch 13 – Exercise 01B.sav**) is the same as the first data set except the *Age* variable has been recoded from a continuous variable that contained the actual ages to a categorical variable, now coded as Pediatric/Adult, using the following recoding criteria:

- If Age < 18, then recode as $0 =$ Pediatric
- If Age ≥ 18, then recode as $1 =$ Adult

The corresponding modification has been made to the codebook:

Variable: Age
Definition: Predictor variable: Age
Type: Categorical (0 = Pediatric, 1 = Adult)

Exercise 13.2

To better comprehend the characteristics of patients who may be susceptible to developing a rash from Drug A, a nurse gathers data on patients who have been prescribed this medication. Since it is known that taking Drug B, which is commonly prescribed with Drug A, may cause complications, the study enquires about Drug B usage. Additional variables of interest include the duration of the dosage and the patient's age.

Data set: **Ch 13 – Exercise 02A.sav**

Codebook

Variable: Rash
Definition: Outcome variable: Did the patient develop a rash?
Type: Categorical (0 = No rash, 1 = Rash)

Variable: Drug_B
Definition: Predictor variable: Is the patient also taking Drug_B?
Type: Categorical (0 = Taking Drug B, 1 = Not taking Drug B)

Variable: Duration
Definition: Predictor variable: Number of days the patient has been taking Drug A
Type: Continuous

Variable: Age
Definition: Predictor variable: Age
Type: Continuous

a. Write the hypotheses.

b. Run each criterion of the pretest checklist (sample size, normality, multicollinearity) and discuss your findings.

c. Run the logistic regression analysis and document your findings (odds ratios and Sig. [*p* value], hypotheses resolution).

d. Write an abstract under 200 words detailing a summary of the study, the logistic regression analysis results, hypothesis resolution, and implications of your findings.

Repeat this exercise using data set: **Ch 13 – Exercise 02B.sav.**

Exercise 13.3

A nurse on the quality improvement team has gathered data from three surgical facilities—Northview Surgical Center, South Hills Hospital, and Central Health Clinic—to determine the factors associated with surgical complications.

Data set: **Ch 13 – Exercise 03A.sav**

Codebook

Variable: Complications
Definition: Outcome variable: Did the patient experience surgical complication(s)?
Type: Categorical (0 = No surgical complications, 1 = Surgical complications)

Variable: Inpatient
Definition: Predictor variable: Was the surgery inpatient?
Type: Categorical (0 = Inpatient, 1 = Outpatient)

Variable: Facility
Definition: Predictor variable: Surgical facility
Type: Categorical (0 = Northview Surgical Center, 1 = South Hills Hospital, 2 = Central Health Clinic)

Variable: Laparoscopic
Definition: Predictor variable: Laparoscopic surgery
Type: Categorical (0 = Laparoscopic, 1 = Not laparoscopic)

a. Write the hypotheses.

b. Run each criterion of the pretest checklist (sample size, normality, multicollinearity) and discuss your findings.

c. Run the logistic regression analysis and document your findings (odds ratios and Sig. [*p* value], hypotheses resolution).

d. Write an abstract under 200 words detailing a summary of the study, the logistic regression analysis results, hypothesis resolution, and implications of your findings.

Repeat this exercise using data set: **Ch 13 – Exercise 03B.sav.**

Exercise 13.4

A nurse who oversees emergency training is investigating the factors pertaining to resuscitation survival at Acme Hospital.

Data set: **Ch 13 – Exercise 04A.sav**

Codebook

Variable: Survival
Definition: Outcome variable: Did the patient survive resuscitation?
Type: Categorical (0 = Did not survive, 1 = Survived)

Variable: Gender
Definition: Predictor variable: Gender
Type: Categorical (0 = Female, 1 = Male)

Variable: Race
Definition: Predictor variable: Race
Type: Categorical (0 = African American, 1 = Asian, 2 = Caucasian, 3 = Latino, 4 = Other)

Variable: Prior_ resuscitation
Definition: Predictor variable: Did the patient require prior resuscitation during this hospitalization?
Type: Categorical (0 = No, 1 = Yes)

Variable: Age
Definition: Predictor variable: Age
Type: Continuous

Variable: LOS
Definition: Predictor variable: Length of stay
Type: Continuous

a. Write the hypotheses.
b. Run each criterion of the pretest checklist (sample size, normality, multicollinearity) and discuss your findings.
c. Run the logistic regression analysis and document your findings (odds ratios and Sig. [*p* value], hypotheses resolution).
d. Write an abstract under 200 words detailing a summary of the study, the logistic regression analysis results, hypothesis resolution, and implications of your findings.

Repeat this exercise using data set: **Ch 13 – Exercise 04B.sav.**

Exercise 13.5

The charge nurse at a dialysis center wants to investigate the characteristics of patients who missed an appointment last month to help focus treatment adherence strategies. In addition to data from patient's records, the nurse administers the Acme Depression Scale to each patient.

Data set: **Ch 13 – Exercise 05A.sav**

Codebook

Variable:	Appointments
Definition:	Outcome variable: Did the patient keep all dialysis appointments last month?
Type:	Categorical (0 = Kept all appointments, 1 = Did not keep all appointments)

Variable:	Gender
Definition:	Predictor variable: Gender
Type:	Categorical (0 = Female, 1 = Male)

Variable:	Race
Definition:	Predictor variable: Race
Type:	Categorical (0 = African American, 1 = Asian, 2 = Caucasian, 3 = Latino, 4 = Other)

Variable:	SES
Definition:	Predictor variable: Socioeconomic status
Type:	Categorical (0 = Lower class, 1 = Middle class, 2 = Upper class)

Variable:	Age
Definition:	Predictor variable: Age
Type:	Continuous

Variable:	Dialysis_time
Definition:	Predictor variable: Total length of time on dialysis (in months)
Type:	Continuous

Variable:	Depression
Definition:	Predictor variable: Score on Acme Depression Scale
Type:	Continuous (0 = Low depression . . . 30 = High depression)

a. Write the hypotheses.

b. Run each criterion of the pretest checklist (sample size, normality, multicollinearity) and discuss your findings.

c. Run the logistic regression analysis and document your findings (odds ratios and Sig. [*p* value], hypotheses resolution).

d. Write an abstract under 200 words detailing a summary of the study, the logistic regression analysis results, hypothesis resolution, and implications of your findings.

Repeat this exercise using data set: **Ch 13 – Exercise 05B.sav.**

Exercise 13.6

A nurse on the palliative care team wants to better comprehend the attributes of those who opt for hospice care when it is clinically offered and those who do not.

Data set: **Ch 13 – Exercise 06A.sav**

Codebook

Variable: Palliative_care
Definition: Outcome variable: Did the patient opt for hospice care?
Type: Categorical (0 = Refused hospice, 1 = Accepted hospice)

Variable: Gender
Definition: Predictor variable: Gender
Type: Categorical (0 = Female, 1 = Male)

Variable: Race
Definition: Predictor variable: Race
Type: Categorical (0 = African American, 1 = Asian, 2 = Caucasian, 3 = Latino, 4 = Other)

Variable: Disease
Definition: Predictor variable: Primary diagnosis
Type: Categorical (0 = AIDS, 1 = Cancer, 2 = Cardiac, 3 = Dementia, 4 = Pulmonary, 5 = Stroke, 6 = Other)

Variable: Religion
Definition: Predictor variable: Religion
Type: Categorical (0 = Atheist, 1 = Buddhist, 2 = Catholic, 3 = Hindu, 4 = Jewish, 5 = Other)

Variable: Age
Definition: Predictor variable: Age
Type: Continuous

a. Write the hypotheses.

b. Run each criterion of the pretest checklist (sample size, normality, multicollinearity) and discuss your findings.

c. Run the logistic regression analysis and document your findings (odds ratios and Sig. [*p* value], hypotheses resolution).

d. Write an abstract under 200 words detailing a summary of the study, the logistic regression analysis results, hypothesis resolution, and implications of your findings.

Repeat this exercise using data set: **Ch 13 – Exercise 06B.sav.**

NOTE: This data set is the same as the first one, but the following variables have been recoded as such (*Cancer* is now the reference category for the *Disease* variable):

Variable: Disease
Definition: Predictor variable: Primary diagnosis
Type: Categorical (0 = Cancer, 1 = AIDS, 2 = Cardiac, 3 = Dementia, 4 = Pulmonary, 5 = Stroke, 6 = Other)

Exercise 13.7

A nurse on the Patient Care Committee wants to better comprehend the attributes of those who opt for DNR (do not resuscitate) orders and those who do not.

Data set: **Ch 13 – Exercise 07A.sav**

Codebook

Variable: DNR
Definition: Outcome variable: Patient's DNR status
Type: Categorical (0 = Not DNR, 1 = DNR)

Variable: Gender
Definition: Predictor variable: Gender
Type: Categorical (0 = Female, 1 = Male)

Variable: Race
Definition: Predictor variable: Race
Type: Categorical (0 = African American, 1 = Asian, 2 = Caucasian, 3 = Latino, 4 = Other)

Variable: Disease
Definition: Predictor variable: Primary diagnosis
Type: Categorical (0 = AIDS, 1 = Cancer, 2 = Cardiac, 3 = Dementia, 4 = Pulmonary, 5 = Stroke, 6 = Other)

Variable: Religion
Definition: Predictor variable: Religion
Type: Categorical (0 = Atheist, 1 = Buddhist, 2 = Catholic, 3 = Hindu, 4 = Jewish, 5 = Other)

Variable: Age
Definition: Predictor variable: Age
Type: Continuous

a. Write the hypotheses.
b. Run each criterion of the pretest checklist (sample size, normality, multicollinearity) and discuss your findings.
c. Run the logistic regression analysis and document your findings (odds ratios and Sig. [*p* value], hypotheses resolution).
d. Write an abstract under 200 words detailing a summary of the study, the logistic regression analysis results, hypothesis resolution, and implications of your findings.

Repeat this exercise using data set: **Ch 13 – Exercise 07B.sav.**

Exercise 13.8

A nurse in the Infection Control Department wants to investigate the characteristics of those who develop nosocomial infections.

Data set: **Ch 13 – Exercise 08A.sav**

Codebook

Variable: Nosocomial_infection
Definition: Outcome variable: Did the patient develop a nosocomial infection?
Type: Categorical (0 = No infection, 1 = Infection)

Variable: Gender
Definition: Predictor variable: Gender
Type: Categorical (0 = Female, 1 = Male)

Variable: Age
Definition: Predictor variable: Age
Type: Continuous

Variable: Ward
Definition: Predictor variable: Ward
Type: Categorical (0 = ICU, 1 = CCU, 2 = 1A, 3 = 1B, 4 = 2A, 5 = 2B)

Variable: LOS
Definition: Predictor variable: Length of stay in hospital (in days)
Type: Continuous

Variable: Surgery
Definition: Predictor variable: Did the patient have surgery?
Type: Categorical (0 = Surgery, 1 = No surgery)

a. Write the hypotheses.

b. Run each criterion of the pretest checklist (sample size, normality, multicollinearity) and discuss your findings.

c. Run the logistic regression analysis and document your findings (odds ratios and Sig. [*p* value], hypotheses resolution).

d. Write an abstract under 200 words detailing a summary of the study, the logistic regression analysis results, hypothesis resolution, and implications of your findings.

Repeat this exercise using data set: **Ch 13 – Exercise 08B.sav.**

Exercise 13.9

The Patient Safety Board has recruited you to determine the factors associated with patient falls during hospitalization.

Data set: **Ch 13 – Exercise 09A.sav**

Codebook

Variable: Fall
Definition: Outcome variable: Did the patient fall?
Type: Categorical (0 = No fall, 1 = Fell)

Variable: Gender
Definition: Predictor variable: Gender
Type: Categorical (0 = Female, 1 = Male)

Variable: Age
Definition: Predictor variable: Age
Type: Continuous

Variable: Ward
Definition: Predictor variable: Ward
Type: Categorical (0 = 1A, 1 = 1B, 2 = 2A, 3 = 2B)

Variable: LOS
Definition: Predictor variable: Length of stay in hospital (in days)
Type: Continuous

Variable: Surgery
Definition: Predictor variable: Did the patient have surgery?
Type: Categorical (0 = Surgery, 1 = No surgery)

a. Write the hypotheses.

b. Run each criterion of the pretest checklist (sample size, normality, multicollinearity) and discuss your findings.

c. Run the logistic regression analysis and document your findings (odds ratios and Sig. [*p* value], hypotheses resolution).

d. Write an abstract under 200 words detailing a summary of the study, the logistic regression analysis results, hypothesis resolution, and implications of your findings.

Repeat this exercise using data set: **Ch 13 – Exercise 09B.sav.**

Exercise 13.10

The Transplant Committee wants to gain a better understanding of those who opt to be an organ donor.

Data set: **Ch 13 – Exercise 10A.sav**

Codebook

Variable:	Organ_donor
Definition:	Outcome variable: Is the person an organ donor?
Type:	Categorical (0 = Not organ donor, 1 = Organ donor)
Variable:	Gender
Definition:	Predictor variable: Gender
Type:	Categorical (0 = Female, 1 = Male)
Variable:	Age
Definition:	Predictor variable: Age
Type:	Continuous
Variable:	Religion
Definition:	Predictor variable: Religion
Type:	Categorical (0 = Atheist, 1 = Buddhist, 2 = Catholic, 3 = Hindu, 4 = Jewish, 5 = Other)
Variable:	SES
Definition:	Predictor variable: Socioeconomic status
Type:	Categorical (0 = Lower class, 1 = Middle class, 2 = Upper class)

a. Write the hypotheses.

b. Run each criterion of the pretest checklist (sample size, normality, multicollinearity) and discuss your findings.

c. Run the logistic regression analysis and document your findings (odds ratios and Sig. [*p* value], hypotheses resolution).

d. Write an abstract under 200 words detailing a summary of the study, the logistic regression analysis results, hypothesis resolution, and implications of your findings.

Repeat this exercise using data set: **Ch 13 – Exercise 10B.sav.**

PART VI

Data Handling

This chapter demonstrates supplemental techniques in SPSS to enhance your capabilities, versatility, and data-processing efficiency.

Chapter 14: Supplemental SPSS Operations explains how to generate random numbers, sort and select cases, recode variables, import non-SPSS data, and practice appropriate data storage protocols.

CHAPTER 14

Supplemental SPSS Operations

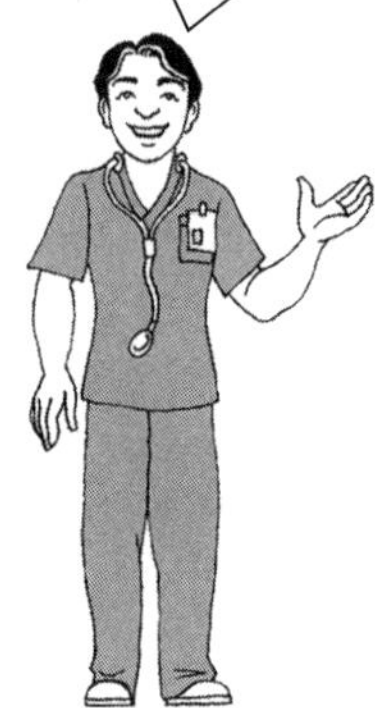
SPSS can perform additional useful functions.

- Generate Random Numbers
- Sort Cases
- Select Cases
- Recode Variables
- Import Data
- SPSS Syntax

Never trust a computer you can't throw out a window.

—Steve Wozniak

LEARNING OBJECTIVES

Upon completing this chapter, you will be able to:

- Perform extended SPSS operations to enhance your capabilities, versatility, and data-processing efficiency
- Generate a list of random numbers to your specifications
- Perform single and multilevel sorting
- Select cases using multiple criteria
- Recode variables
- Import data from external sources: Excel and ASCII files
- Practice safe data storage protocols
- Comprehend the basics of the SPSS Syntax language

OVERVIEW—SUPPLEMENTAL SPSS OPERATIONS

The data sets that have been provided thus far have been crafted to work as is in the SPSS environment, but as you become more statistically proficient, your research curiosity and scientific creative thinking are likely to further develop. You may want to analyze data of your own, examine data from other non-SPSS sources, or run more elaborate statistical analyses. This chapter explains some of the most useful supplemental SPSS features and functions to help you work more productively.

Data Sets

This chapter includes examples involving the following files:

- Ch 14 – Example 01 – Hospital Census.sav
- Ch 14 – Example 02 – Smoking Cessation.sav
- Ch 14 – Example 03 – Excel Data.xls
- Ch 14 – Example 04 – Comma Delimited Data.txt

The codebook for each data set will be presented with each demonstration.

Generating Random Numbers

In Chapter 2, the *Simple Random Sampling* section discussed the need to randomly select 30 individuals from a sample frame of 1,000 potential participants. Flipping a coin to make these selections is clearly out of the question; instead, we can use SPSS to generate this list of random numbers:

1. On the *Variable View* screen, create a numeric variable to contain the 30 random numbers that we will have SPSS generate; we will call it *RandNum* (Figure 14.1).

Figure 14.1 Create a numeric variable (*RandNum*) to contain the random numbers.

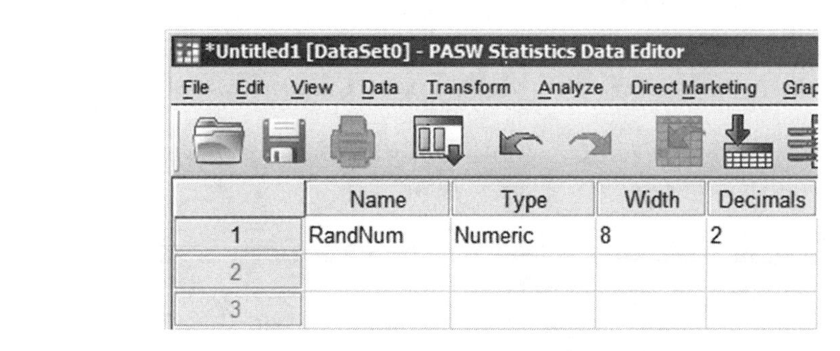

2. Switch to the *Data View* screen and put a *0* (or any number) in the *RandNum* column at record 30 (Figure 14.2).

Figure 14.2 Enter any number at record 30 for *RandNum* (so SPSS will know how long the list should be).

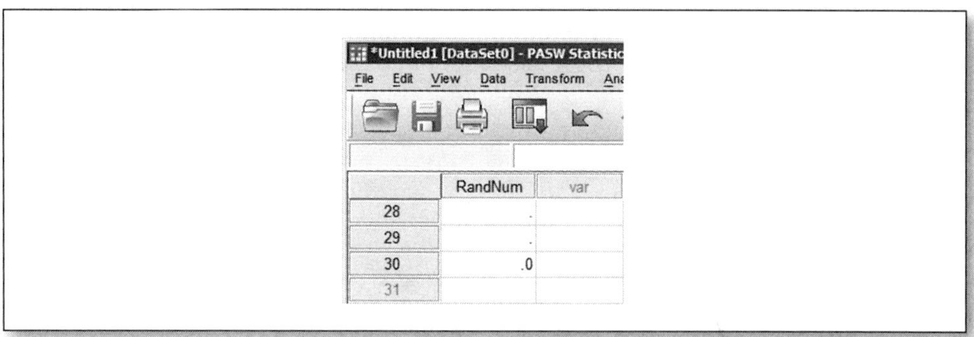

3. Click on *Transform, Compute Variable* (Figure 14.3). This will take you to the *Compute Variable* menu.

Figure 14.3 Click on *Transform, Compute Variables.*

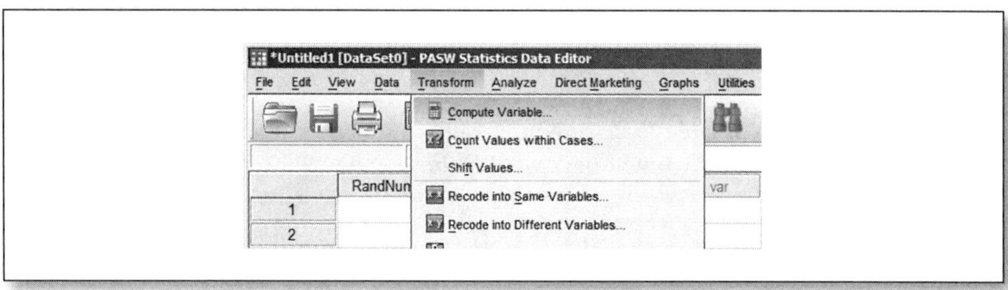

4. On the *Compute Variable* menu, in the *Target Variable* window, enter *RandNum;* in the *Numeric Expression* window, enter *rnd(rv.uniform(1,1000))* (Figure 14.4).

This tells SPSS to place the random values in the *RandNum* variable. Now to demystify the *rnd(rv.uniform(1,1000))* expression:

- *rnd* means round the result to the nearest integer; if you wanted the random numbers to include decimal digits, you could enter *rv.uniform(1,1000).*
- *rv.uniform* means "random values, uniform," wherein each number has an equal chance of being selected.
- *(1,1000)* specifies the minimum (1) and maximum (1,000) values.

Figure 14.4 On the *Compute Variable* menu, in the *Target Variable* window, enter *RandNum;* in the *Numeric Expression* window, enter *rnd(rv.uniform(1,1000))*.

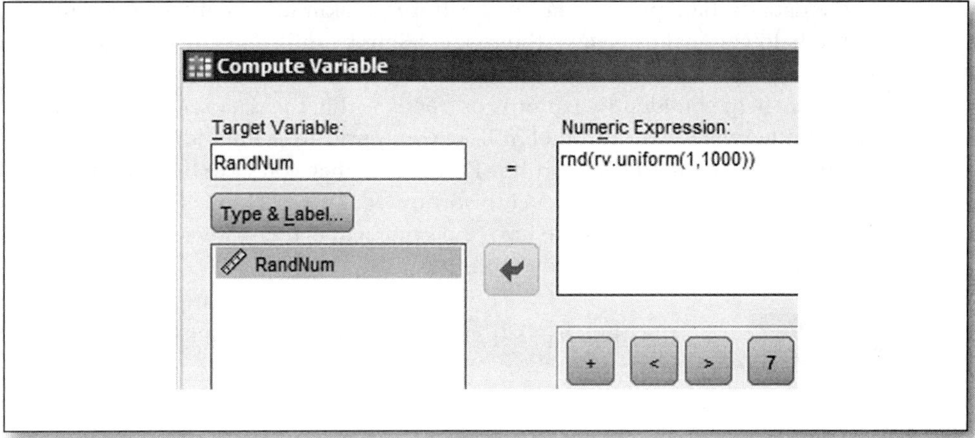

5. Click on the *OK* button. If you are then asked if you wish to *Change existing variable?,* click on the *OK* button.

6. The *Data View* screen should now show 30 random numbers in the *RandNum* column (Figure 14.5).

Figure 14.5 *Data View* screen with resulting random numbers for *RandNum*.

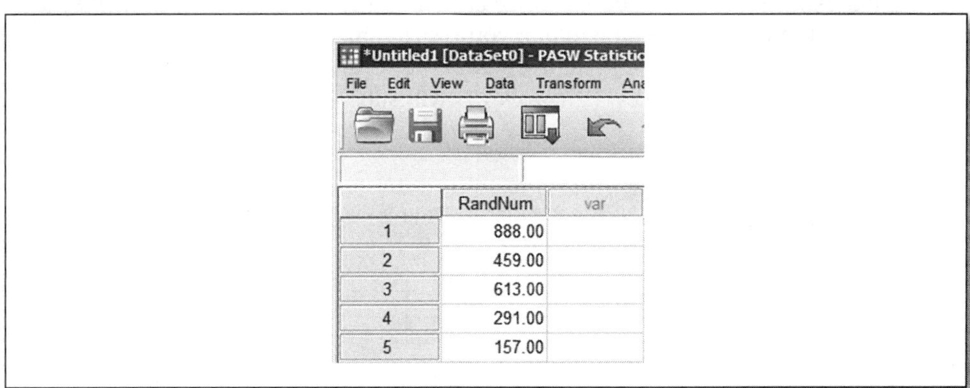

	RandNum	var
1	888.00	
2	459.00	
3	613.00	
4	291.00	
5	157.00	

NOTE: Naturally, your results will produce a different set of random numbers.

The random-number generator does not keep track of repeats among these numbers; hence, you may want to order more random numbers than you actually need so that you can discard duplicates.

Sort Cases

As you have probably noticed, the order of the data on the *Data View* screen has no effect on the statistical outcomes, but at times you may find it useful to inflict some order on the data. In data processing, the term *sort* is akin to alphabetizing; you can sort the data to help you make sense of them. You might be interested in those who scored highest or lowest on a particular variable to better conceptualize the data set; inflicting such order may help you identify patterns or trends within the data set that may not have been evident otherwise—you can then follow your curiosity with additional statistical tests.

SPSS supports multilevel sorting. This means that you could specify the first level to sort by *Name* and the second level to sort by *Age* (you can specify as many levels as you need). So if two or more people have the same name, the system would then look to age to finalize the sorting sequence (Table 14.1).

Table 14.1 Data Sorted by *Name* (Level 1), Then by *Age* (Level 2).

Name	Age
Adrian	15
Blake	12
Blake	27
Blake	38
Cary	19

The default is to sort the variable at each level in *ascending* order (from lowest to highest); alternatively, you can specify that you want to sort in *descending* order (from highest to lowest). For example, if you specify that Level 1 is *Name* ascending and Level 2 is *Age* descending, the system will sort the data with the names arranged from A to Z, but if there is a tie at Level 1 (*Name*), it will subsort those records by *Age*, from highest to lowest (Table 14.2).

Table 14.2 Data Sorted Ascending by *Name* (Level 1), Then Descending by *Age* (Level 2).

Name	Age
Adrian	15
Blake	38
Blake	27
Blake	12
Cary	19

Data Set

1. Load the following data file: **Ch 14 – Example 01 – Hospital Census.sav.** This data set contains the patient census for Acme Hospital. Notice, the records are initially arranged by *Room* number.

Codebook

Variable: Room
Definition: Patient's room number
Type: Continuous

Variable: Ward
Definition: Patient's ward
Type: Categorical

Variable: Patient
Definition: Patient's name (Last name, First initial)
Type: Alphanumeric

Variable: Age
Definition: Patient's age
Type: Continuous

Variable: Gender
Definition: Patient's gender (1 = Female, 2 = Male)
Type: Categorical

Variable: Doctor
Definition: Patient's primary care physician (Last name, First initial)
Type: Alphanumeric

Variable: AdmittingDx
Definition: Patient's admitting diagnosis
Type: Alphanumeric

Variable: LOS
Definition: Length of stay
Type: Continuous

Variable: Note
Definition: Notes regarding the patient's condition
Type: Alphanumeric

2. Suppose you want to identify the patients with the longest length of stay (*LOS*) on each *Ward;* this would involve a two-level sort:

    Level 1: *Ward* (ascending)

    Level 2: *LOS* (descending)

3. Click on *Data, Sort Cases* (Figure 14.6).

Figure 14.6 To sort data, click on *Data, Sort Cases.*

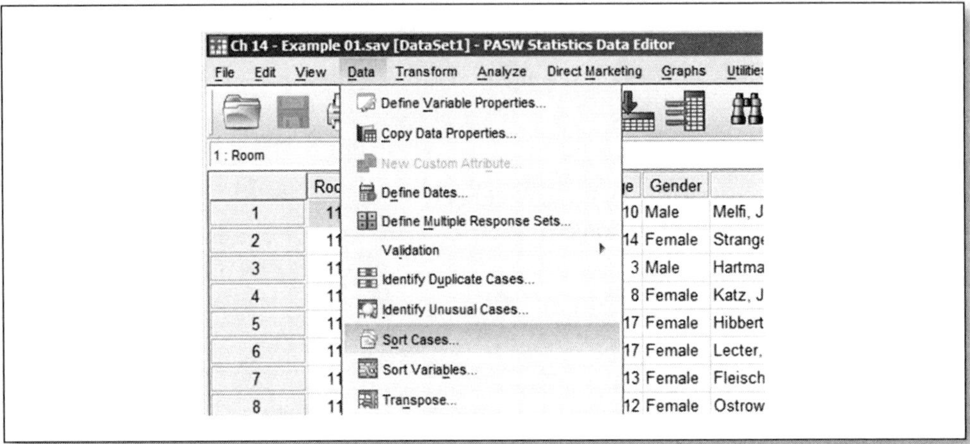

4. On the *Sort Cases* menu (Figure 14.7), move *Ward* from the left window to the *Sort by* window, and click on *Ascending.*
5. Move *LOS* from the left window to the *Sort by* window and click on *Descending.*
6. Notice that once a variable is in the *Sort by* window, you can click on a variable to drag it up and down the list, thereby altering the sorting levels. You can also change the *Sort Order* for a variable by clicking on the variable, then selecting *Ascending* or *Descending.*
7. Click on *OK,* and the system will sort the records (rows).

Figure 14.7 *Sort Cases* menu indicates a two-level sort: first by *Ward* (in *Ascending* order), then by *LOS* (in *Descending* order).

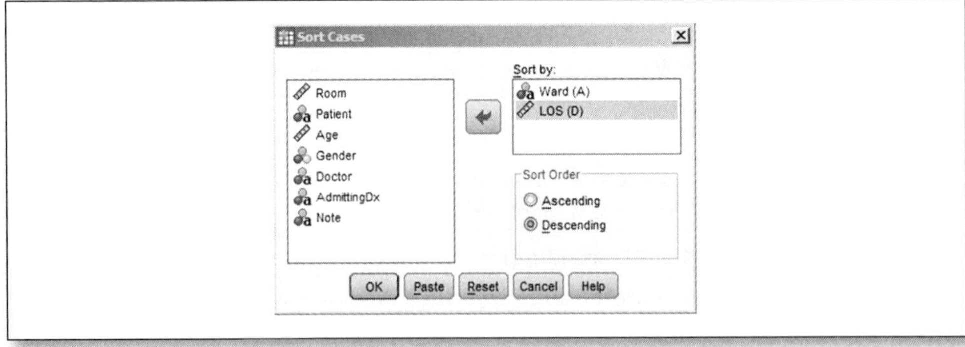

8. Observe the order of the data on the *Data View* screen (Figure 14.8).

Figure 14.8 Two-level sort—*Ward* (ascending), then by *LOS* (descending).

*Ch 14 - Example 01.sav [DataSet1] - PASW Statistics Data Editor

File Edit View Data Transform Analyze Direct Marketing Graphs Utilities Add-ons Window Help

35 : Gender 2 | Visible: 9 of 9 Variables

	Room	Ward	Patient	Age	Gender	Doctor	AdmittingDx	LOS	Note
1	1104	1A	Lamm, R	8	Male	Katz, J	Infected L big toe	11	Contact isolation
2	1102	1A	Rosenblatt, K	14	Female	Strangelove, V	Seizure	9	NPO
3	1106	1A	Hayes, E	17	Female	Lecter, H	Appendicitis	9	
4	1107	1A	Whitaker, A	13	Female	Fleischman, J	Bowel obstruction	7	
5	1114	1A	Gray, A	11	Female	Honeydew, B	Seizure	7	
6	1103	1A	Nemhart, Y	3	Female	Hartman, E	Shortness of breath	6	
7	1111	1A	Wilkerson, F	14	Male	Zorders, D	Abdominal pain	6	
8	1115	1A	Rose, E	12	Male	Hackenbush, H	Infected wound	5	Contact isolation
9	1116	1A	Campbell, J	15	Male	Fine, L	Lupus	5	
10	1101	1A	Swatt, J	10	Female	Melfi, J	Septicemia	4	
11	1112	1A	Carter, M	6	Female	Winchester, C	Tonsillitis	3	
12	1105	1A	Milner, M	17	Female	Hibbert, J	Syncope episode	2	
13	1108	1A	Harret, L	12	Female	Ostrow, C	Tonsillitis	2	
14	1109	1A	Martin, P	17	Female	Steinberg, L	Pneumonia	1	
15	1110	1A	Frank, M	14	Female	Kauffman, D	Subcutaneous tissue infections	1	
16	1113	1A	York, K	16	Male	Soran, T	Fractured R femur	1	

Notice that as we specified, all of the entries for *Ward 1A* moved to the top of the list (in ascending order), and the rows (within Ward 1A) are subsorted by LOS (in descending order) (Figure 14.8). Below all of the data for *Ward 1A* are the records for *Ward 1B,* with the highest *LOS* at the top of that *Ward.*

Try sorting the database using different sorting criteria on other variables and observe the resulting order of the records after each sort. Note that all of the rows will migrate per the specified sorting parameters whether they are slashed out or not. For example, if you had used the *Select Cases* feature to exclude some cases from analyses and then executed a sort, *all* of the rows, including those that are slashed out, would be included in the sort (and they would remain slashed out).

This example involved a two-level sort (first ascending by *Ward,* then descending by *LOS*), but not all sorts need to be multilevel; if you are interested in seeing the data sorted by a single variable, simply specify that one variable and the order (ascending or descending) and the system will process it.

Select Cases

In prior chapters, we have used the *Select Cases* (icon) to run the pretest checklist for various statistical tests, which has enabled us to process statistics for one group at a time. The *Select Cases* function is also capable of choosing data using more complex selection criteria.

For example, you may wish to perform statistical analyses only on *Males who are at least 50 years old.*

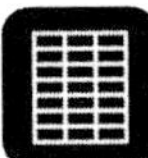

Data Set

1. Load the following data file (unless it is already loaded): **Ch 14 – Example 01 – Hospital Census.sav.**
2. Click on the *Select Cases* icon.
3. In the *Select group,* click on the *If condition is satisfied* button.
4. Click on the *If* button. This will take you to the *Select Cases: If* menu; in the large box at the top, enter the following selection criteria: *Gender = 2* and *Age >= 50* (Figure 14.9).

NOTE: These criteria include *Gender* = 2 since the *Gender* variable has the following labels assigned to it: 1 = *Female*, 2 = *Male*.

Figure 14.9 *Data View* screen showing values (not labels).

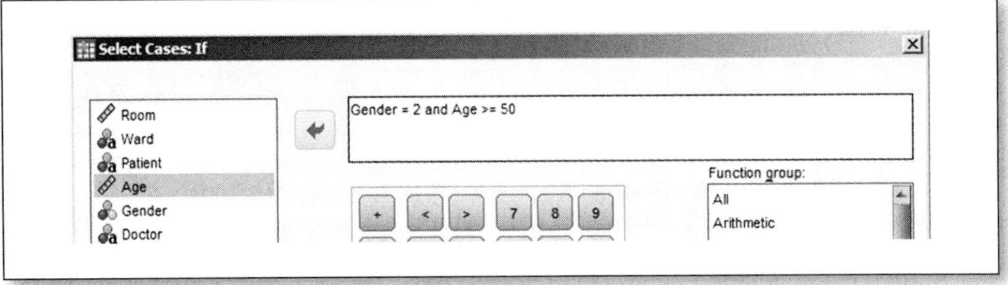

5. Click on the *Continue* button; this will take you back to the *Select Cases* menu.
6. Click on the *OK* button.
7. Go to the *Data View* screen.
8. Notice that all records are slashed out except for the *Males* who are at least 50 years old. Now you can proceed with whatever statistical analysis you wish to perform on the selected (not slashed-out) records.

Try some other case selection criteria and observe which records are affected on the Data View screen:

- *Age* < 18 and *Gender* = 1
- *Room* > 1999 and *Room* < 3000
- *Doctor* < "G"
- *Patient* > "C" and *Patient* <= "R"
- *Age* > 17 and *LOS* > 3

You have probably surmised some of the coding syntax from the examples above; just to clarify a few things:

- Single and compound *and/or* logic is supported.
- Commonly used logical relationships are symbolized as follows:

=	Equal to
<>	Not equal to
<	Less than
>	Greater than
<=	Less than or equal to
>=	Greater than or equal to

Although the system supports *not* logic, negative logic can be confusing; try to build your selection criteria using *and/or* parameters.

When your selection criteria involve alphanumeric (string) variables, be sure to wrap quotation marks around your parameter(s) (e.g., *Doctor* < "G"); otherwise, the processor will think you are referring to a variable named *G*.

Recoding—Example 1

Occasionally, you may wish to change the way a variable is presented in a data set. For example, in the current database, *Age* is a continuous variable that ranges from 3 to 91, but suppose you wanted to use a *t* test to compare the LOS (length of stay) of pediatric (age < 18) to adult (age > 18) patients; you would need a categorical variable to designate which group (pediatric vs. adult) each record belonged to based on *Age*. This is accomplished via *recoding*. We will leave *Age* (a continuous variable) intact, but we can use the *Recode into Different Variables* function to create the new variable, *Age2* (a categorical variable), which will be based on *Age* using the following (two) criteria:

If *Age* < 18, then *Age2* = 1.

If *Age* >= 18, then *Age2* = 2.

Remember: ">=" notation is computer language for "greater than or equal to." After the *recode* function generates the values for *Age2,* we will assign the following value labels to *Age2* to provide clarity:

1 = Pediatric

2 = Adult

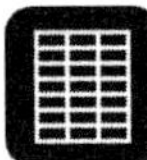

Data Set

1. Load the following data file (unless it is already loaded): **Ch 14 – Example 01 – Hospital Census.sav.**
2. Click on *Transform, Recode into Different Variables* (Figure 14.10).

Figure 14.10 Click on *Transform, Recode into Different Variables.*

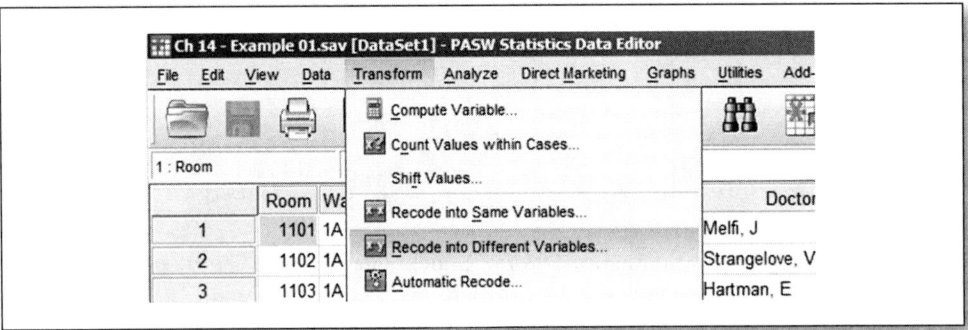

3. On the *Recode into Different Variables* menu, move *Age* from the left window into the *Numeric Variable -> Output Variable* window (Figure 14.11).
4. Enter *Age2* in the *Output Variable, Name* box.
5. Click on the *Change* button.

Figure 14.11 *Recode into Different Variables* menu.

6. So far, you have indicated that the (continuous) variable *Age* will be recoded into the new (categorical) variable *Age2*. Now you need to indicate how age will be recoded into *Age2*. Click on the *Old and New Values* button.

7. Notice that there are a variety of recoding options; we will use a simple method. In the *Old Value* area, select *Range,* and enter *1 through 17* (Figure 14.12). In the *New Value* area, select *Value* and enter *1*. Then click on the *Add* button.

This tells the processor to look within the *Age* variable, and for any record with an *Age* between 1 and 17 (inclusive), write a *1* in that record in the *Age2* variable (without changing the contents of the *Age* variable).

Figure 14.12 *Recode into Different Variables: Old and New Values* menu, recoding *Age* 1–17 to *Age2* as 1.

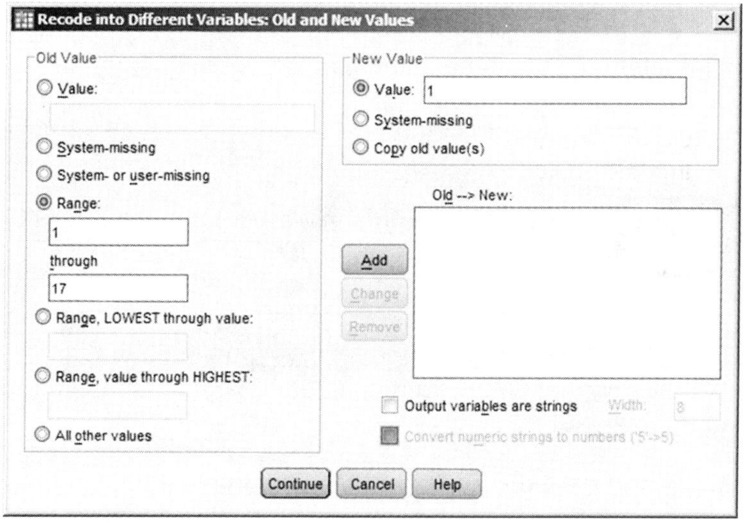

8. In the *Old Value* area, select *Range,* and enter *18 through 99*. In the *New Value* area, select *Value* and enter *2*. Then click on the *Add* button (Figure 14.13).

This tells the processor to look within the *Age* variable, and for any record with an age between 18 and 99 (inclusive), write a 2 in that record in the *Age2* variable (without changing the contents of the *Age* variable).

9. At this point, the *Old --> New* window shows the recoding criteria (Figure 14.14).

Figure 14.13 *Recode into Different Variables: Old and New Values* menu, recoding *Age* 18–99 to *Age2* as 2.

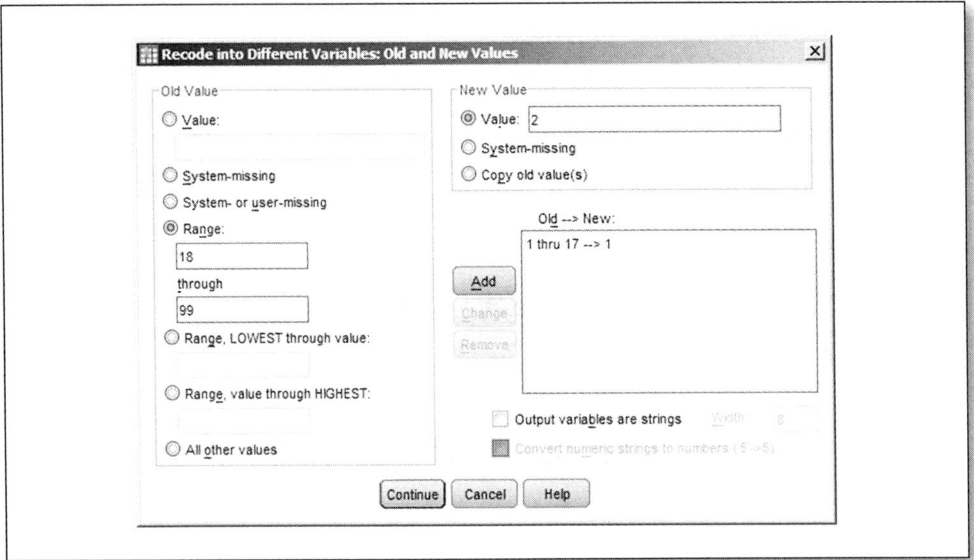

Figure 14.14 *Recode into Different Variables: Old and New Values* menu: criteria that will be used recode *Age* to *Age2*.

Recode into Different Variables: Old and New Values
Old Value
Value:
System-missing
System- or user-missing
Range:
through
Range, LOWEST through value:
Range, value through HIGHEST:
All other values
New Value
Value:
System-missing
Copy old value(s)
Old --> New:
1 thru 17 --> 1
18 thru 99 --> 2
Add
Change
Remove
Output variables are strings
Width:
8
Convert numeric strings to numbers ('5'->5)
Continue
Cancel
Help

10. Click on the *Continue* button; this will return you to the *Recode into Different Variables* menu.
11. Click on the *OK* button, and the recoding will process.
12. Go to the *Data View* screen, and notice that the new variable *Age2* is populated with 1s and 2s based on the *Age* for each record.
13. To finalize the process, go to the *Variable View* screen and specify the corresponding *Value Labels* for *Age2* (*1* = *Pediatric*, *2* = *Adult*) (Figure 14.15).

NOTE: On the *Data View* screen, you may need to scroll to the right to see the (new) *Age2* variable.

Figure 14.15 Assign *Value Labels* to *Age2* (1 = *Pediatric*, 2 = *Adult*).

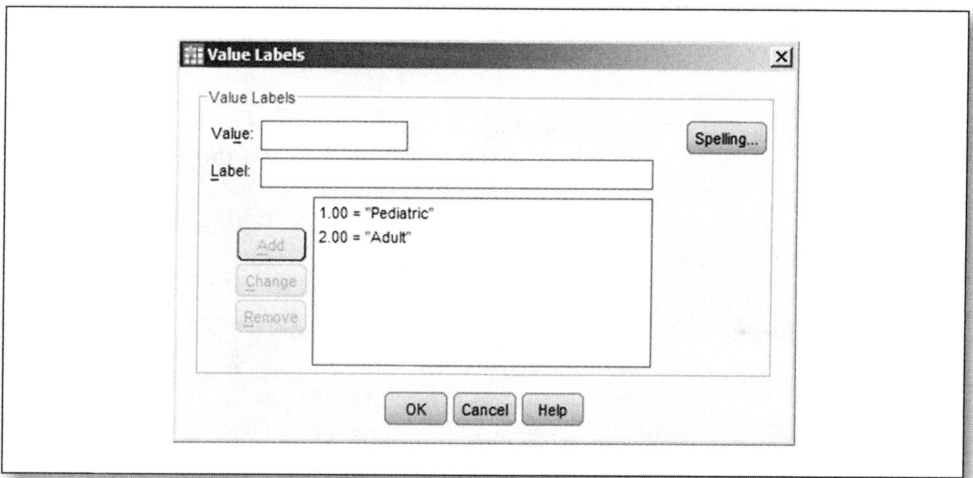

Recoding—Example 2

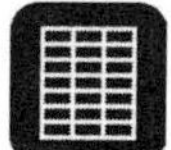

Data Set

Load the file: **Ch 14 – Example 02 – Smoking Cessation.sav** (this is a copy of **Ch 13 – Example 01 – Logistic Regression.sav**).

Codebook

Variable:	Gender
Definition:	Gender
Type:	Categorical (1 = Female, 2 = Male)

Variable: Race
Definition: Race
Type: Continuous (0 = African American, 1 = Asian, 2 = Caucasian, 3 = Latino, 4 = Other)

Variable: Age
Definition: Age
Type: Continuous

Variable: Income
Definition: Income (in dollars)
Type: Continuous

Variable: Cigarettes
Definition: Average number of cigarettes participant smokes per day
Type: Continuous

Variable: Smoking
Definition: Current smoking status
Type: Continuous (0 = Still smoking, 1 = Quit smoking)

As mentioned briefly in Chapter 13: Logistic Regression, recoding enables you to examine variables in a variety of ways. In this data set, the *Race* variable is coded as such:

Race
0 = African American 1 = Asian 2 = Caucasian 3 = Latino 4 = Other

This coding scheme means that when the *Race* variable is included in a logistic regression model, *African American* will constitute the reference category since it is coded as 0 (per the alphabetical arrangement of the categories within the *Race* variable). As such, all of the resulting odds ratios for *Race* will be computed in terms of comparisons to *African Americans*. Recoding enables you to designate a different *Race* (e.g., *Other*) as the reference category (category 0).

To summarize, the goal is to use the *Recode into Different Variables* function to

- *Recode Race* (wherein ***African American* = 0** and ***Other* = 4**) into a new variable (*Race_O*) wherein ***Other = 0*** and ***African American* = 4**
- Copy all the other category codes within *Race* (1 = Asian, 2 = Caucasian, 3 = Latino) as is to *Race_O*
- Leave the original *Race* variable intact (Figure 14.16):

Figure 14.16 Recoding *Race* (without altering *Race*) to create *Race_O.*

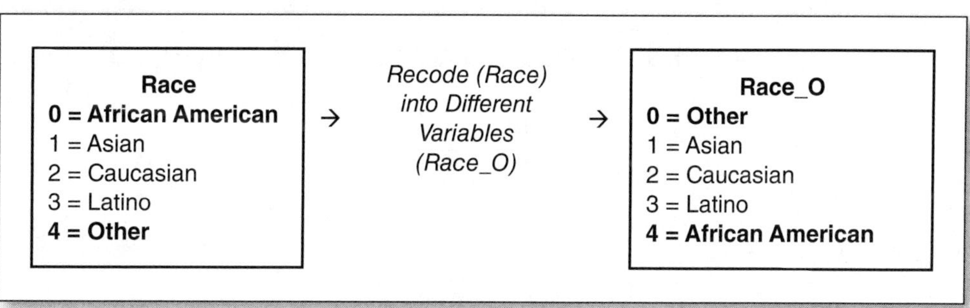

1. Click on *Transform, Recode into Different Variables* (Figure 14.17).

Figure 14.17 Click on *Transform, Recode into Different Variables.*

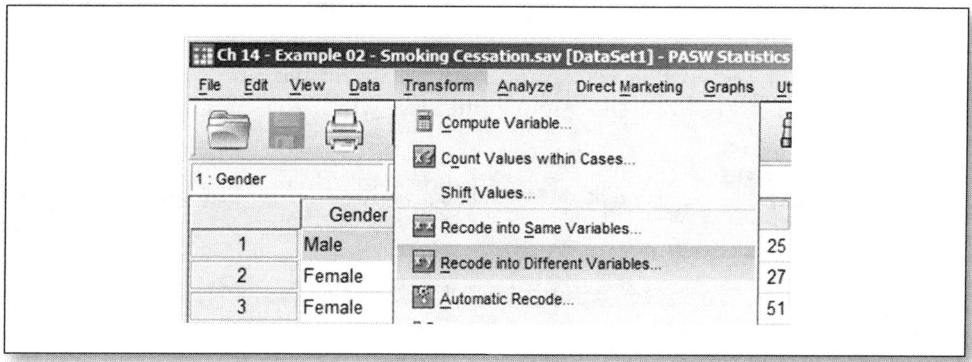

2. On the *Recode into Different Variables* menu, move *Race* into the *Numeric Variable –> Output Variable:* box.
3. In the *Output Variable, Name* box, type in *Race_O* (which stands for *Race* with *Other* as 0—the reference category).
4. Click on *Change.*
5. Click on *Old and New Values.*
6. In the *Old Value, Value* box, enter 0, and in the *New Value/Value box,* enter 4 (this will recode *African Americans* to 4 in the *Race_O* variable) (Figure 4.18).

Figure 14.18 Define recoding: *Change old value* (*Race* = 0) to *New Value* (*Race_O* = 4).

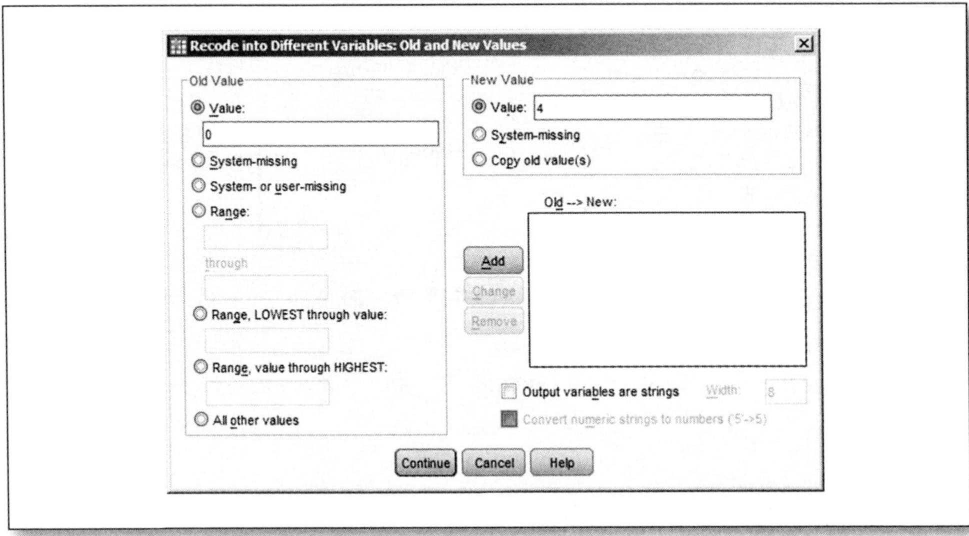

7. Click on *Add*.

8. In the *Old Value, Value* box, enter 4, and in the *New Value, Value* box, enter 0 (this will recode *Other* to 0 in the *Race_O* variable) (Figure 4.19).

Figure 14.19 Define recoding: *Change old value* (*Race* = 4) to *New Value* (*Race_O* = 0).

Recode into Different Variables: Old and New Values
Old Value
Value:
4
System-missing
System- or user-missing
Range:
through
Range, LOWEST through value:
Range, value through HIGHEST:
All other values
New Value
Value: 0
System-missing
Copy old value(s)
Old --> New:
0 --> 4
Add
Change
Remove
Output variables are strings
Width: 8
Convert numeric strings to numbers ('5'->5)
Continue
Cancel
Help

9. Click on *Add.*

10. To copy the other values from *Race* to *Race_O* as is, click on *Old Value/All other values.*

11. Click on *New Value, Copy old value(s)* (Figure 14.20).

Figure 14.20 Define recoding: *Change old value* (*Race* = 0) to *New Value* (*Race_O* = 2).

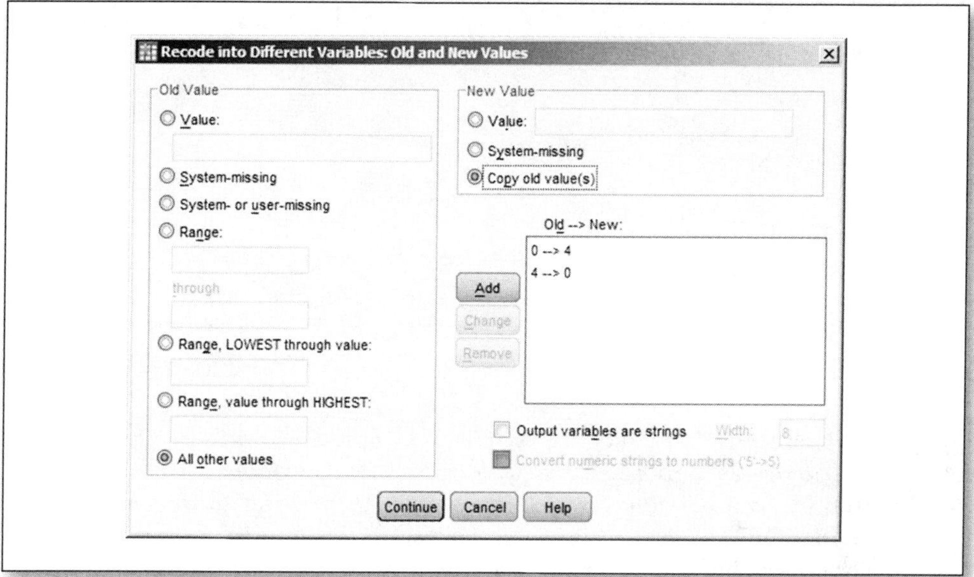

12. Click *Add.* The menu should resemble Figure 14.21, indicating that *0* will be recoded as *4, 4* will be recoded as *0,* and everything *ELSE* will be *Copied* as is: 1 will be recoded as 1, 2 will be recoded as 2, and 3 will be recoded as 3.

13. Click *Continue;* this will return you to the *Recode into Different Variable* menu.

14. On the *Recode into Different Variable* menu, click *OK.*

15. To finalize the process, go to the *Variable View* menu and make the following modifications to configure the properties of the (new) *Race_O* variable:

    a. Set *Width* to 20

    b. Set *Decimals* to 0

    c. Set *Align* to Right

    d. Set *Measure* to Nominal

    e. Set *Values* to 0 = Other, 1 = Asian, 2 = Caucasian, 3 = Latino, 4 = African American

Figure 14.21 Final recoding definitions.

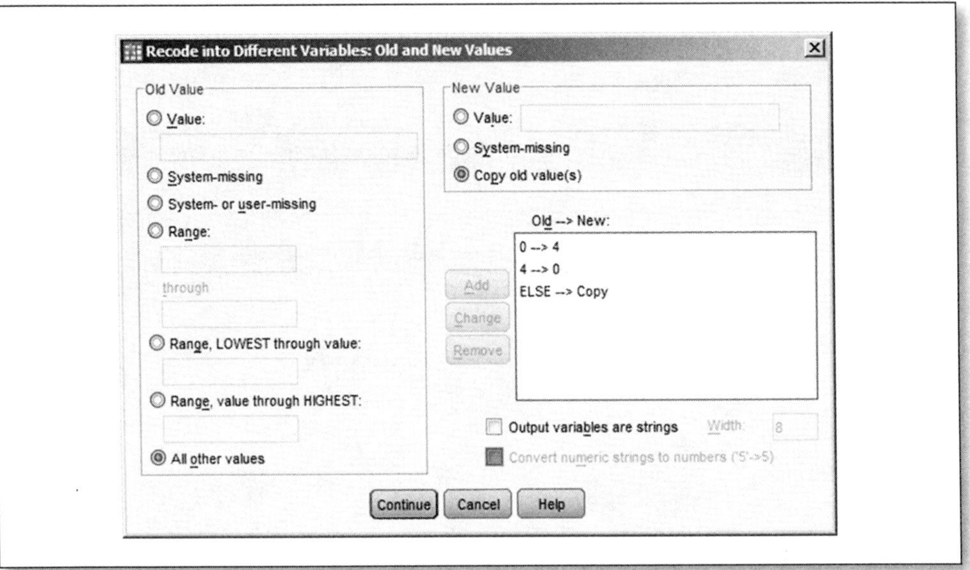

Notice that in both of the *Recoding* examples, we opted to *Recode into Different Variables* as opposed to *Recode into Same Variables*. This choice preserved the original variables, which enables us to perform further analyses on them. Had we used *Recode into Same Variables*, the original values would have been overwritten; hence, the source data would be compromised. In addition, if an error had occurred during the recoding process, the (source) variable would have been corrupted, and hence it would not be possible to reattempt the recoding procedure. As a rule, when recoding, use the *Recode into Different Variables* option to keep your source data intact.

Importing Data

So far, all data we have used have been prepared to operate properly in SPSS, but as you might expect, there is a world of worthy data not necessarily in SPSS format. When the data are only available on paper, naturally you will have to enter the data manually. Fortunately, more and more data are available in a digital form; even if the data are not in SPSS format, SPSS is equipped with some fairly versatile data import features designed to promptly load non-SPSS data into the SPSS environment for processing.

The two most common forms of non-SPSS data are Microsoft Excel and ASCII (pronounced *ask-key*) files, also known as *text* files; once you see how to import data from these two sources, you should be able to reason your way through importing other data formats.

The import data feature in SPSS tends to vary somewhat from version to version. If there is a discrepancy between the instructions in this section and how your version of SPSS operates, then consult the Help menu in your software and search for *import* or *import data.*

Importing Excel Data

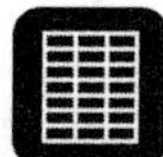

Data Set

The data set that will be imported into SPSS is **Ch 14 – Example 03 – Excel Data.xls.**

SPSS contains an import utility that enables you to load data from multiple (non-SPSS) sources, including Excel. The Excel file that we will be importing contains 101 rows; the first row contains the variable name for each column (*ID, Age, Score*), followed by 100 records, each with three variables (columns):

Codebook

Variable: ID
Definition: Identification number
Type: Alphanumeric

Variable: Age
Definition: Age
Type: Continuous

Variable: Score
Definition: Exam score
Type: Continuous

The first row of the Excel file that you will be importing has the variable names at the top of each column; this will be useful when it comes to the import process. If these names were not present, you could still proceed with the import, but you would need a codebook to know how to label the variables after the file has been imported.

1. Click on *File, Open, Data* (Figure 14.22). This will take you to the *Open File* menu (Figure 14.23).
2. On the *Open Data* menu (Figure 14.23) for *Files of type,* select *Excel;* this will narrow the file list to Excel worksheets only.
3. In the large file list window, select **Chapter 14 – Example 03 – Excel Data.xls** and click on the *Open* button. This will take you to the *Opening Excel Data Source* menu (Figure 14.24).
4. In this case, in the *Opening Excel Data Source* menu (Figure 14.24), the defaults are correct: Since the Excel worksheet has the variable names at the top of each column, the corresponding checkbox (*Read variable names from the first row of*

Figure 14.22 To begin import process, click on *File, Open, Data.*

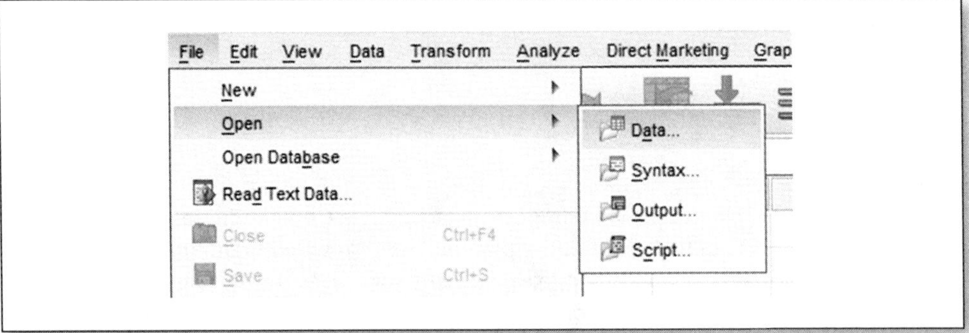

Figure 14.23 *Open Data* menu; for *Files of type,* select *Excel,* and for *File name,* select **Ch 14 – Example 03 – Excel Data.xls.**

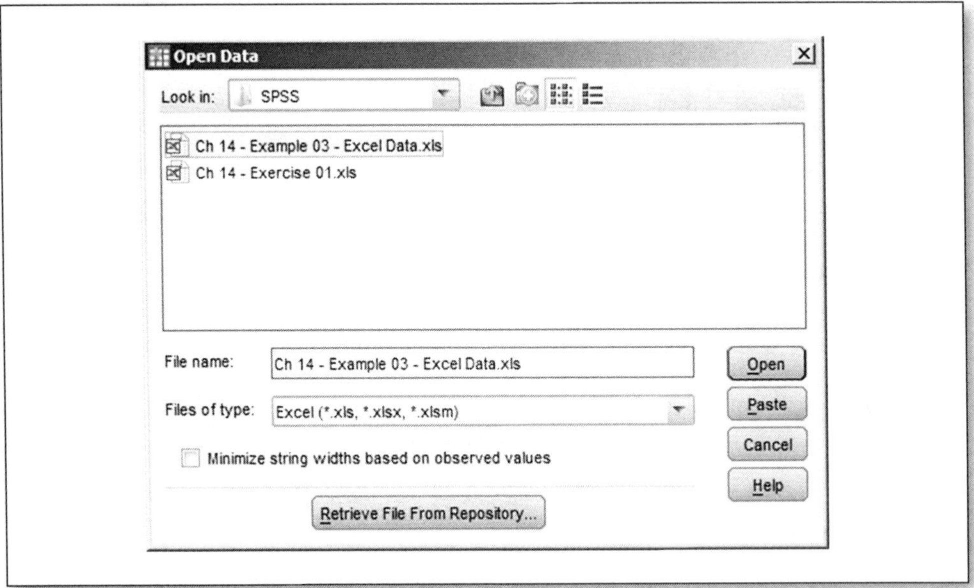

data) is checked. If the variable names are not included as the first row in the Excel sheet, then uncheck that box.

5. The input utility also identified the worksheet and cells involved correctly: *Sheet1 [A1:C101].* Click on the *OK* button.

Figure 14.24 *Opening Excel Data Source* menu.

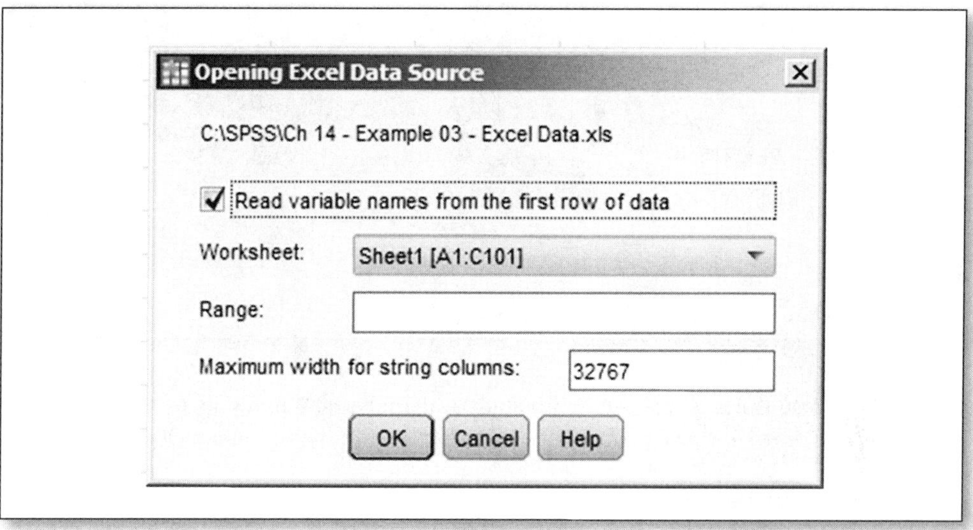

6. SPSS will process the import; notice that the system loaded the Excel file, and the variable names have been assigned accordingly (Figure 14.25).

Figure 14.25 *Data View* screen after Excel file import.

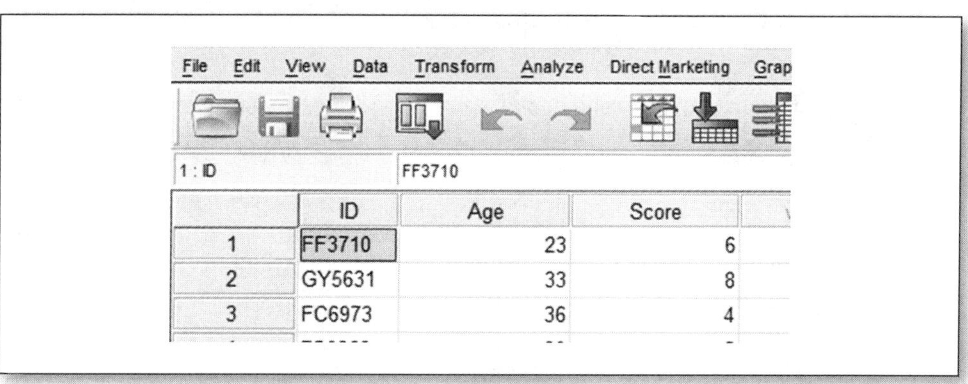

7. To further verify that the import worked properly, switch to the *Variable View* screen (Figure 14.26). Notice that *ID* has been brought in as a string variable since it contains alphanumeric characters, and *Age* and *Score* have been correctly configured as numeric variables.

Figure 14.26 *Variable View* screen after Excel file import.

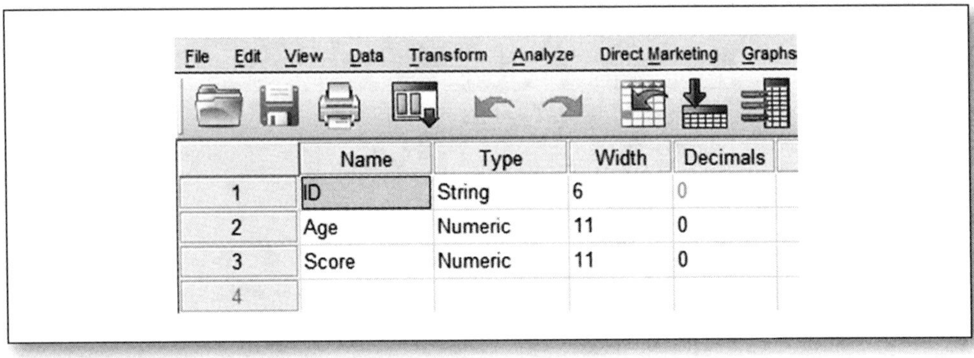
File Edit View Data Transform Analyze Direct Marketing Graphs
Name Type Width Decimals
1 ID String 6 0
2 Age Numeric 11 0
3 Score Numeric 11 0
4

8. You can now proceed with statistical analyses. When you are ready to save the file, the system will write it out as an SPSS file unless you specify otherwise.

Importing ASCII Data

ASCII stands for *American Standard Code for Information Interchange;* it is basically a generic, plain text file, not associated with any particular software package. ASCII filenames typically have a *.txt* (text), *.csv* (Comma Separated Values), or, less often, an *.asc* (ASCII) suffix (e.g., *Experiment18.txt, Test_Scores_Cycle_23.csv, DistrictA.asc*). The data in such files are traditionally arranged with one record per row; the variables within each row are usually separated by a delimiter character, such as a comma or other symbol (Figure 14.27). Alternatively, some files do not use delimiters to separate variables; instead, they use a fixed number of characters per variable, producing columns of data padded with spaces (Figure 14.28).

Figure 14.27 Comma-delimited ASCII data.

```
ID,Age,Score
DE7015,72,5
LP4964,35,6
PF9120,51,6
HC4109,49,10
EH8610,66,3
RV3966,31,3
JZ4866,61,8
```

Figure 14.28 Fixed-column ASCII data.

ID	Age	Score
DE7015	72	5
LP4964	35	6
PF9120	51	6
HC4109	49	10
EH8610	66	3
RV3966	31	3
JZ4866	61	8

Since delimited files are more common, this example will involve a comma-delimited ASCII file.

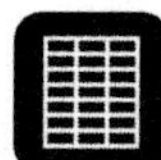

Data Set

The data set that will be imported into SPSS are **Ch 14 – Example 04 – Comma Delimited Data File.txt.**

1. Click on *File, Open, Data* (Figure 14.29). This will take you to the *Open File* menu (Figure 14.30).

Figure 14.29 To begin import process, click on *File, Open, Data.*

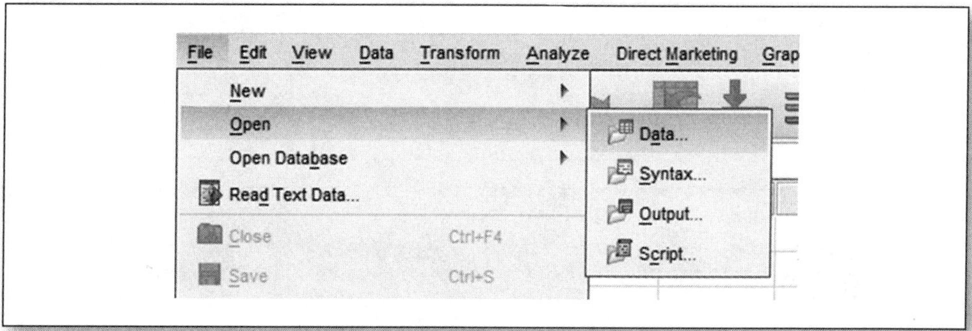

2. On the *Open Data* menu (Figure 14.30) for *Files of type,* select *Text;* this will narrow the file list. If the file name has a suffix other than *.txt,* then at the *Files of type* option, select *All Files.*

3. On the large file list window, select **Ch 14 – Example 04 – Comma Delimited Data.txt** and click on the *Open* button. This will take you to the *Text Import Wizard—Step 1 of 6* menu (Figure 14.31).

4. On the *Text Import Wizard—Step 1 of 6* menu, click on the *Next* > button. This will take you to the *Text Import Wizard—Step 2 of 6* menu (Figure 14.32).

5. On the *Text Import Wizard—Step 2 of 6* menu, since this is a comma-delimited data set, for the *How are your variables arranged?* question, select *Delimited.*

   For the *Are variable names included at the top of your file?* question, select *Yes.* Then, click on the *Next* > button; this will take you to the *Text Import Wizard—Step 3 of 6* menu.

6. On the *Text Import Wizard—Steps 3–5* menus, the defaults are all appropriate. Click on the *Next* > button for each of these menus until you reach the *Text Import Wizard—Step 6 of 6* menu.

Figure 14.30 *Open Data* menu; for *Files of type,* select *Text (*.txt, *.dat),* and for *File name,* select **Ch 14 – Example 04 – Comma Delimited Data.txt.**

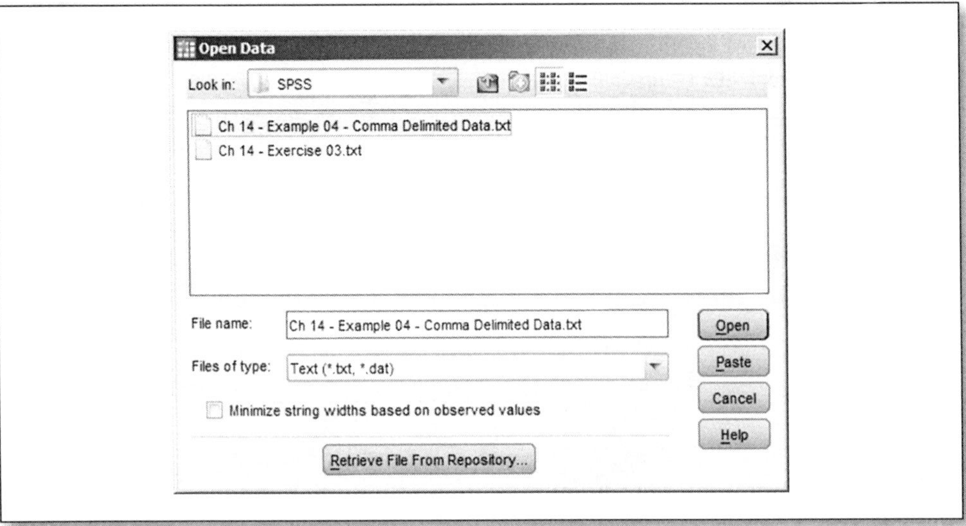

Figure 14.31 *Text Import Wizard—Step 1 of 6* menu.

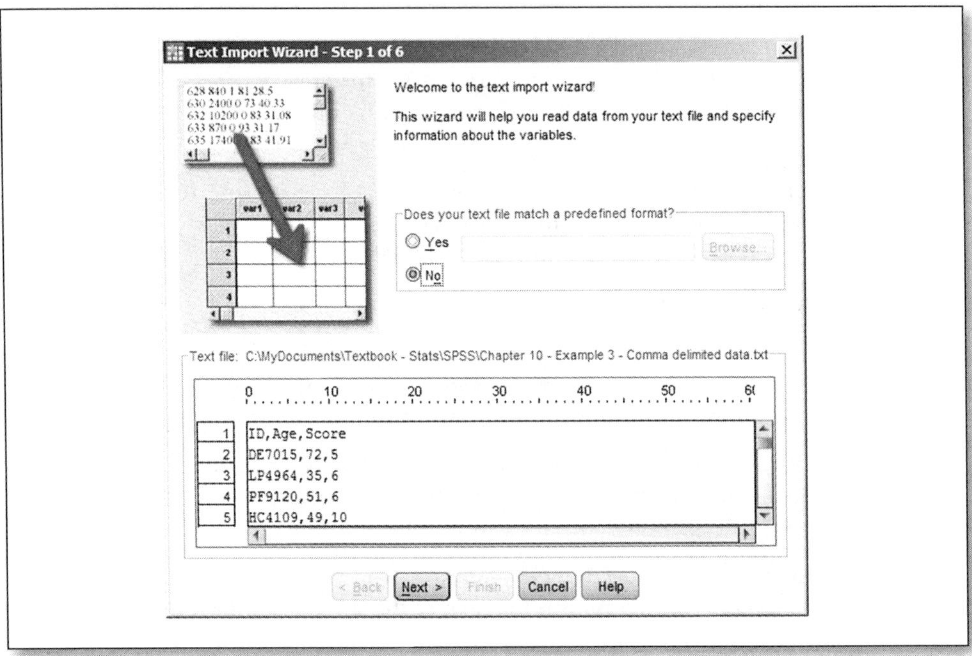

Figure 14.32 *Text Import Wizard—Step 2 of 6* menu.

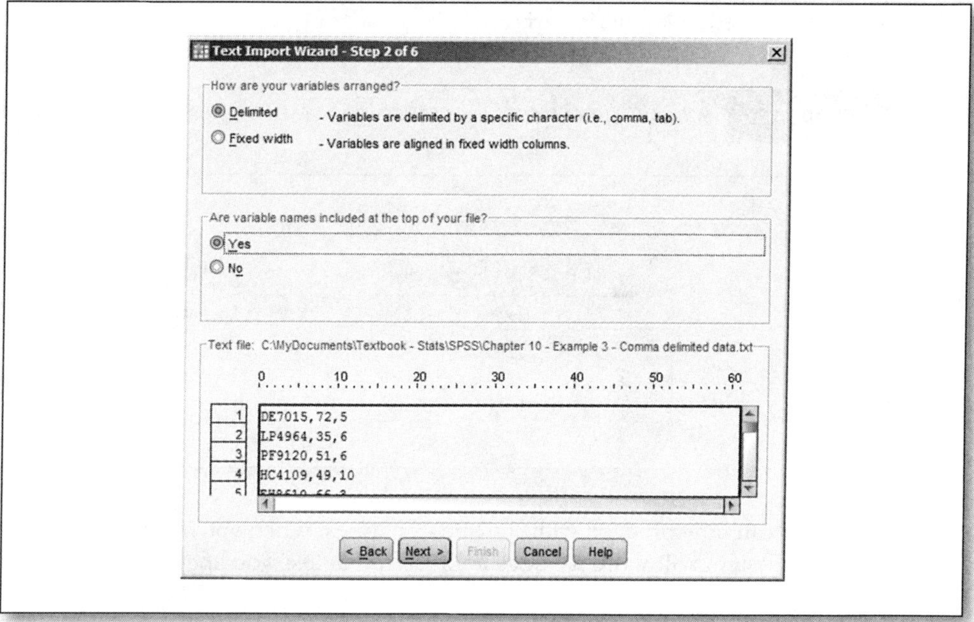

7. On the *Text Import Wizard—Step 6 of 6* menu, click on the *Finish* button.
8. SPSS will process the import; notice that the system loaded the ASCII comma-delimited text file, with the variable names assigned accordingly (Figure 14.33).

Figure 14.33 *Data View* screen after text file import.

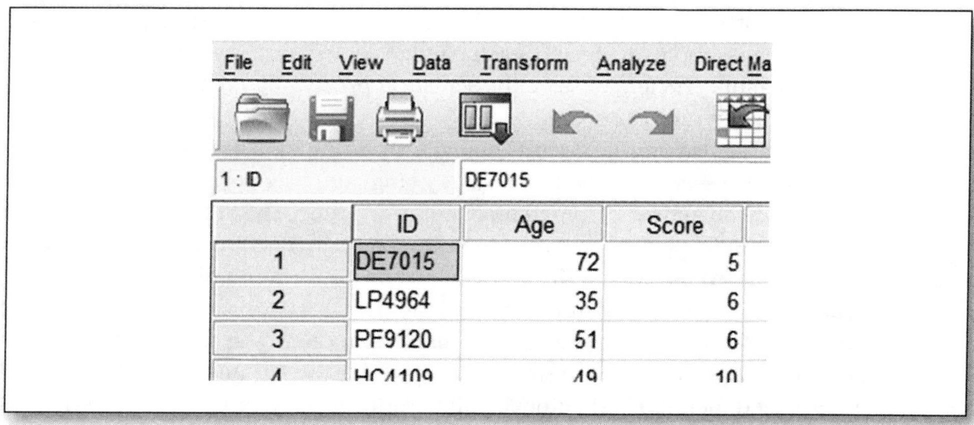

9. To further verify that the import worked properly, switch to the *Variable View* screen (Figure 14.34). Notice that *ID* has been brought in as a string variable since it contains alphanumeric characters, and *Age* and *Score* have been correctly configured as numeric variables.

Figure 14.34 *Variable View* screen after text file import.

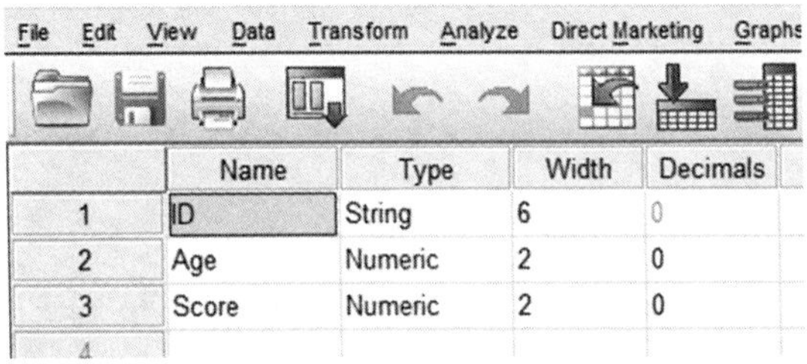

File Edit View Data Transform Analyze Direct Marketing Graphs

	Name	Type	Width	Decimals
1	ID	String	6	0
2	Age	Numeric	2	0
3	Score	Numeric	2	0
4				

10. You can now proceed with statistical analyses. When you are ready to save the file, the system will write it out as an SPSS file unless you specify otherwise.

If the data that you are importing contain categorical variables coded as numbers (e.g., 1 = *Yes*, 2 = *No*), it would be to your advantage to gather as much codebook information as you can, so you can assign the appropriate data labels for each such variable.

SPSS Syntax

The convenient point-and-click menu system that we have used to operate SPSS is ideal for the kind of statistical processing that we have performed in this book, wherein each data set is processed just once.

In instances involving complex analyses that will be run repeatedly (e.g., weekly/monthly reports on an evolving database), there is an alternative to clicking through multiple menus, hoping to specify each parameter perfectly every time. In such instances, it would be more efficient to store the statistical processing commands in a program that could be reliably run on demand.

Historically speaking, SPSS was initially implemented before the advent of menu-driven software—as such, the SPSS Syntax language was developed, wherein statistical processing commands were typed in, one line at a time. The SPSS Syntax language is still a part of the SPSS system, but you do not necessarily need to learn an entire programming language to use it.

You may have noticed that on most of the menus, there is a *Paste* button next to the *OK* button. Whereas *OK* executes the instructions that you specified on the menu(s) immediately, *Paste* does not; instead *Paste* assesses the parameters that you specified on the associated menu(s) and automatically produces the equivalent SPSS Syntax code.

For example, suppose you wanted to produce descriptive statistics and a histogram with a normal curve for the variable *Age*. You would begin at the *Analyze, Descriptive, Statistics, Frequencies* menu (Figure 14.35).

Next, on the *Statistics* (sub)menu, you would specify the descriptive statistics that you want processed (Figure 14.36), and on the *Charts* (sub)menu, you would order the corresponding histogram with normal curve (Figure 14.37).

Figure 14.35 *Frequencies* menu (for descriptive statistics).

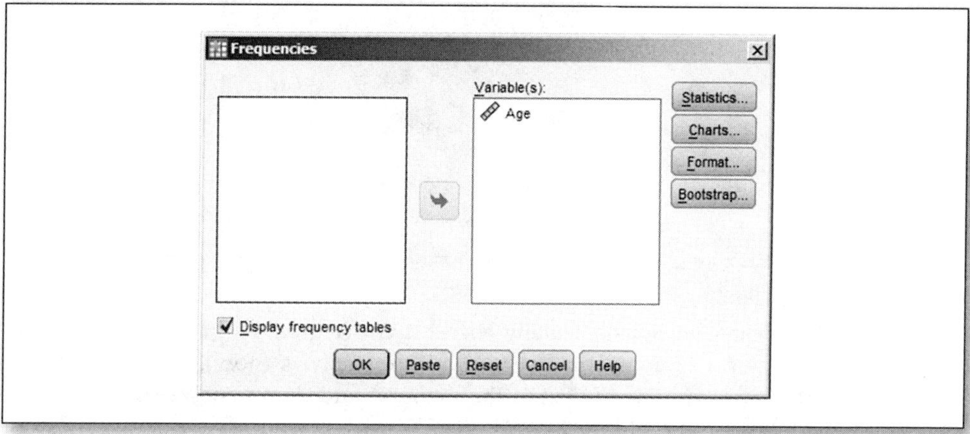

Figure 14.36 *Frequencies Statistics* menu.

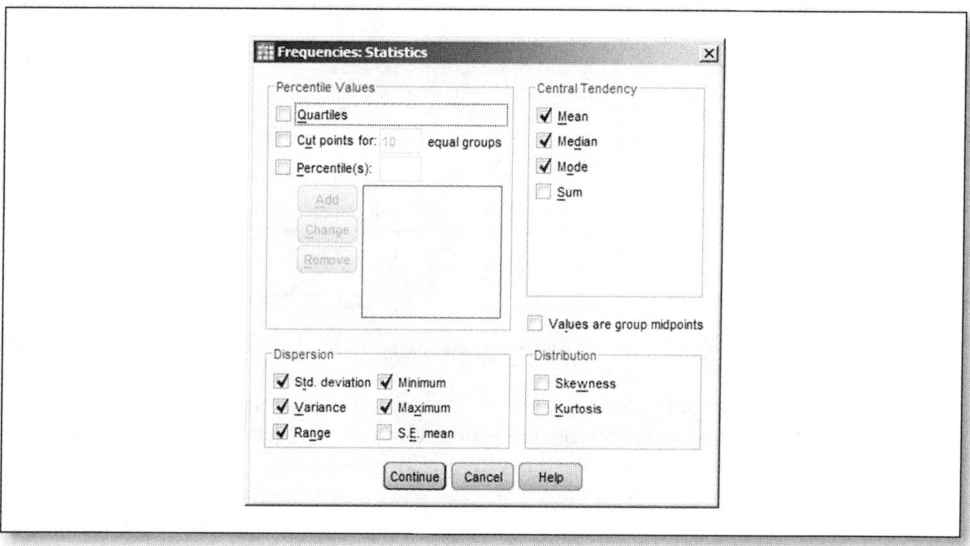

Figure 14.37 *Frequencies Charts* menu.

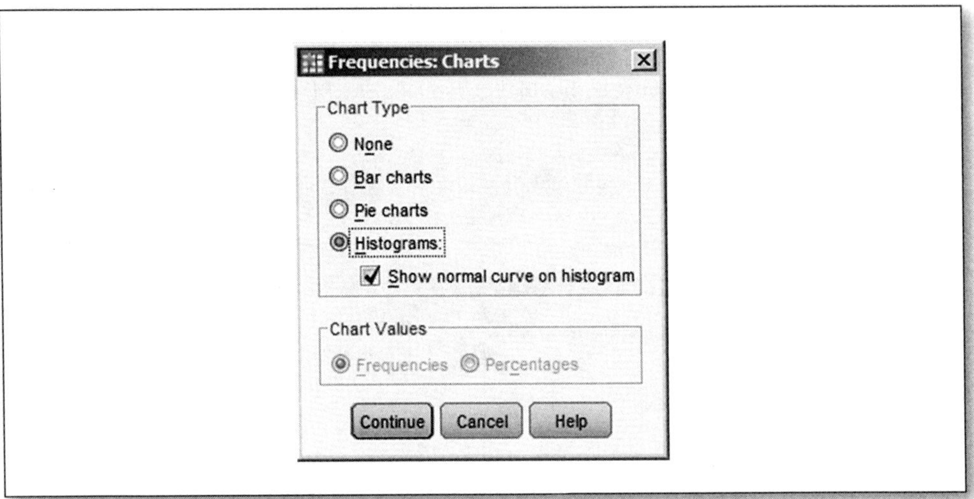

At this point, we would usually click on *OK* (Figure 14.35) to run the analysis, but instead, click on *Paste*. Instead of running the analysis (now), *Paste* tells the system to assess the parameters specified in the menu(s) and then generate the equivalent block of SPSS Syntax code (Figure 14.38):

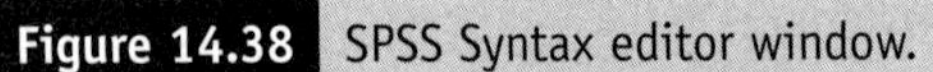

Figure 14.38 SPSS Syntax editor window.

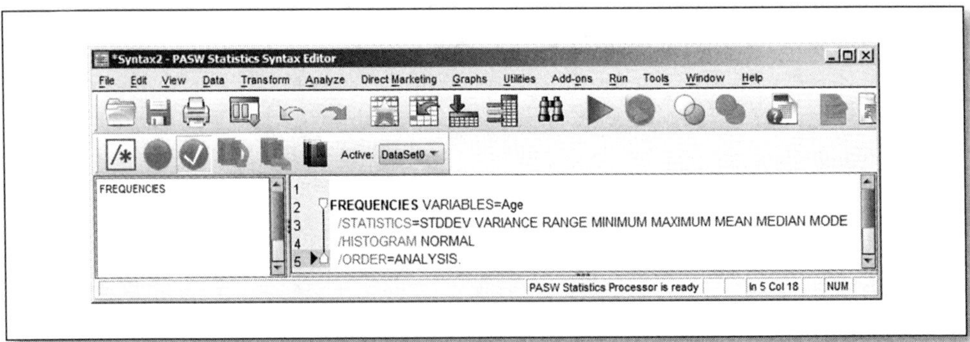

Each time you click on the *Paste* button, SPSS makes this menu-to-Syntax conversion and adds the lines of Syntax programming code to the bottom of the accumulating Syntax file—essentially, you are building a Syntax program, one block of code at a time.

When you save the Syntax code, it will be assigned the *.sps* suffix to the file name; (e.g., *Monthly_Rx_Analysis.sps*) you have probably already noticed that SPSS data files have the *.sav* file name suffix.

Using a Syntax file to run analyses spares you from having to visit multiple menus and specify the parameters each time. To run this code, highlight the lines that you want processed (in this case, all of the lines), and then click on the *Run* (▶) icon.

Most but not all menus in SPSS contain the *Paste* button; hence, if you opt for the SPSS Syntax language to run your analyses, occasionally you may need to do some manual editing or coding. The SPSS Syntax language is a fully developed programming language that extends well beyond the blocks of code that you can generate by clicking on the *Paste* button.

For a more comprehensive guide detailing the commands and functions available in the SPSS Syntax language, a useful introductory manual is *How to Use SPSS Syntax: An Overview of Common Commands* by Manfred te Grotenhuis and Chris Visscher.

GOOD COMMON SENSE

It is good practice to save an unedited master copy of your source data sets (e.g., *File_Name[MASTER].sav*) and only perform your analysis on a work-copy of the file (e.g., *File_Name[WORK].sav*).

Even for the most careful person, data loss or data corruption is just an accidental keystroke away. Try to avoid deleting records; a better practice is to use *Select Cases* to rule them out of the analyses.

If you have source data (e.g., survey cards, written records, recordings, etc.), keep them intact and stored in a secured fashion. It is generally considered good practice not to destroy or discard source media just because the information has been entered into a database; you may need to refer to such materials over the course of your investigation (e.g., to resolve discrepancies, verify that some anomalous data are coded properly, etc.). Occasionally, such references to source materials take place during the analytic process as outliers, and other reasonably questionable data begin to emerge in reports or in visual inspection of the coded data.

All hardware fails at some point; therefore, it is good practice to keep secured/encrypted up-to-date backups of data files in at least two safe locations (e.g., a copy at home and another copy at work), unless your research protocol prohibits this. The rational for two sites is to offer additional protection against unforeseen adverse events at a site (e.g., fire, water damage, natural disaster, theft, electrical problems, etc.).

Some research protocols specify how long the research team is required to retain the source data (e.g., surveys, field notes, recordings, etc.). The time frame may range from days to years. The research protocol may also indicate how such data are to be disposed of on the specified expiration date (e.g., shredding, purging media, transfer to a secured storage site, etc.) so as to facilitate participant confidentiality. As a responsible researcher, be sure you fully understand and adhere to these protocols.

Key Concepts

- Generating random numbers
- Sorting cases
  - Ascending
  - Descending
- Selecting cases
- Recoding
- Importing data
- SPSS Syntax
- Data management
  - Master file
  - Work file
  - Data handling
  - Data storage
  - Data disposal

Practice Exercises

Exercise 14.1

You have been given an Excel data set containing patient's blood pressure readings.

Data set: **Ch 14 – Exercise 01.xls**

Codebook

Variable:	Patient ID
Definition:	Patient's identification number
Type:	Continuous
Variable:	Systolic
Definition:	Systolic blood pressure (mmHg)
Type:	Continuous
Variable:	Diastolic
Definition:	Diastolic blood pressure (mmHg)
Type:	Continuous

a. Import the Excel file: **Ch 14 – Exercise 01.xls** into SPSS.

b. Recode *Systolic* into a new variable called *BP_Category* using the following criteria:

   - If *Systolic* is less than 121, then code *BP_Category* as 1.
   - If *Systolic* is 121–140, then code *BP_Category* as 2.
   - If *Systolic* is 141–160, then code *BP_Category* as 3.
   - If *Systolic* is over 160, then code *BP_Category* as 4.

c. Set the following *Value Labels* for *BP_Category:*

   - 1 = *Normal*
   - 2 = *Prehypertension*
   - 3 = *Hypertension Stage 1*
   - 4 = *Hypertension Stage 2*

d. For all patients with *Hypertension Stage 1,* produce descriptive statistics for *Systolic;* include a histogram with the normal curve.

e. For all patients with *Hypertension Stage 2,* produce descriptive statistics for *Systolic;* include a histogram with the normal curve.

Exercise 14.2

You have been given a sample frame with record numbers ranging from 852 through 5,723; the research team wants to gather a 2% sample (n = 97). Use SPSS to generate this list of random numbers.

Exercise 14.3

You have been requested to compute statistics involving patients' appointment keeping.

Data set: Import the ASCII, comma-delimited data set: **Ch 14 – Exercise 03.txt** into SPSS.

Codebook

Variable: Journal
Definition: Journal number for each scheduled appointment
Type: Continuous

Variable: Clinic
Definition: Clinic of the patient's appointment (1 = Primary care, 2 = Physical therapy, 3 = Dialysis, 4 = Mental health)
Type: Categorical

Variable: Appt
Definition: Appointment status (1 = On time, 2 = Late, 3 = Rescheduled, 4 = Canceled, 5 = No show)
Type: Continuous

a. Set the *Value Labels* for *Clinic* and *Appt* as specified above.

b. Run a chi-square analysis to produce a bar chart that shows the *Appointment* results for each *Clinic.*

Exercise 14.4

For this exercise, we will use the hospital census data that were used to demonstrate *Sorting* in this chapter.

Data set: **Ch 14 – Exercise 04.sav**

Codebook

Variable: Room
Definition: Patient's room number
Type: Continuous

Variable: Ward
Definition: Patient's ward
Type: Categorical

Variable: Patient
Definition: Patient's name (Last name, First initial)
Type: Alphanumeric

Variable: Age
Definition: Patient's age
Type: Continuous

Variable: Gender
Definition: Patient's gender (1 = Female, 2 = Male)
Type: Categorical

Variable: Doctor
Definition: Patient's primary care physician (Last name, First initial)
Type: Alphanumeric

Variable: AdmittingDx
Definition: Patient's admitting diagnosis
Type: Alphanumeric

Variable: LOS
Definition: Length of stay
Type: Continuous

Variable: Note
Definition: Notes regarding the patient's condition
Type: Alphanumeric

a. Sort the data by *Doctor* in ascending (A to Z) order, and print the database.
b. Sort the data by *Ward* in ascending order (A to Z), with a secondary sort by *LOS* in descending order (highest to lowest), and print the database.

Exercise 14.5

Prior to enrolling in an advanced nursing skills recertification in-service, those who score 80 or higher on a preexam are granted recertification; those with scores under 80 are required to take the recertification course.

Data set: **Ch 14 – Exercise 05 & 06.sav**

Codebook

Variable: *Stafft_ID*
Definition: Participant's identification number
Type: Continuous

Variable:	Score
Definition:	Participant's pretest score
Type:	Continuous

a. Use the *Recode* (*into different variable*) function to create a new variable (*PassFail*) (based on *Score*) that identifies those who passed (scored 80 or higher) and those who failed (scored under 80).

b. Run descriptive statistics for *Score* for those who passed.

c. Run descriptive statistics for *Score* for those who failed.

Exercise 14.6

Repeat *Exercise 5,* this time set the passing *Score* to 70.

Exercise 14.7

A clinic would like you to process the (numeric) data gathered from the *Patient Satisfaction Survey Cards:*

Data set: **Chapter 14 – Exercise 07.sav**

Codebook

Variable:	Satisfaction
Definition:	Patient's nursing satisfaction score
Type:	Continuous
Variable:	Comment
Definition:	Patient's comments regarding his or her clinical experience
Type:	Alphanumeric

Patient Satisfaction Survey Card

How satisfied are you with the quality of the care that you received today?

☐	☐	☐	☐
Very unsatisfied	Unsatisfied	Satisfied	Very satisfied

Please provide any comments about your experience in our clinic today:

a. Recode *Satisfaction* into a new (different) variable called *Quality* using the following criteria:

   - If *Satisfaction* is 1 or 2, then code *Quality* as 1.
   - If *Satisfaction* is 3 or 4, then code *Quality* as 2.

b. Set the following *Value Labels* for *Quality:*

   - 1 = *Negative*
   - 2 = *Positive*

c. Run descriptive statistics for *Satisfaction;* include a histogram with normal curve.

d. Run descriptive statistics for *Quality;* include a bar chart.

Exercise 14.8

Explain what is meant by a *master file* and the rationale for safely preserving it.

Exercise 14.9

Explain what is meant by a *work file* and the rationale for performing analyses on it.

Exercise 14.10

Data safety and confidentiality are essential in the realm of research and analysis. Discuss the rationale and techniques for appropriate data handling, data storage, and data disposal.

Glossary

!: See *Factorial*

% formula: See *Percent*

.sas file extension: .sas files contain SPSS syntax code (programs)

.sav file extension: .sav files contain SPSS data sets

α error: See *Type I error*

α value: See *Alpha value*

β error: See *Type II error*

Δ%: See Delta %

Alpha value: The cutoff score for the p value; alpha is typically set to .05, wherein p values $\leq .05$ suggest statistically significant finding(s)

Alternate hypothesis (H_1): The hypothesis that states that the treatment effect will be significant; the score for the control group will be different from the score for the treatment group

ANCOVA: Analysis of covariance is similar to ANOVA, except results are adjusted per the identified confounding variable (covariate)

ANOVA: Analysis of variance is similar to the t test, except it compares all pairs of groups (G_1:G_2, G_1:G_3, G_2:G_3)

ANOVA repeated measures: Similar to the paired t test, except it compares scores from all pairs of time points (T_1:T_2, T_2:T_3, T_1:T_3)

Area sampling: A probability sampling technique typically used to draw proportional random samples from multiple domains (e.g., blocks spanning a community)

ASCII: American Standard Code for Information Interchange (a generic/alphanumeric data file)

Availability sampling: See *Convenience sampling*

Bar chart: A graphical representation of the numbers contained within a categorical variable, consisting of a bar chart

Bimodal: Two numbers are tied for the most common number contained within a continuous variable (both numbers are equally frequent within the variable)

Box's *M* test: See *Homogeneity of variance-covariance (Box's* M *test)*

Categorical variable: A variable that contains a discrete value (e.g., Gender = Female/Male)

Causation: Correlation demonstrating that one variable influenced the outcome of another by meeting three criteria: (1) association/correlation, (2) temporality, and (3) nonspurious relationship

Chi-square: Indicates if there is a statistically significant difference between two categorical variables

Cluster sampling: See *Area sampling*

Comma delimited data: A data set wherein a comma (,) separates the variables

Confounding variable: A variable or factor, other than the independent variable (IV), that influences the dependent (outcome) variable (DV)

Continuous variable: A variable that contains a number along a continuum (e.g., Age = 0 . . . 100)

Control group: The group that receives either no treatment or treatment as usual (TAU) to serve as a comparison against the group(s) that receive the (experimental) treatment

Convenience sampling: A nonprobability sampling technique wherein those who are readily available are recruited as research participants

Correlation: Indicates the strength of the relationship between two continuous variables gathered from each participant/data record

Correlation strength: Correlations nearer to −1 or +1 suggest stronger correlations than correlations nearer to 0

Covariate: See *Confounding variable*

Crosstabs: A statistical table that contains results based on column : row

Data disposal: Pertains to when and how data (electronic and other) are to be disposed of (e.g., secure reformat/erasure of electronic media, shredding paper, relocating media to secured facility)

Data set: A table of alphanumeric information prepared for statistical processing

Data storage: Pertains to where and how data (electronic and other) are securely kept

Data view: SPSS screen wherein the actual information contained in the SPSS data set is viewed/edited

Delta %: Also represented as "Δ%," expressing the change percentage in a variable: $\Delta\% = (\text{New} - \text{Old}) \div \text{Old} \times 100$

Descriptive statistics: A summary of a variable using figures and graphs that can characterize continuous or categorical variables

Dichotomous: A categorical variable that contains two values (e.g., Gender: Female/Male)

Disproportionate stratified sampling: A probability sampling technique wherein the percentage of items/participants selected from each stratum does not match the percentage in the population

Experimental group: The group(s) that receives the (experimental) treatment, which will be compared to the control group

External validity: The extent to which the results of the sample can be generalized to the overall population from which the sample was drawn

Factorial: Also represented as "!", a probability calculation wherein a number is multiplied by all of the integers between 1 and the specified number (e.g., $3! = 1 \times 2 \times 3$, which equals 6)

GIGO: Acronym: "Garbage In, Garbage Out" pertains to the necessity of entering and processing quality data to produce quality results

H_0: See *Null hypothesis*

H_1: See *Alternate hypothesis*

Histogram with normal curve: A graphical representation of the numbers contained within a continuous variable, consisting of a bar chart with a bell-shaped curve superimposed on it

Historical confound: Threat to internal validity that is most relevant to longitudinal designs (e.g., *t* test, ANOVA repeated measures), wherein events outside the experimental procedure may act as confounding variables

Homogeneity of regression slopes: A pretest criterion for ANCOVA that evaluates the similarity of the regression slopes among the independent variables (IVs)

Homogeneity of variance: Similarity of variance (SD^2) among two or more variables

Homogeneity of variance-covariance (Box's *M* test): A pretest criterion for MANOVA that evaluates the similarity of the covariances among the independent variables (IVs)

Homoscedastic: See *Homoscedasticity*

Homoscedasticity: The arrangement of points on a scatterplot wherein most of the points are in the middle of the distribution

Hypothesis resolution: Using the statistical results to determine which hypothesis came true

Importing data: Transforming data that were initially coded in a foreign format to accurately load into an application

Incremental monitoring (O X O X O): A research design that can be used with ANOVA repeated measures to assess the effectiveness of a treatment on an ongoing basis

Interval variable: A continuous variable wherein the values are equally spaced and can be negative (e.g., bank account balance)

Kruskal-Wallis test: Similar to ANOVA, but used when data distribution does not meet normality criteria

Levene statistic: See *Homogeneity of variance*

Linearity: Points on a scatterplot align in a (fairly) straight line

Logistic regression: Indicates the odds that a variable predicts one of two possible outcomes

Mann-Whitney *U* test: Similar to the *t* test, but used when data distribution does not meet normality criteria

MANOVA: Multiple analysis of variance is similar to ANOVA, except instead of results revealing between-group differences for one (outcome) variable, the results reflect differences between groups for a combined (blended) set of variables

Master file: The source data set that is typically not edited or worked on

Mauchly's test of sphericity: A pretest criterion for ANOVA repeated measures that evaluates the similarity of the variances of the independent variables (IVs) across the specified time points

Maximum: The highest number contained within a continuous variable

Mean: The average of the numbers contained within a continuous variable

Median: The center number contained within the sorted list (lowest to highest) of a variable

Minimum: The lowest number contained within a continuous variable

Mode: The most common number contained within a continuous variable

Moderate correlation: A pretest criterion for MANOVA, wherein the (bivariate) correlation among the independent variables (IVs) should be between −.9 and −.3 or between .3 and .9

Multicollinearity: A strong (bivariate) correlation among the predictor variables, wherein $r > \pm.7$ (some statisticians use ±.8 or ±.9 as the cutoff)

Multimodal: More than two numbers are tied for the most common number contained within a continuous variable (the numbers are equally frequent within the variable)

Multiple regression: A statistical process that determines the percentage that continuous and/or categorical predictor variables have in terms of predicting the value of a (single) continuous outcome variable

Multistage cluster sampling: See *Area sampling*

***n*:** The total number (count) of elements contained within a variable for a sample

***N*:** The total number (count) of elements contained within a variable for a population

Negative correlation: Among the specified pair of scores, one variable increases as the other decreases

Nominal variable: A categorical variable wherein the values have no sequence (e.g., Color = Red, Green, Blue)

Nonprobability sample: A sample wherein each item/participant does not have an equal chance of being selected to partake in the research procedure

Normal curve: See *Histogram with normal curve*

Normality: See *Normal curve*

Null hypothesis (H_0): The hypothesis that states that the treatment effect will be null; the score for the control group will be the same as the score for the treatment group

O O X O (design): See *Stable baseline and treatment effect (O O X O)*

O X O design: See *Pretest/treatment/posttest*

O X O O (design): See *Treatment effect and sustainability (O X O O)*

O X O X O (design): See *Incremental monitoring (O X O X O)*

Ordinal variable: A categorical variable wherein the values have a sequence (e.g., Meal = Breakfast, Lunch, Dinner)

***p*:** See p *value*

***p* value:** A score generated by inferential statistical tests to indicate the likelihood that the differences detected would emerge by chance alone

Paired *t* test: Indicates if there is a statistically significant difference between the pretest and posttest (T1:T2), for continuous variables

Paste: The Paste button assesses the parameters specified on the associated menu(s) and produces the equivalent block of SPSS Syntax code

Pearson correlation: See *Regression*

Percent: A method for expressing a fraction in terms of 100 (% = Part ÷ Total × 100)

Pie chart: A graphical representation of the numbers contained within a categorical variable, consisting of a circle wherein each "pie slice" represents the proportion of each category

Polychotomous: A categorical variable that contains more than two values (e.g., Meal: Breakfast/Lunch/Dinner)

Population: All of the members/records (see *Sampling*)

Positive correlations: The specified pair of scores tends to increase or decrease concurrently

Power calculations: Formulas that provide estimates specifying optimal sample size

Pretest/posttest design: See *Pretest/treatment/posttest*

Pretest/treatment/posttest: Longitudinal design model, typically using a single group, wherein a pretest is administered, followed by the treatment, followed by the posttest, which involves (re)administering the same instrument/metric used at the pretest to detect the effectiveness of the treatment

Pretest checklist: Assumptions regarding the characteristics of the data that must be assessed prior to running a statistical test

Probability sample: A sample wherein each item/participant has an equal chance of being selected to partake in the research procedure

Proportionate stratified sampling: A probability sampling technique wherein the percentage of items/participants selected from each stratum matches the percentage in the population

Pseudo-R^2: Typically refers to Cox and Snell or Nagelkerke statistics, which are an estimate of the total variability accounted for in a logistic regression model

Purposive sampling: A nonprobability sampling technique wherein each potential participant must meet multiple criteria

Quota sampling: A nonprobability sampling technique wherein the total number of participants is specified prior to starting the data collection process; data collection continues until the specified number of participants is achieved

***r*:** See *Regression*

R^2: The total predictive value of a multiple regression or logistic regression model

Random assignment: Randomly assigning members to (control/experimental) groups reduces the likelihood of creating biased/unbalanced groups

Random numbers: Figures that have no predictable sequence

Range: The maximum–minimum

Ratio variable: A continuous variable wherein the values are equally spaced and cannot be negative (e.g., Age)

Recoding: Systematically altering the way a variable is represented in a data set

Regression: Indicates the direction of the relationship between two continuous variables gathered from each participant/data record

Regression line: The line drawn through a scatterplot that shows the average pathway through those points

Representative sample: A sample that is proportionally equivalent to the population

Research question: The inquiry that forms the basis for the hypotheses construction, analyses, and documentation of results

Sample: A sublist of the sample frame or population specifying those who will actually partake in the research procedure

Sample frame: A sublist of the population that could be accessed to comprise the sample

Sampling: The process of gathering a (small) portion of the population data to better comprehend the overall population, or a portion of the population with specific characteristics

Sampling bias: Any procedure/incident/factor that interferes with the process of gathering a representative sample

Scatterplot: A graphical representation of a bivariate correlation

***SD*:** See *Standard deviation*

Sidak test: A test used to detect pairwise score differences wherein the groups have unequal *n*s; typically used as an ANOVA post hoc test

Simple random sample: A probability sampling technique wherein a set number of participants are randomly selected from a sample frame

Simple time-series design: See *Pretest/treatment/posttest*

Skewed distribution: A nonnormal (asymmetrical) distribution within a continuous variable wherein most of the numbers are either high or low

Snowball sampling: A nonprobability sampling technique wherein the researcher requests each participant to provide referral(s) to other potentially suitable participants

Sort cases: See *Sorting*

Sorting: Arranging items in ascending or descending sequence

Spearman correlation: Assesses the similarly two sequenced lists

Spearman rank correlation coefficient: See *Spearman correlation*

Spearman's rho: See *Spearman correlation*

SPSS Syntax: A language used to code and run SPSS statistical programs

Stable baseline and treatment effect (O O X O): A research design that can be used with ANOVA repeated measures to assess the stability of the baseline and treatment effectiveness

Standard deviation: A statistic that indicates the amount of similarity/diversity among the numbers contained within a variable

Stratified sampling: A probability sampling technique wherein the sample frame is split into two or more strata (lists) (e.g., Females/Males), and then random selections are made from each stratum (list)

Syntax: See *SPSS Syntax*

Systemic sampling: A probability sampling technique wherein periodic selections of items/participants are made

***t* test:** Indicates if there is a statistically significant difference between the two groups (G_1:G_2) containing continuous variables

Treatment effect and sustainability (O X O O): A research design that can be used with ANOVA repeated measures to assess the sustainability of a treatment

Treatment group: See *Experimental group*

Tukey test: A test used to detect pairwise score differences wherein the groups have equal *ns*; typically used as an ANOVA post hoc test

Type I error: Occurs when the findings indicate that there is a statistically significant difference between two variables (or groups) ($p \leq .05$) when, in fact, on the whole, there actually is not, meaning that you would erroneously reject the null hypothesis

Type II error: Occurs when the findings indicate that there is no statistically significant difference between two variables (or groups) ($p > .05$) when, in fact, on the whole, there actually is, meaning that you would erroneously accept the null hypothesis

Unique pairs formula: Computes the total number of comparisons that can be made when groups are gathered two at a time (G = total number of groups); unique pairs = $G! \div (2 \times (G - 2)!)$

Variable view: SPSS screen wherein the attributes (properties) for each variable are defined

Variance: The standard deviation squared (variance = SD^2)

Wilcoxon test: Similar to the paired *t* test but used when data distribution (posttest − pretest) does not meet normality criteria

Work file: The Work file is typically a copy of the Master file that statistical analyses/recoding is carried out on

Index